# Musculoskeletal Disorders:
# A Practical Guide
# for Diagnosis and Rehabilitation

# Musculoskeletal Disorders: A Practical Guide for Diagnosis and Rehabilitation

Edited by

## Ralph M. Buschbacher, M.D.

Clinical Assistant Professor
Indiana University Medical Center
Indianapolis, Indiana

Staff Physician
Richard L. Roudebush Veterans Administration Medical Center
Indianapolis, Indiana

Consulting Physician
Lifelines Children's Rehabilitation Hospital
Indianapolis, Indiana

With 23 contributing authors

**Andover Medical Publishers**

Boston   London   Oxford   Singapore   Sydney   Toronto   Wellington

# Dedication

To Richard Edlich, M.D., scholar, teacher, and friend. Through your encouragement and by setting an example you have inspired so many to succeed. On behalf of those who have benefited from your mentorship, I thank you.

and

To Lois, Michael, and Peter for their patience and support.

# Contents

## PART THREE / SPECIAL ISSUES

# Contributing Authors

JACK BRAUTIGAM, P.T., A.T.C.
  Clinical Director
  Morgantown Physical Therapy Associates
  Morgantown, West Virginia
STEVEN E. BRAVERMAN, M.D.
  Major, U.S. Army
  Director, Inpatient Services
  Physical Medicine and Rehabilitation Service
  Walter Reed Army Medical Center
  Washington, District of Columbia
  Assistant Professor of Neurology
  Uniformed Services University of Health Sciences
  Bethesda, Maryland
PHILLIP R. BRYANT, D.O.
  Chairman, Department of Physical Medicine and
  Rehabilitation
  Children's National Medical Center
  Washington, District of Columbia
LOIS P. BUSCHBACHER, M.S., M.D.
  Clinical Assistant Professor
  Indiana University Medical Center
  Department of Physical Medicine and
  Rehabilitation
  Indianapolis, Indiana
  Hook Rehabilitation Center
  Indianapolis, Indiana
RALPH BUSCHBACHER, M.D.
  Clinical Assistant Professor
  Indiana University Medical Center
  Indianapolis, Indiana
ANDREA R. CONTI, D.O.
  Medical College of Virginia
  Richmond, Virginia
CHRISTINA DALMADY-ISRAEL, PHARM.D.
  Assistant Professor
  Department of Pharmacy and Pharmaceutics
  Virginia Commonwealth University/Medical

College of Virginia School of Pharmacy
  Richmond, Virginia
THOMAS FLORIAN, M.D., D.C.
  Fort Smith Rehabilitation Hospital
  Fort Smith, Arkansas
SUSAN A. FOREMAN, M.ED., A.T.C., M.P.T.
  Assistant Athletic Trainer
  Instructor, Curry School of Education
  University of Virginia
  Charlottesville, Virginia
JOE H. GIECK, ED.D., A.T.C., P.T.
  Head Athletic Trainer
  University of Virginia
  Associate Professor, Curry School of Education
  Assistant Professor, Department of Orthopedics
  and Rehabilitation
  University of Virginia
  Charlottesville, Virginia
BARBARA KOCH, M.D.
  Associate Physiatrist
  Associate Professor
  Department of Medicine and Pediatrics
  Children's National Medical Center
  Washington, District of Columbia
JOHN LEARD, P.T., A.T.C.
  Curriculum Director, Athletic Training
  West Virginia University
  Morgantown, West Virginia
DENISE L. MASSIE, A.T.C.
  Athletic Trainer, West Virginia University
  Coordinator, Education and Research
  Morgantown Physical Therapy Associates
  Morgantown, West Virginia
BARBARA E. MCNEIL, M.D.
  Department of Physical Medicine and Rehabilitation
  Medical College of Virginia
  Richmond, Virginia

ROBERT P. NIRSCHL, M.S., M.D.
Medical Director, The Nirschl Orthopedic and Sportsmedicine Clinic
Medical Director and Orthopedic Consultant
Virginia Sportsmedicine Institute
Arlington, Virginia

PATRICIA PAYNE, P.T.
Senior Physical Therapist
Research Therapist
Motion Analysis Laboratory
Children's Hospital
Richmond, Virginia

MICHAEL D. ROBINSON, M.D.
Captain, U.S. Army
Director, Outpatient Clinic
Physical Medicine and Rehabilitation Service
Walter Reed Army Medical Center
Washington, District of Columbia
Assistant Professor of Neurology
Uniformed Services University of Health Sciences
Bethesda, Maryland

SHARON GEER RUSSO, M.S., P.T.
Clinical Supervisor, Physical Therapy
Woodrow Wilson Rehabilitation Center
Fishersville, Virginia

ETHAN N. SALIBA, PH.D., A.T.C., P.T., S.C.S.
Associate Athletic Trainer
Assistant Professor, Curry School of Education
Instructor, Department of Orthopedics and Rehabilitation
University of Virginia
Charlottesville, Virginia

LESLIE SCHUTZ, M.D.
Clinical Assistant Professor
Indiana University Medical Center
Department of Physical Medicine and Rehabilitation
Indianapolis, Indiana
Hook Rehabilitation Center
Indianapolis, Indiana

JANET SOBEL, R.P.T.
Director of Rehabilitation
Virginia Sportsmedicine Institute
Arlington, Virginia

SANDY TIMOK, P.T.
Director of Physical Therapy
Children's Hospital
Richmond, Virginia

MARY J. WELLS, PH.D.
Assistant Professor
Assistant Director
Rehabilitation Psychology and Neuropsychology
Department of Physical Medicine and Rehabilitation
Medical College of Virginia
Richmond, Virginia

ROBERT WILDER, M.D.
The Nirschl Orthopedic and Sportsmedicine Clinic
Arlington, Virginia

# Foreword

WANTED: A good book on musculoskeletal disorders that's easy to read and understand.

No physician, regardless of specialty, can completely avoid treating the musculoskeletal system. All physicians from dermatologists to psychiatrists are called on from time to time to treat such common musculoskeletal problems as low back pain. You cannot avoid them because they are so common. For example, low back pain is second only to the common cold as a reason for visits to physicians.

When medical students and residents want to learn about the musculoskeletal system and its problems from a source that is written in a concise and easy-to-read manner, they unfortunately have precious few alternatives. Most sources on the subject are written by expert clinicians who write excellent books, but who cannot seem to remember how difficult it is to get that first grasp on the musculoskeletal system. Ralph Buschbacher and his collaborators in this book have endeavored to meet this need. They have designed the book for the medical student, the resident, or any physician who is unfamiliar with the musculoskeletal system and who needs a book to get them "up to speed" as rapidly as possible. Therapists and athletic trainers will also find the book to be very helpful, especially Part I, Principles of Musculoskeletal Rehabilitation.

One of the beauties of this book is that while it is written in deceptively plain English, its content is sophisticated. Most will find the book very readable, despite the fact that it is chock full of facts for those seeking clinically usable current knowledge in the diagnosis and treatment of musculoskeletal problems.

The book does have its limitations. For example, its intentional brevity does not permit coverage of all the controversial issues on each musculoskeletal problem or topic. However, to satisfy those readers who want further information, carefully selected additional reading sources for in-depth coverage are listed at the end of each chapter.

This is a great beginning book on the musculoskeletal system and the rehabilitation dimension of musculoskeletal disorders. It will bring the physician or therapist to a new level of competence and confidence in treating these problems and will whet your appetite for further study. Bon appetit!

Randall L. Braddom
Indianapolis, Indiana

# Preface

To me, musculoskeletal medicine is the most enjoyable medical subspecialty. Yet, it is an often-ignored area in today's "high tech" medical environment. It requires careful history taking and physical examination and a comprehensive knowledge of the human musculoskeletal anatomy. It is not generally emphasized during medical training, yet it encompasses complaints and conditions that every clinician will encounter.

The purpose of this book is twofold: first, to provide useful information to the clinician who sees patients with musculoskeletal disorders but does not have extensive formal training in the area. The second is to bring together physicians, therapists, and trainers, so that all can speak the same language without misunderstandings.

In medical school much emphasis is placed on diseases of the internal organs, pharmacology, genetics, and surgery. Little time is devoted to learning about the musculoskeletal function of the body or how the musculoskeletal system can become deranged. Yet such disorders are probably the most common complaints among otherwise healthy people. It is common for patients, family, and friends to ask the physician, "Why does it hurt when I do this?" All too often an otherwise excellent clinician does not have a clue as to why it hurts. This book addresses those deficits. It helps guide the reader to a level of proficiency in understanding musculoskeletal disorders that is sufficient for treating most such disorders. It also provides appropriate guidelines for further study.

All too often a therapist discusses a medical problem with a physician and betrays a lack of understanding of the problem. The physician in turn discusses therapy decisions with an equally apparent lack of knowledge. In both cases, the clinician is attempting to speak "on the other's turf." This book attempts to bridge the gap between the various medical disciplines by teaching a common "language" and understanding of the basics of musculoskeletal medicine. It explains what each discipline does, how it does it, and how the services of that discipline can best be utilized. For instance, Chapter 8 describes what electromyography can do and when it is helpful. Chapter 9 describes some of the common "hands-on" approaches of physical therapy. We hope this will lead to a more harmonious interaction among professionals in the musculoskeletal arena.

When musculoskeletal issues are ignored, patients rightly feel shortchanged. If patients are told that their problems are due to "old age" or if they are told to quit otherwise enjoyable activities or work because of a certain complaint, they feel frustrated. A proper understanding of the musculoskeletal system helps to address those issues and helps the clinician to improve the quality of life for many patients.

Ralph Buschbacher
Indianapolis, Indiana

## Acknowledgments

I wish to thank Sue Arden for her support and diligence in helping me prepare this manuscript.

She is truly a joy to work with. Thanks also to Jenny Sehen for her help.

Mary Beatty of the Hunter-McGuire VA Medical Center and Dave Gregory of the Richard L. Roudebush VA Medical Center deserve special praise for their fine artwork, which helps this book "come alive."

Randall L. Braddom, M.D., has been a tremendous help with his advice and guidance, and I owe him a great deal for taking the time to help.

Last, I wish to thank each of the contributors to this book for the excellent work they have done. They are to be commended.

# PART ONE

## Principles of Musculoskeletal Rehabilitation

# Chapter 1
# Anatomic Terminology

RALPH BUSCHBACHER

As practitioners of musculoskeletal medicine, we must all be able to communicate with one another in a predictable and reproducible manner. It does not really help us to know that a patient is having trouble moving the thumb up or down unless we know which direction is "up" for the thumb. Is the hand being held with the palm up or palm down? Is the patient sitting or lying down? Unless we know the answers to these questions and until we have a common standard reference point, we cannot be sure that we are speaking the same language. And yes, anatomy is virtually a separate language, full of its own rules, quirks, and exceptions.

## Anatomic Position

A standard reference position has been adopted for describing body position, and it is depicted in Figure 1-1. The reference person stands straight with toes and palms facing forward. The reference person can be divided into three planes, the sagittal, coronal, and transverse planes, also shown in Figure 1-1 A-C. The midsagittal plane splits the person into left and right halves. Other sagittal planes can be imagined off center but parallel to the midsagittal one. The transverse plane cuts the body into upper and lower segments, and the coronal plane creates a front and a back portion. When I move my arm in the sagittal plane I am moving it

forward in the direction of my nose. When I move it in the coronal plane my arm is moving sideways, away from my body.

Since the terms up and down have different meanings depending on whether or not one is standing or lying down, the use of these terms is discouraged. Instead *cranial* (to the skull) and *caudal* (to the tail) are preferred. Another less exact way of saying the same thing would be *superior* and *inferior*. Cephalad (to the head) is also used. The back is referred to as the *dorsal* or *posterior* surface, while the belly surface is *anterior* or *ventral*. The palm of the hand is the *volar* surface, while the back of the hand is *dorsal*. Somewhat confusingly, the top of the foot is referred to as the *dorsum*, while the sole is the *plantar* surface.

When describing relationships between body parts, the term *medial* is used to mean closer to the midsagittal plane. *Lateral* refers to areas farther from this plane. Thus the shoulder is lateral to the head. When describing the hand or foot this is sometimes confusing. For instance, technically the little finger side of the hand is medial to the thumb side. To avoid confusion, the thumb side is often referred to as the *radial* surface, while the little finger side is called the *ulnar* surface. The sides are named after their respective bones in the forearm, the radius and the ulna. The midline of the hand is described as passing through the middle finger. The midline of the foot goes through the second toe.

*Proximal* and *distal* are terms commonly used. They refer to position on the limbs. The hand is

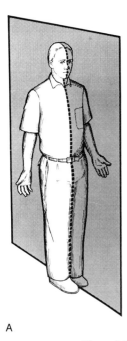
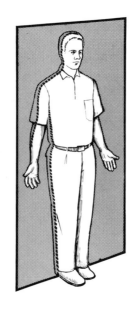
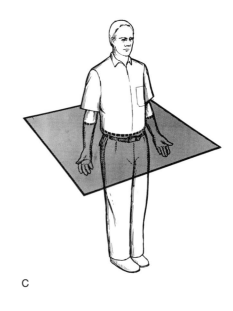

A

C

**Figure 1-1.** Planes of the body: *A*, saggital plane; *B*, coronal plane; *C*, transverse plane.

distal to the elbow and the knee is proximal to the foot. The belly button is neither proximal nor distal to the nose; they are both midsagittal, although the nose is the more cranially located.

## Body Motions

Describing joint motions can be difficult, even for an experienced clinician (Figure 1-2). *Flexion* is usually defined as motion that decreases the angle of a joint, such as bending the elbow. *Extension* is the reverse motion. When the joint is extended past its normal resting position this is sometimes called *hyperextension*. For instance, reaching forward to grasp a steering wheel involves flexion at the shoulder. Moving the arm back to the side involves extension, while reaching to the back pocket requires hyperextension.

*Abduction* is defined as moving the body part away from midline, in the coronal plane, as one would do to spread the arms or legs. *Adduction* is the opposite motion. This becomes complicated when describing finger and toe motions. Since the midline of the hand has been defined as passing through the middle finger, abduction is any deviation away from this line. Thus moving the little

finger medially is actually the same as abducting it. The middle finger cannot be adducted. It is either abducted radially or ulnarly. Since this confuses almost everyone, many people just skip these terms and say the finger was moved in an ulnar or a radial direction, but understanding these terms is necessary to properly grasp the functions of the intrinsic hand muscles.

The anatomic position of the hand is with the thumb held close to the rest of the hand with its pad facing parallel to the plane of the palm. Thus the thumb flexes toward the palm, in a direction perpendicular to flexion of the fingers. When the thumb is moved in the opposite direction, it is called extension. Moving the thumb directly away from the palm is called abduction while the reverse is adduction. The last hand motions to be defined are *opposition* and *reposition*. Opposition is when the thumb and little fingers are brought toward each other so that they touch at the tips. Reposition is the movement returning them to their anatomic positions.

*Circumduction* is the motion of swinging a joint in a circle, for example, tracing a circle with the arm. It is actually a combination of flexion, extension, abduction, and adduction.

*Rotation* is the motion of turning, for instance of the spine. *Internal* rotation and *external* rotation

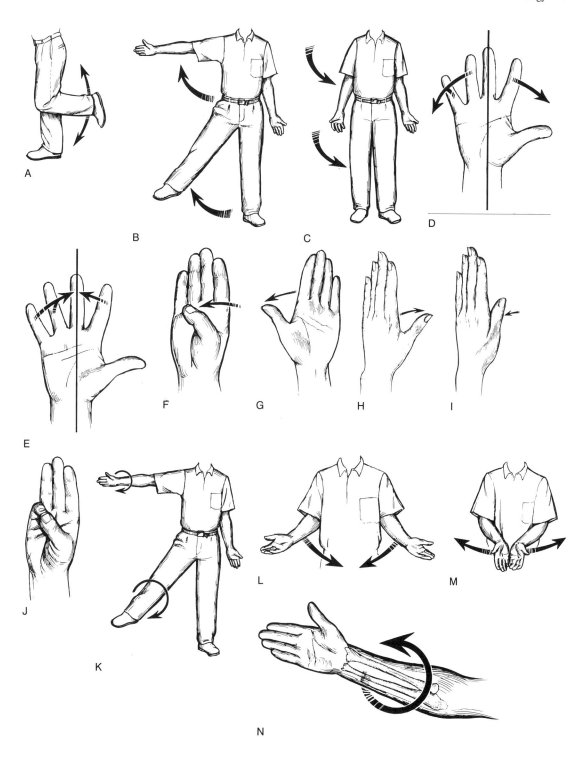

**Figure 1-2.** Body motions: *A*, flexion (up) and extension (down); *B*, abduction; *C*, adduction; *D*, finger abduction; *E*, finger adduction; *F*, thumb flexion; *G*, thumb extension; *H*, thumb abduction; *I*, thumb adduction; *J*, opposition; *K*, circumduction; *L*, internal rotation; *M*, external rotation; *N*, supination. See text for definitions.

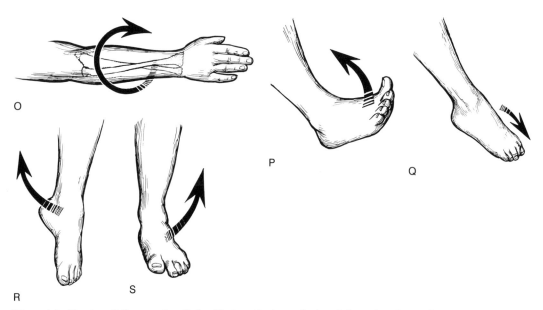

**Figure 1-2.** *(Continued) O,* pronation; *P,* dorsiflexion; *Q,* plantarflexion; *R,* inversion; *S,* eversion. See text for definitions.

refer mainly to motion at the hips and shoulders. Moving the hands to clap them together involves internal rotation. External rotation is the opposite motion. This can be confusing in the hip since internal rotation with the hip flexed actually causes the foot to swing out laterally.

Motions of the forearm are described from a position with the elbows bent 90 degrees and held at the side. Turning the palm up is called *supination*. Turning it down is called *pronation*. These terms are also used in the foot, although here supination is defined as a combination of *inversion* (moving the heel medially) and forefoot adduction. Pronation involves *eversion* (moving the heel laterally) and forefoot abduction. Obviously the foot is not flexible enough to carry out much of these motions, but supination is the motion of turning the sole upward, similar to the palm-upward position of the hand. Pronation is the opposite.

Describing motion in terms of flexion and extension at the ankle can be tricky. For this reason, when the foot is bent downward, as if to stand up on the toes it is called *plantar flexion*. Pulling the foot up toward the shin is called *dorsiflexion*.

*Protraction* means that a body part is being moved forward, for instance the shoulder blade (scapula) when the back is rounded. *Retraction* is the opposite, as in pinching the shoulder blades together. *Elevation* is raising a part cranially, as in shrugging the shoulder; *depression* is the reverse. *Upward rotation* of the shoulder blade is the motion involved in abducting the arm, while *downward rotation* occurs during adduction.

The last common terms used to describe body positions are *valgus* and *varus*. These refer to static position, not movements. Valgus means that the distal part of the joint is pointing laterally. For instance, a knock-kneed person has excessive valgus at the knee (some valgus here is normal). Also a great toe bunion usually involves valgus at the great toe. Varus refers to a distal part of a joint that deviates medially, for instance, a bow-legged stance.

### Suggested Readings

Jenkins DB: *Hollinshead's Functional Anatomy of the Limbs and Back*, 6th ed. Philadelphia: WB Saunders, 1991.

# Chapter 2
# Basic Tissue Organization and Function

RALPH BUSCHBACHER

## Connective Tissue

Connective tissue makes up the bulk of the body's mass. It includes all cellular and extracellular elements that are not directly functioning as organs. For instance, all bones and cartilage are connective tissues. Fascia and tendons that hold muscles together are connective tissue. Fat is a connective tissue and, in a sense, so is blood. Connective tissue permeates all the body organs and gives them their shape.

A common misconception is that connective tissue is inert and acellular. On the contrary, connective tissue contains highly active cells that are involved in everything from making collagen to storing fat to mediating inflammation. What makes connective tissue unique is that these cells secrete substances that carry out the functions of the tissue extracellularly (except for adipose tissue which stores fat intracellularly).

### Cell Functions

The major intrinsic cells of connective tissue are fibroblasts, chondrocytes, osteogenic cells, and adipocytes. Fibroblasts are involved in tissue modeling and repair. They can move to sites of damage and create scar tissue. They secrete structural proteins, glycosaminoglycans, connecting proteins, and degradative enzymes. They are constantly breaking down and remodeling the fibrous tissues of the body. Adipocytes store fat. They are also involved in some endocrine functions but do not offer any structural support. Chondrocytes and osteogenic cells, the cells of cartilage and bone, are discussed later.

The extrinsic cells of connective tissue include the cells that fight infection and mediate inflammation. They include neutrophils, basophils, eosinophils, monocytes, lymphocytes, and macrophages. These cells move freely from blood to extracellular fluids and migrate to the sites where they are needed. They ingest foreign particles and release enzymes that can fight infection, but also damage parts of the body.

### Structural Proteins

The major structural fibers of the body are collagen, elastin, reticulin, and proteoglycans.

*Collagen*. This is the most abundant protein in the body. It is created as a precursor molecule which is secreted by fibroblasts, chondrocytes, and osteoblasts. The precursor molecules bind together to form very tough chains. Collagen fibers have great tensile strength but readily deform when bent. They are strongest when aligned in parallel with other collagen fibers as in tendons and ligaments. There are special types of collagen produced depending on which tissue the collagen is made in.

*Elastin.* As its name implies, this protein is more elastic than collagen. Its fibers are arranged in a flexible network that is easily deformed in many directions. It is prevalent in some ligaments and in blood vessels to allow deformation without rupture. Its tensile strength is obviously less than that of collagen.

*Reticulin.* This building block is arranged as a sheet of tough fibers. It resists deformation in the plane of the sheet but not in other directions.

Proteoglycans are discussed later under Cartilage.

### Dense Versus Loose Connective Tissue

The two major categories of connective tissue are dense and loose (also known as areolar) connective tissue. The tendons and fascia are composed of dense connective tissue. Loose connective tissue is found between body parts that move. For instance, some of the tendons of the wrist are in contact with each other. To keep them from sticking together they are separated by a thin layer of loose connective tissue. The loose tissue allows movement between muscles, between muscles and bone, and around joints. When a body part is injured or immobilized, the loose tissue gradually becomes dense. This is what causes joint contractures and reduced mobility—a true case of "use it or lose it."

### Skeletal System

#### Bones

Bone is made of a protein matrix, mainly collagen, which is mineralized by calcium crystals. Collagen gives bone its toughness, while the calcium provides hardness. There are two types of bone, cortical (or compact) and trabecular (cancellous or spongy). The outside shell of bone is made of cortical bone. Cortical bone also makes up the long hollow tube of long bones, known as the diaphysis. Trabecular bone looks like a hard sponge with open cells contained in a bone meshwork. It exists inside the ends of long bones and between layers of cortex in all other bones. The mesh of the bone is aligned to provide optimal strength in the direction of force and it is usually abundant beneath the cartilage of weight-bearing joint surfaces.

During growth, the long bones of the limbs contain a zone of cartilage, the epiphyseal plate, which divides the area of trabecular bone into an inner metaphysis and an outer epiphysis. The cartilage of the epiphyseal plate grows outward toward the epiphysis, while it is calcified on the metaphyseal side. This allows the bone to grow in length. When the calcification catches up to the cartilage reproduction, the epiphyseal plate fuses and growth ceases. Bones grow in thickness by adding layers of cortical bone to the outside. To keep the bone from becoming too heavy, part of the inner cortical bone is removed. This provides optimal strength with less weight. The inner hollow part of the bone, the medullary cavity, is filled with either fat or bone marrow. The structure of a long bone is depicted in Figure 2-1.

Some bones, such as those of the skull, deviate from the long bone pattern. They are formed by calcification of an embryonic membrane, which results in an inner and outer cortex with no epiphysis.

As with all connective tissue, bone is not inert. It contains cells that are interconnected with each other and with blood vessels of the bone in what is known as the haversian system (Figure 2-1). Small arteries travel the length of the bone and support the cells within a small radius of their path. Many arteries run in a parallel fashion creating numerous independent haversian systems which are all packed together much like a handful of uncooked spaghetti noodles. These small cylinders slide up and down on one another and allow the bone to deform ever so slightly.

There are three types of bone cells: osteoblasts, osteocytes, and osteoclasts. Osteoblasts live on the outer layer of the bone, in a membranous sheath called the periosteum. The periosteum is necessary for bone growth and healing. It is very tough but can actually be peeled from the bone. When bone is fractured, the periosteum reacts, and osteoblasts lay down new bone to heal the disrupted site. Osteocytes are osteoblasts that have been trapped inside the haversian system. They keep the bone deposition and bone resorption processes in balance. Osteoclasts are cells that break down bone.

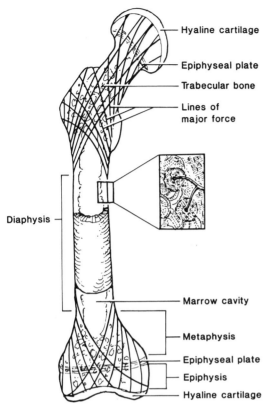

Hyaline cartilage

Epiphyseal plate

Trabecular bone

Lines of
major force

Diaphysis

Marrow cavity

Metaphysis

Epiphyseal plate

Epiphysis

Hyaline cartilage

**Figure 2-1.** The structure of a long bone. Cutout depicts the Haversian system of cortical bone nutrition.

The dynamic equilibrium of bone can be changed by stresses. Regular weight bearing increases the net deposition of bone relative to resorption in order to increase bone mass to a new, stronger equilibrium. When bones are not stressed, bone mass slowly decreases and leads to a weaker bone. This weakening may predispose a person to fracturing the bone. Hormones play a role in regulating the dynamic equilibrium of bone, which is why postmenopausal women may develop osteoporosis (see Chapter 23).

## Cartilage

Cartilage is more rigid than fibrous tissue but less so than bone. It resists compressive and bending forces somewhat, but deforms just enough not to get damaged. There are a number of types of cartilage, and the location of each depends on the function that it is carrying out.

The most common type of cartilage, hyaline cartilage, lines the ends of bones to provide smooth joint surfaces. Bone rubbing on bone would quickly wear out, but the hyaline cartilage allows joints to move with almost no friction and very little wear and tear. (Similar material also forms part of the center, the nucleus pulposus, of the intervertebral disks.) This cartilage is made mostly of collagen, proteoglycans, and water. Proteoglycans are made of bristle-comb type structures held onto a core of hyaluronic acid. The bristles are full of sugar chains that attract water. The actual chains make up very little of the substance of the cartilage, but they attract enough water to keep the cartilage turgid. Randomly arranged collagen fibers hold the cartilage together and keep it from expanding under the pressure of the water it contains. When weight is borne it presses water out of the cartilage and disks. (This is why during a day of sitting and standing the body loses about ¾ inch of its height.) When weight is removed from the joints, water is pulled back in, and with it come the nutrients that the cartilage cells, the chondrocytes, require. Chondrocytes, unlike bone, have no blood vessels to supply them. Thus the inflow and outflow of nutrients and waste that come from using the joints are the only way these cells can survive. When joints are immobilized too long the cartilage suffers and may deteriorate. Hyaline cartilage contains no nerves; thus pain is not felt directly in the cartilage.

Another type of cartilage is fibrocartilage. It is tougher than hyaline cartilage and forms the outer layer of the intervertebral disks, the annulus fibrosis. Other forms of cartilage, such as in the trachea, provide support for soft tissues. In the nose and ears this cartilage contains elastin to provide flexibility.

## Joints

There are three classes of joints: synarthrodial, amphiarthrodial, and diarthrodial. Synarthrodial, or fibrous joints, allow very little movement. The bones are held tightly together, as in the sutures of the skull. A variant of the synarthrosis, the syndesmosis, is a membranous connection, such as between the radius and ulna in the forearm. Here much movement is allowed in rotation, but the membrane is very effective at transmitting force from the distal radius to the proximal ulna.

Amphiarthrodial joints are cartilaginous connections between bones. They allow some bending to occur but do not serve as centers of motion. Examples include the rib cartilages and the intervertebral disks.

Diarthrodial joints are also known as synovial joints. They are what one usually thinks of when talking about joints. They are the primary centers of motion between bones in the body. The surfaces of opposing bones in a synovial joint are lined by hyaline cartilage. The rest of the joint is lined by a synovial membrane which secretes joint fluid. Surrounding the synovial membrane is a small fatty layer which contains blood vessels and a few nerves, and an outer joint capsule which is a tough membrane richly innervated by pain fibers. Normally, the synovial membrane secretes only a small amount of fluid into the joint. This fluid is highly viscous and lubricates the joint. It also supplies nutrients to the hyaline cartilage. When a joint is injured, blood or inflammatory fluid builds up inside the joint. This stretches the capsule and stimulates the pain fibers in the capsule, leading to the familiar swollen, tender, painful joint.

The purpose of synovial joints is to allow mobility and function. Thus, they often have little intrinsic stability. The stability of these joints is usually provided by extrinsic ligaments, muscles, and by reinforced areas of the joint capsule.

There are six types of synovial joints (see Figure 2-2).

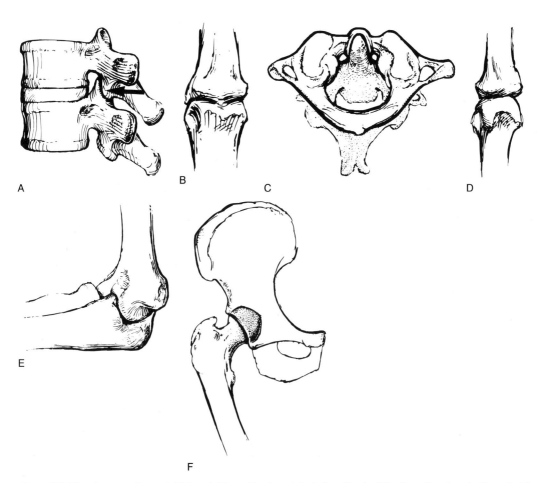

**Figure 2-2.** The six types of synovial joint. *A*, Plane (the facet joint); *B*, sellar (saddle shaped surfaces); *C*, trochoid (pivot); *D*, condylar; *E*, ginglymus (hinge); *F*, spheroid (ball and socket).

1. *Plane joints:* These are gliding joints found in the hands and feet, between the intervertebral facets, and between the patella and the femur. They usually move in one major plane only.
2. *Sellar (saddle) joints:* The opposing bones of these joints are concave in one direction and convex in the other. They are found in the carpometacarpal joint of the thumb and allow motion in many directions.
3. *Trochoid (pivot) joints:* As their name implies, these joints involve a pivoting of one bone on another. Examples are the proximal radioulnar joint in the forearm and the atlantoaxial joint in the neck. They allow motion only in the plane of rotation.
4. *Condylar joints:* These joints contain a relatively convex surface on one bone (the more proximal one) and a concave surface on the opposing bone. Classic examples are the metacarpophalangeal joints of the hand. The knee is also considered a condylar joint. A variant of the condylar type is the ellipsoid joint, such as in the radiocarpal articulation of the wrist.
5. *Ginglymus (hinge) joints:* These joints move in only one axis, flexion and extension. They are found in the elbow and in the fingers and toes.
6. *Spheroid (ball and socket) joints:* These joints allow the most movement in multiple directions. They are found in the hip and shoulder. Obviously, a deep ball and socket joint such as the hip is much more stable than a shallow one, an example of which is the shoulder.

Besides these true joints of the body, there are other functional joints, such as the scapulothoracic joint which is an articulation between the scapula (shoulder blade) and the chest wall. It is not lined by cartilage but does have a type of synovial lining, a bursa.

### Bursae

These structures are not truly part of the skeletal system but are similar to joints and therefore discussed here. Besides lubricating the scapulothoracic joint, there are numerous other sites of bursae in the body. Bursa means purse, and it is a small sac containing only a small amount of fluid. The fluid is indistinguishable from synovial fluid. Like

joints, bursae are lined by an inner membrane and an outer capsule. They lie in areas of potential friction, such as between bones and ligaments or between bones and skin. Like joints, they can become inflamed and swollen. Common examples of this are a swollen prepatellar bursa at the knee, housemaid's knee, or olecranon bursitis at the elbow, known as "student's elbow." Both of these conditions occur from leaning on the bursa too much.

### Ligaments

Very few joints of the body are intrinsically stable just from the way their bones fit together. Almost all require some sort of external stabilizers. During motion, this stabilization is accomplished by muscles and ligaments. Ligaments are composed of densely packed collagen fibers, and they hold bones together. Some ligaments contain elastin also. This allows them to stretch within certain limits without rupturing. The location of the ligaments is determined by the function of the joint. For instance, in hinge joints, the ligaments are found at the sides. This allows flexion and extension to occur but provides side-to-side stability.

## The Muscular System

### Cellular Organization

There are three types of muscle: skeletal, smooth, and cardiac. Smooth muscle is found in the abdominal organs and in blood vessels. Cardiac muscle is found only in the heart. The remainder of this section deals only with the remaining muscle type, skeletal muscle.

Skeletal muscle makes up a large part of the body's bulk and gives it much of its characteristic shape. It gives our bodies the ability to move and is normally under totally voluntary control.

Muscles are made up of individual muscle cells, the myofibers, which are surrounded by a membrane called the endomysium. Groups of myofibers, called fascicles (or bundles) are surrounded by a membrane called the perimysium, and groups of fascicles make up the whole of the muscle and are surrounded by a fascia, the epimysium. The epimysium and perimysium give muscle its shape, and the endomysium contains blood vessels and nerves that run to the myofibers themselves (Figure 2-3).

Within a myofiber are parallel groups of rodlike contractile units called myofibrils, which in turn are made up of smaller interwoven myofilaments. Myofilaments are the building blocks of the contractile unit and are what allows a muscle to be shortened or lengthened.

The functional repeating contractile unit, the sarcomere, is made up of actin and myosin protein filaments. The actin and myosin filaments interweave much like the fingers of two hands held together fingertip to fingertip. As these filaments slide toward each other, the muscle shortens and motion occurs (Figure 2-4). What causes the sliding to occur is a deformation of myosin that pulls it up along the actin. It is triggered by the release of calcium onto the myofilaments. This occurs when the electrical impulse from the nerve controlling the muscle spreads to the muscle membrane. Maximum tension is possible when the muscle is at or slightly longer than its resting length (Figure 2-4).

There are dozens to hundreds of sarcomeres lining up along the length of a muscle, and when they all contract, they pull the whole muscle together. This is a process that consumes stored energy and produces heat. The contractile parts of muscle can shorten by about 50% of their length.[1]

### Tendons

The contractile portions of muscles connect to bones by way of tendons at their ends. Tendons, like ligaments, are made up of densely packed, parallel collagen fibers. They have great tensile strength. Some tendons, such as in the forearm, are very long while others are short. In the forearm this adaptation allows the more bulky muscles of the arm to pass into the hand as thin tendons.

### Neurologic Control

Muscle is controlled by nerve impulses coming from the brain or spinal cord. These nerves branch apart so that each myofiber is innervated by a single nerve cell. One nerve may branch and innervate as few as two or three myofibers (as in the laryngeal muscles) or as many as 2000 myofibers (as in the gastrocnemius).[1] The ratio of an axon to the average number of muscle cells it innervates is called the innervation ratio. A muscle can obviously be more precisely controlled when each nerve supplies only a few muscle cells. The strength of a muscle's contraction can be regulated both by how many nerve/muscle units are being activated and by the rate at which they are activated.

Within each muscle the majority of the fibers are involved in generating strength and motion. They are called the extrafusal fibers. There are also

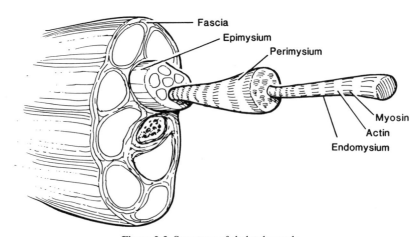

**Figure 2-3.** Structure of skeletal muscle.

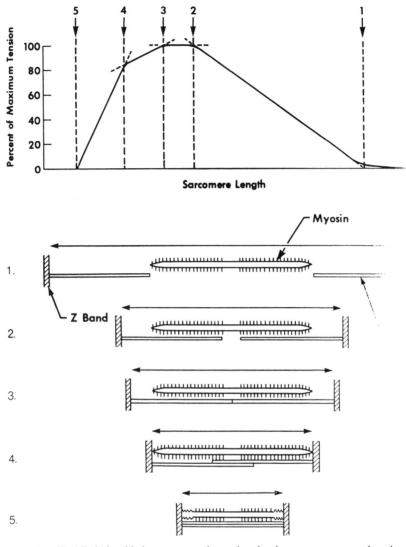

**Figure 2-4.** *(Top)* Relationship between muscle tension development, sarcomere length, and actin-myosin interaction. Maximum tension is possible when the muscle is at or slightly longer than its resting length. *(Bottom)* A schematic depiction of actin-myosin overlap. (Joynt RL: Therapeutic exercise. In DeLisa JA (ed): *Rehabilitation Medicine: Principles and Practice*. Philadelphia: JB Lippincott, 1988:346–371. Reproduced with permission.)

a few fibers dedicated to the control and fine tuning of the muscle. These are called the intrafusal or muscle spindle fibers. The muscle spindles are small organs of intrafusal muscles which are richly innervated. They are arranged in parallel with the extrafusal fibers and measure the change in length and rate of change in length of the muscle. These nerve fibers are involved in generating the muscle stretch (deep tendon) reflexes, such as the knee jerk reflex. They are also involved in spasticity in spinal cord and other injuries.

The intrafusal fibers and muscle spindles are often targets of therapeutic intervention in disease states. If they can be manipulated, the patient can sometimes be helped. This will be described in later chapters.

Muscle cells usually run the length of the muscle and attach to tendons at either end. The tendons in turn anchor the muscles to bones. Within the tendons is another group of nerve endings, the Golgi tendon organ, which is arranged in series with the extrafusal fibers. These nerves signal the brain and spinal cord when excessive tension is being placed on the tendon and relax the muscle to prevent it from being damaged.

### Muscle Fiber Types

There are two major classes of muscle fibers: type I and type II (Table 2-1). Type I fibers are small, slow twitch, and fatigue resistant. They contain large amounts of oxygen-carrying and metabolizing proteins, which makes them better at performing prolonged, low-intensity, endurance-type work. Muscles that are used for long periods of time, such as postural muscles, contain a large percentage of type I fibers. The muscles of long distance runners and other endurance athletes have a relatively large proportion of this type of fiber. When muscles are called to action, the first fibers to fire are type I. More forceful or rapid movement brings the type II fibers into play.

Type II fibers are larger, faster twitch, and fatiguable. They contain more glycolytic enzymes, which enables them to generate large amounts of force for short periods of time. They are found in muscles used for short powerful bursts, and they make up a large portion of the muscles of weight lifters and sprinters.

Type II fibers are sometimes subdivided into type IIa and type IIb. Type IIa fibers contain more oxidative endurance-type enzymes, which places them in an intermediate position between type I fibers and type IIb fibers. While in animals some muscles contain virtually exclusively one fiber type or the other, human muscles are a mixture of both types. Thus while some muscles contain relatively more type I or type II fibers, they all contain at least a fair amount of each type.

The fiber type of a muscle cell is decided by the nerve cell that innervates it. Thus all the muscle fibers innervated by a type I nerve cell are type I. The same holds true for a type II nerve cell. Ordinarily, muscle fibers cannot be converted from type I to type II or vice versa.

### Muscle Hypertrophy

The numbers of type I and type II fibers do not change with growth and may increase only minimally as a result of exercise.[2] What makes muscles larger is growth from within the muscle cells, called hypertrophy. Weightlifting, for instance, will increase the amount of actin and myosin within the myofibers, mainly those of type II. Thus, the relative cross-sectional area of type II muscle fibers increases. Similarly, marathon training increases the relative cross-sectional area of type I muscle fibers, but the total number of type I fibers does not change.

### Functional Considerations

All muscles generate the same amount of force per cross-sectional area, about 3.6 kg/cm$^2$. This holds true for everyone, from the power weight lifter to the ballerina. Obviously, the power weight lifter attempts to improve his performance by increasing his muscular cross-sectional area. Each extra square centimeter increases his force by 3.6 kg.

Muscles in different locations serve different purposes. Some are called on to generate large forces over small distances. Others must move the

**Table 2-1.** Muscle Fiber Types and Properties

|  | Type 1 | Type IIa | Type IIb |
|---|---|---|---|
| Speed | Slow twitch | Fast twitch | Fast twitch |
| Fatiguability | Fatigue resistant | Relatively fatigue resistant | Fatiguable |
| Metabolism | Oxidation | Oxidation | Glycolysis |
| Size | Small | Medium | Large |
| Function | Endurance, posture | Intermediate | Brief bursts of power |
| Recruitment | Recruited first | Intermediate | Recruited last |

body quickly with less force. Such specialization is allowed by the varying lever arms and shapes of the muscles, even though their force/square centimeter does not vary. When a muscle inserts close to a joint, it has a short lever arm. It can move the limb over a large distance but with relatively less force than if inserted farther from the joint. The biceps brachii muscle is a good example of this. It inserts close to the elbow joint and moves the forearm over a large distance. To make up for its disadvantage in leverage it must hypertrophy to a large size.

Muscle shapes and fiber orientation are a very important way that the body allows muscle form to fit its function. Imagine a "tug-of-war" in which there was no rope, where each participant pulled on the shoulders of the person in front of him or her. Obviously, a team would only be as good as its weakest player. Adding a rope allows each participant to contribute to his or her ability. In a muscle the rope is the tendon and varying the way fibers pull on the "rope" changes their contribution.

In some muscles most or all of the fibers run parallel to each other. Examples might include some of the finger flexors or the gluteus maximus. Each myofiber runs the whole length of the muscle, and since an active sarcomere can shorten by about 50% of its length, such a parallel arrangement offers the maximum movement possible. The cross-sectional area devoted to developing force is equal to the cross-section of the muscle.

When the fibers attach to the tendon at an angle, it is called a unipennate or bipennate (fusiform) design (Figure 2-5). Various combinations of a pennate design exist, depending on the three-dimensional shape of the muscle, but all have in common the principle of angled fibers. Each fiber

no longer runs the whole length of the muscle. Thus the shorter fibers, contracting to 50% of their length and inserting on the tendon at an angle, move the muscle a shorter distance than in the parallel design. Since more fibers are pulling though, the effective cross-sectional area is increased and the muscle gains strength (Figure 2-6).

## Nervous System

### Cell Functions

The nervous system is the fundamental control unit of the body. It is organized to receive information from the environment and body by way of specialized receptors, process this information, and control the muscles and organs. With this mission, it is clear that the cells of the nervous system must transmit information from one to the other and to the muscles, sometimes over great distances. The cells of the nervous system are called neurons. Neurons have a cell body which supports branches called dendrites and axons. A single neuron may have many dendrites, and their function is to gather information from other neurons. Axons, of which there is only one per neuron, transmit impulses away from the cell to other neurons or to muscles. The method of impulse transmission is by means of an electrical wave which passes down the length of the axon. A single axon may branch to supply many other nerves or muscle cells, but once the axon fires all of its branches must fire (Figure 2-7). A motor nerve plus all the muscle fibers that it innervates is called a motor unit.

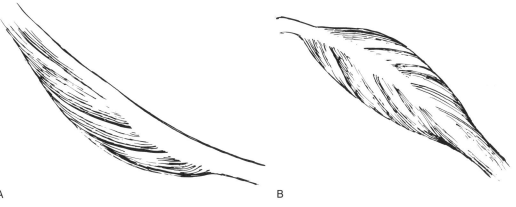

A                                    B

**Figure 2-5.** *A*, Unipennate muscle form; *B*, bipennate form.

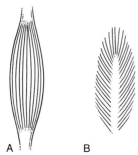

**Figure 2-6.** *A*, Parallel muscle fiber arrangement. *B*, Pennate muscle design. The primary reason for muscle fibers to be longer is so that they can pull over a longer distance. All fibers, both long and short, pull with the same force, although the shorter fibers pull over a shorter distance.

Functionally this means that parallel muscles exert less force than pennate muscles of the same mass. For instance, one may imagine that both muscles in *A* and *B* have the same mass, but that the parallel muscle has 9 schematically depicted fibers, while the pennate muscle has 38. The pennate muscle exerts 38/9, or approximately 4.2 times the force of the parallel muscle (modified by the angle of insertion).

Individual nerves are surrounded by a membrane called the endoneurium. Nerves are grouped into fascicles which are surrounded by a perineurium. Groups of fascicles make up a peripheral nerve which is surrounded by a connective tissue sheath called the epineurium (Figure 2-8).

### *Impulse Conduction*

All cell membranes have a charge difference across them. This charge difference is maintained by energy consumption. When certain sodium ion channels open, they cause a reversal of this charge to occur. The reversal, called depolarization, affects neighboring sodium channels, causing them to open, and so the charge reversal passes down the length of the axon as an electrical signal. This electrical signal is the way that nerves gather information from the body and how they communicate with each other. When the signal reaches other nerves or muscles it causes the membrane of the nerve or muscle to depolarize, thus passing on the information.

Some nerves carry information over only a few millimeters' distance. Others travel all the way from the toes to the spinal cord. In order to increase their speed and efficiency nerves are insulated by layers of fatty cells in what is called the myelin sheath. In peripheral nerves the myelin sheath is created by Schwann cells. All axons in a nerve are myelinated, but some much more so than others. Heavily myelinated axons carry information quickly but are relatively thick. If all axons were heavily myelinated, nerves would be too thick to be practical. Therefore the types of information that the brain does not need to know about right away are carried in relatively unmyelinated nerve fibers.

### *Central Nervous System*

The nervous system can be divided into two parts: the central nervous system, which consists of the brain and spinal cord (Figure 2-9), and the peripheral nervous system, which includes all the rest of the neural tissues. The brain has an outer layer of cells, the cortex, which controls all the basic functions of sensation, motor control, thought processes, and so on. Deeper inside the brain are numerous clusters of cells that process the incoming and outgoing information. The posteroinferior portion of the brain, the cerebellum, is involved in coordinating motor function and balance. The spinal cord is a continuation of the brain that passes down the back within the vertebral column. Since the spinal cord stops growing before the body does, it is shorter than the vertebral column and ends at

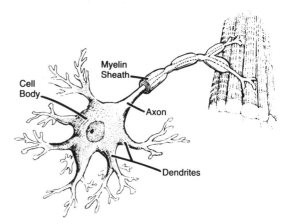

**Figure 2-7.** The motor unit consists of a nerve cell, axon, and the muscle fibers it innervates.

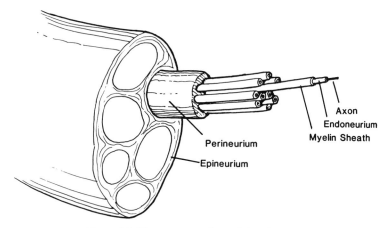

**Figure 2-8.** The structure of a peripheral nerve.

L2. The central nervous system contains most of the nerve cell bodies. Nerve cell bodies that directly control muscles are located in a few groups, called nuclei, of the brain, and in a column down the anterior spinal cord. From these positions they send out 12 pairs of cranial nerves (from the brain) and 31 pairs of spinal nerves to control body movement. The nerve cell bodies of the sensory nerves are located within nuclei in the brain, but in the spinal cord they lie outside the cord itself, near the exit of the spinal nerves from the bony vertebral column. Figure 2-10 depicts a cross-sectional segment of spinal cord. The sensory nerve bodies live in the dorsal root ganglion. Sensory impulses come into the dorsal part of the spinal cord and either pass through it to the brain, cross over, and then enter the brain, or they connect with motor neurons. The motor neurons, called alpha motor neurons, send impulses out the ventral (anterior) roots of the spinal nerves. When incoming signals contact the motor cells, they create a reflex arc, such as the one for the knee jerk reflex.

The brain controls the alpha motor neurons by descending impulses in the corticospinal tracts, also known as the pyramidal tracts. These impulses are heavily modulated by other nuclei and by the cerebellum to provide smooth, coordinated voluntary movement.

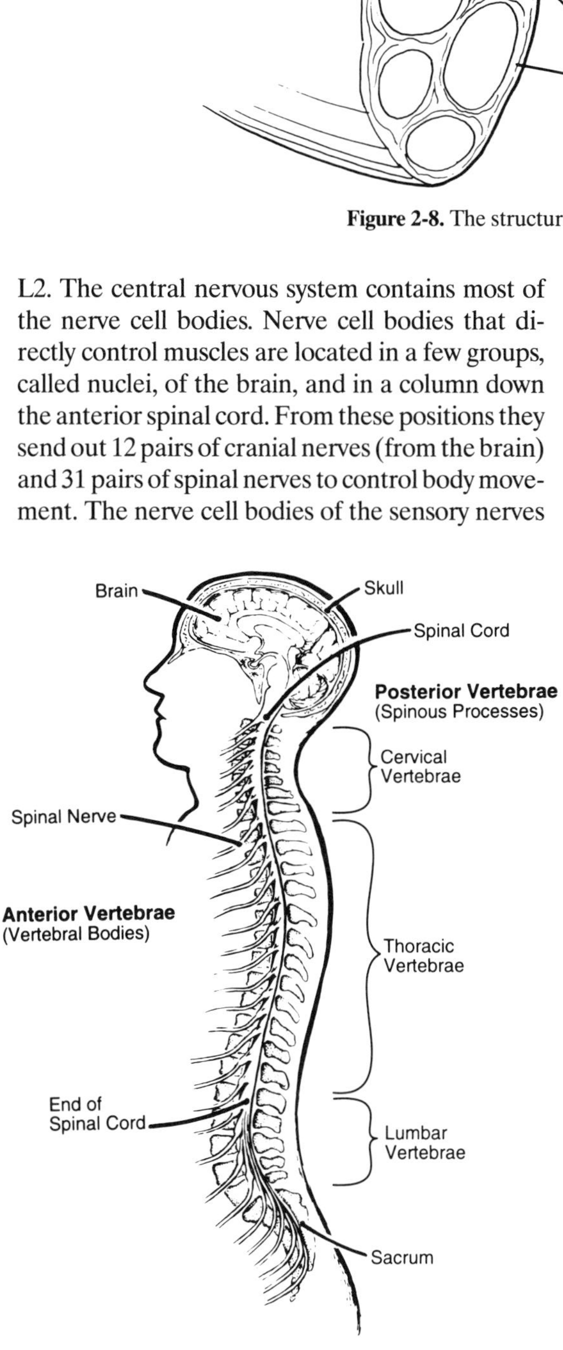

**Figure 2-9.** The central nervous system.

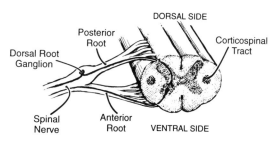

**Figure 2-10.** A cross-sectional slice through the spinal cord depicting the descending motor tract, the corticospinal tract, as well as the afferent and efferent nerve fibers.

### Peripheral Nervous System

Once the dorsal and ventral roots of the spinal nerves join, they exit the vertebral column and become part of the peripheral nervous system. The cranial nerves are also part of the peripheral nervous system.

### Autonomic Nervous System

A part of the nervous system is devoted to regulating body functions such as digestion, heart rate, blood flow, sweating, sexual function, and bladder control.

This complex group of nerves is divided into the somewhat opposite sympathetic nervous system which readies the body for action, and the parasympathetic nervous system which helps maintain body regulatory functions. The autonomic nervous system does not innervate skeletal muscle. It is important to the musculoskeletal system because by altering blood flow, it may cause muscle ischemia and pain.

### Nerve Plexus

After the spinal nerves exit the vertebral column they split into dorsal rami which supply the skin and muscles of the back, and ventral rami which go to the limbs and trunk. During embryonic growth, the ventral rami grow more or less straight out into the growing embryo, but as limbs develop and rotate and as muscles and bones form, the rami become intertwined into bundles of nerves called plexuses. There is a cervical plexus in the neck, a brachial plexus at the arm level (Figure 2-11), and a lumbosacral plexus which goes to the buttocks and legs. In the thoracic region, the spinal nerves follow the ribs and thus do not form a plexus.

The nerves of the brachial and the lumbosacral plexuses innervate the muscles of the limbs and the skin in a well-known and reproducible pattern. By examining the muscles in the limbs, an injury to the plexus may be localized to a specific site. The skin of the body, like the muscles, is innervated in a more or less standard fashion. The strips of skin innervated by specific spinal levels are called dermatomes (see Chapter 11). Dermatomes overlap somewhat, but in conditions such as spinal cord

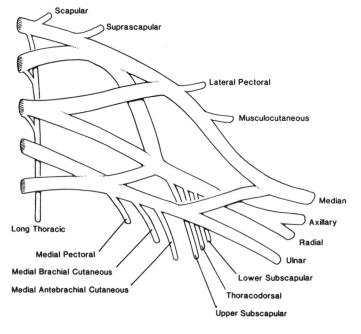

**Figure 2-11.** The brachial plexus consists of nerve roots branching and exchanging branches to form the peripheral nerves.

Scapular
Suprascapular
Lateral Pectoral
Musculocutaneous
Median
Axillary
Radial
Ulnar
Lower Subscapular
Thoracodorsal
Upper Subscapular
Medial Antebrachial Cutaneous
Medial Brachial Cutaneous
Medial Pectoral
Long Thoracic

injury, abnormal dermatomal sensation may be used to identify the level of injury. In conditions of nerve root irritation (e.g., radiculopathy) the muscles and skin involved can be used to determine the level of damage, often by electrodiagnostic evaluation as well as physical examination.

## Points of Summary

1. Connective tissue is a dynamic cellular substance whose extracellular matrix determines its properties.
2. Type I muscle fibers are slow twitch, fatigue resistant, oxidative cells, while type II fibers are fast twitch, fatiguable and glycolytic.
3. Pennate muscles develop high force over a short distance. Parallel muscles generate lower force over a longer distance.
4. Alpha motor neurons in the spinal cord are the final controlling link to the muscles.
5. The brachial and lumbosacral plexuses are made of intertwining ventral roots of spinal nerves on their way to supplying the limbs.

## References

1. Goodgold J, Eberstein A: *Electrodiagnosis of Neuromuscular Diseases*, 3rd ed. Baltimore: Williams & Wilkins, 1983:1–20.
2. Gonyea WJ, Sale DG, Gonyea FB, et al.: Exercise induced increases in muscle fiber number. *Eur J Appl Physiol* 1986;55:137–141.

## Suggested Readings

Jenkins DB: *Hollinshead's Functional Anatomy of the Limbs and Back*, 6th ed. Philadelphia: WB Saunders, 1991.

Jiminez SA: The connective tissues: structure, function, and metabolism. In Schumacher HR Jr (ed): *Primer on the Rheumatic Diseases*, 9th ed. Atlanta: Arthritis Foundation, 1988:6–14.

Simkin PA: Joints: Structure and function. In Schumacher HR Jr (ed): *Primer on the Rheumatic Diseases*, 9th ed. Atlanta: Arthritis Foundation, 1988:18–23.

# Chapter 3
# Tissue Injury and Healing

RALPH BUSCHBACHER

## Types of Musculoskeletal Injuries

### Macrotrauma

Tissue damage can be classified by etiology as due to either macrotrauma or repetitive microtrauma. Macrotrauma is acute damage due to some strong force. It can be seen in athletic injuries such as ankle sprains or in falls or accidents. When macrotrauma occurs, the patient is usually aware of the incident that caused it, and he or she usually has an abrupt onset of pain as a result. Macrotrauma can be due to either direct trauma to the area in question or indirect transmission of force to that area. An example would be a clavicular fracture caused by a forceful blow to the clavicular bone (direct) in contradistinction to a clavicular fracture caused by a fall on an outstretched arm (indirect). Older people, inactive or osteoporotic individuals, and those who have had previous injuries are more likely to sustain macrotraumatic injury, sometimes from seemingly minor incidents.

### Repetitive Microtrauma

This is caused by overuse from repetitive motion, stress, or stretching. After minor injury, the body needs time to heal. If instead of healing, the damaged areas are restressed and reinjured, the healing process becomes pathologic, with chronic inflammation, weakness, stress fractures, and abnormal calcification resulting. At the microscopic level collagen fiber failure is occurring. If left untreated, repetitive microtrauma may weaken body tissues to such an extent that macrotraumatic injury is likely, if not inevitable. Examples include rotator cuff tendonitis and chronic degenerative disk disease.

## Stages of Healing

After injury there are three stages of healing: inflammation, repair, and remodeling.

### Inflammation

When body tissues are injured there may be bleeding, clot formation, swelling, and a cellular reaction. Initially the cellular reaction consists of an influx of macrophages and other cells that mediate inflammation. They increase blood flow and ingest particulate matter. Within about 3 to 5 days fibroblasts proliferate and produce collagen fibers.

### Repair

In early repair, collagen begins to take the place of the fibrin clot which is broken down and resorbed. The collagen is oriented at random and has very little structural strength.

### *Remodeling*

Beginning about 1 to 2 weeks after injury, the collagen scar begins to remodel. The randomly oriented fibers are gradually broken down, and longitudinally arranged fibers take their place. Thus the collagen is reoriented in the directions in which it is needed, and the tissue slowly regains its strength. This whole process takes months to years before it is complete.

## Maximizing Repair Success

Repetitive microtrauma is an overuse cycle in which tissue repair is not allowed to catch up with injury. It is essentially chronically stuck in the inflammatory stage of healing. Since inflammation itself can weaken connective tissue by up to 50% of its strength, the overuse often ends in a rupture of the tissue. Thus to maximize healing, adequate rest is essential.

In macrotraumatic injuries, such as sprains, there is usually a tissue defect that needs to be filled. If it becomes filled with disorganized collagen fibers it will not have much strength, yet this is exactly what happens if the tissue is immobilized for a prolonged time after injury.[1] When small amounts of longitudinal stress are placed on the healing area, the collagen fibers become properly aligned and heal stronger (Figure 3-1). Thus it is clear that prolonged immobilization is contraindicated after injury.

Inflammation is a necessary part of the early healing process. If it goes on for too long, however, it becomes detrimental. Therefore, control of inflammation is desirable in the subacute stages of healing. Nonsteroidal antiinflammatory medications are helpful, and occasionally steroid medications need to be used to reduce inflammation. Steroids, however, actually inhibit healing if given too early, in the first days of inflammation.

Healing depends somewhat on the age of the individual; older people may heal more slowly. It also depends on the individual's general nutrition, health, and vascular supply. When possible these factors should be optimized.

## Special Considerations

### *Tendon and Ligament Injury*

Tendons and ligaments are mostly made up of parallel collagen fibers. If they are not mobilized soon after injury (or surgery) they develop adhesions to the surrounding tissues. The loose connective tissue that ordinarily allows the tendons and ligaments to move freely turns to dense fibers that bind to the tendons and ligaments and limit their function. Without stress from active movement, the collagen fibers remain disorganized and strength is reduced.[2-6] Some ligaments, such as those in the back, must stretch to allow proper body motion to occur. They contain elastin fibers. If these ligaments are immobilized and not put through an adequate range of motion, they lose their elastin. This decreases their strength and predisposes them to reinjury.

Ligamentous sprains are often graded as I, II, or III. Grade I injury is a microscopic tearing of the

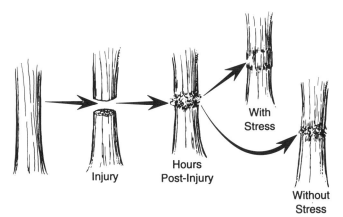

**Figure 3-1.** Normal recovery progression of a tendon after being lacerated. If the tendon is not stressed the collagen scar is unorganized instead of being arranged as parallel fibers.

With Stress

Without Stress

Injury

Hours Post-Injury

ligament which causes pain. Joint stability is normal but ligament testing causes pain. Grade II sprains involve tearing of some of the ligamentous fibers. Stability testing reveals laxity, with increased abnormal joint motion but still with a firm endpoint. Grade III sprains are complete disruptions of the ligaments.

### Muscle Injury

When collagen fibers within muscles are torn, it is called a strain. In conditions of muscle strain or laceration, a scar forms between the disrupted ends much as in tendon or ligament injury. The scar may interrupt the contractile fibers of the muscle, but usually such injuries heal well with little residual dysfunction.

Muscles may also become contused or develop hematomas. Such injury involves a crushing of muscle cells along with local bleeding. During healing this may progress to the development of hard, organized masses or even abnormally placed bone islands within the muscle. If a contused muscle is stressed too soon after injury, this may aggravate the edema and worsen the condition. Thus such traumatic injury should be rested until pain and acute inflammation are largely resolved. Compression and ice are useful acutely to prevent worsening of the damage.

### Joint Injury

Cartilage may be fractured along with bone in a macrotraumatic injury. When this occurs in a joint it often requires surgical fixation. The normal hyaline cartilage cannot repair itself, so a fibrocartilaginous scar is formed within the joint cartilage. This fibrocartilage is not as suited to function in a joint as is hyaline cartilage and, therefore, future pain and degeneration may occur.

When the cartilage of the epiphyseal plate is injured in a growing child it may cause future growth abnormalities. Such an injury should always be ruled out or suspected in a child with painful bone or joint trauma and, if present, requires assessment by an orthopedist.

Degenerative joint disease is primarily due to a degeneration of hyaline joint cartilage. The cause is unknown, but previous injury and genetic predisposition may play a role in its etiology. This is sometimes viewed as normal "wear and tear" of joints and is certainly more prevalent in heavy and older individuals and in weight-bearing joints, but it is unclear why it is painful in some people and not in others. As the cartilage degenerates it tries to repair itself and causes a mild inflammation within the joints involved. It leads to nonuniform cartilage destruction and "spurring" (bony proliferation) of the surrounding bones. Intervertebral disks are often affected.

Cartilage is also destroyed in connective tissue diseases such as rheumatoid arthritis. In these conditions the synovial membrane becomes inflamed and releases enzymes that destroy the cartilage. This leads to uniform cartilage degeneration and swollen painful joints. Range of motion exercise, even when done passively, can aggravate the inflammation of arthritic joints[7] and is to be avoided in the acutely inflamed stages. Care must also be taken not to develop contractures in these joints. Patients attempt to hold their joints in the position of least intraarticular pressure, and if held in this manner for too long they may develop permanent loss of range of motion. The inflammation of joints in connective tissue disease may weaken tendons and ligaments that pass near to the joint. Ruptures of these structures may occur and should be avoided by not overstressing the tendons and ligaments.

### Bone Injury

Bone, as all other connective tissue, can be injured by macrotrauma or repetitive microtrauma. When macrotrauma causes a fracture, the osteoblasts within the periosteum lay down new bone in what is termed a *callus*. The callus is formed and remodeled to provide complete healing of the bone. When bones lose density, called osteoporosis, they are more likely to fracture, but fracture healing occurs just as fast as in normal bones.

Bone normally responds to a greater than average weight-bearing stress by slight resorption or weakening followed by bone buildup to a level stronger than it was before. Thus regular weight-bearing exercise causes bone density to increase and create a stronger bone. When the stressors are excessive and repeated, however, the initial slight resorption is not given enough time to heal, and the bone weakens and develops fracture lines, the so-called stress fracture.

Stress fractures, just like other fractures, cause the periosteum to react in an attempt to heal the defect. It heals if it is given some rest, but if the excessive stress is continued, the fracture worsens. Stress fractures are common, for example in runners who have recently increased their mileage or changed their footwear or terrain.

*Neural Tissue Injury*

While there is some evidence that nerve cells in the brain and spinal cord may be able to repair themselves, for all practical purposes this is essentially a research interest at the present time. In the future we may be able to help these cells recover from injury, but for now, if they are damaged they stay that way. That does not mean, however, that different parts of the central nervous system cannot learn to carry out the functions that were lost. The whole field of neurorehabilitation is designed to help patients work around their deficits to achieve function.

Peripheral nerves are injured in several different ways. Damage may be isolated to the Schwann cells of the myelin sheath. While this may disrupt the flow of information past the damaged area, the myelin usually regenerates and function often recovers with time. Such an injury is seen in the early stages of nerve compression such as carpal tunnel syndrome.

If the compression is not relieved, the axon inside the myelin may die. It deteriorates distal to the compression, but more proximally it is sustained by the cell body which remains unharmed. If such compression is relieved, there may be regrowth of the axon into the tube of myelin it had previously inhabited. Function may recover, but depending on the severity and duration of the compression, with variable success.

When a nerve is cut, the axon distal to the laceration dies. The intact proximal segment attempts to regrow and "sprouts" at its end. Sprouts can sometimes reach the opposite cut end, but since the tube of the axon has been disrupted, such regrowth is often unsuccessful. Microsurgery may help to reattach the ends of cut nerves. Outcome is not usually optimal, but doing nothing is usually worse. Nerve sprouts form a small bulb or growth on the end of the nerve. This bulb, called a neuroma, may be painful. Painful neuromas can be seen after injury or after amputation surgery.

## Points of Summary

1. Musculoskeletal injury occurs from macrotrauma or from repetitive microtrauma.
2. There are three stages of connective tissue healing: inflammation, repair, and remodeling.
3. In healing ligaments or tendons the collagen fibers must be stressed to achieve proper alignment.
4. Muscle strains involve collagen tissue failure and tearing.
5. When hyaline cartilage is injured a fibrocartilaginous scar forms.
6. Bone responds to regular weight-bearing stress by increasing its mass and strength.
7. Cut nerves form distal "sprouts," called neuromas, which are sometimes painful.

## References

1. Buck RC: Regeneration of tendon. *J Pathol Bacteriol* 1953;66:1–18.
2. Tipton CM, Schild RJ, Tomanek RJ: Influence of physical activity on the strength of knee ligaments in rats. *Am J Physiol* 1967;212:783–787.
3. Tipton CM, Matthes RD, Maynard JA, et al.: The influence of physical activity on ligaments and tendons. *Med Sci Sports Exerc* 1975;7:165–175.
4. Noyes FR: Functional properties of knee ligaments and alterations induced by immobilization: A correlative biomechanical and histological study in primates. *Clin Orthop* 1977;123:210–242.
5. Vailas AC, Tipton CM, Matthes RD: Physical activity and its influence on the repair process of medial collateral ligaments. *Connect Tissue Res* 1981;9:25–32.
6. Amiel D, Akeson WH, Harwood FL, et al.: Stress deprivation effect on metabolic turnover of the medial

collateral ligament collagen: A comparison between nine and 12 week immobilization. *Clin Orthop* 1983; 172:265–270.

7. Merritt JL, Hunder GG: Passive range of motion, not isometric exercise, amplifies acute urate synovitis. *Arch Phys Med Rehabil* 1983;64:130–131.

## Suggested Readings

Daniel D, Akeson W, O'Connor J (eds): *Knee Ligaments: Structure, Function, Injury, and Repair.* New York: Raven Press, 1990.

Medoff RJ: Soft tissue healing. *Ann Sports Med* 1987; 3(2):67–72.

# Chapter 4

# Rehabilitation of Musculoskeletal Disorders: The Sports Medicine Approach

RALPH BUSCHBACHER

Musculoskeletal medicine owes a lot to the pioneering efforts of sports medicine physicians, athletes, and trainers who have helped revolutionize treatment in the field. The unproven dogma of treatment in the past consisted of prolonged periods of rest, immobilization, and even casting—often for minor injuries. This treatment was used after childbirth and surgery as well as musculoskeletal injury. We now know that pampering the body is often the worst thing we can do to it. Sports medicine has developed ideas that were controversial, but are now considered mainstream musculoskeletal medicine. The principles that are discussed in this chapter include early mobilization, the importance of proprioceptive exercise, an outline of rehabilitative progression, and preventive intervention.

## Early Mobilization

As discussed in Chapter 3, prolonged immobilization causes connective tissue to shorten, locking the body part into a contracted, nonfunctional structure. Cartilage nutrition suffers, bone density decreases, muscles atrophy, the body loses neural coordination, and cardiorespiratory fitness deteriorates.[1-6]

These events should be prevented whenever possible. Correcting them after they have occurred is time-consuming and frustrating. It takes up to twice as long for muscles and cardiac fitness to recover as it takes to deteriorate. [1,5] Cartilage function may never completely recover, and bone density may take months to years to reach its premorbid level.[6]

As soon as acute inflammation has been controlled, the injured area should be mobilized. This may be done with passive or assisted motion as long as it does not aggravate the problem. Isometric exercises can be used to help maintain muscle mass. Probably most importantly, the rest of the body should not be allowed to deteriorate.

When treating musculoskeletal disorders sometimes immobilization is prescribed, and at other times relative rest is indicated; when possible relative rest is the preferred option.

Immobilization is, of course, necessary after some fractures. It is also useful in acutely inflamed joint conditions, ligament sprains, and tendonitis. It should not be prescribed for more than a few days for tendonitis or ligamentous sprain. It may be necessary for up to 2 weeks in inflamed joints.

Relative rest is meant to let the damaged part of the body function, but to limit performance of aggravating motions. For instance, relative rest in rotator cuff tendonitis might mean refraining only from overhead activities. Other motions are allowed and even encouraged. Deciding when to prescribe relative rest versus immobilization is not always easy. In general, if a joint is stable and not acutely inflamed it is safe to prescribe rest. In conditions such as shoulder dislocation, a short period of sling immobilization may be recommended, although some would argue that even in this case it is not necessary.

One of the most impressive cases for early mobilization has been described by Deyo et al. in the treatment of acute low back strain.[7] They randomized patients to treatment groups that were instructed to remain on bed rest for 2 days or 7 days. Both groups actually stayed in bed for a shorter period than recommended and outcome in both was essentially the same.

## Proprioceptive Exercises

In 1965 Freeman postulated and gave evidence that a proprioceptive defect after ankle sprains caused functional instability of that joint.[8] He felt that ligaments contain nerve endings that inform the brain of the joints' position. If the ligaments are disrupted, this position sense, proprioception, is impaired. Immobilization of the joint allows proprioception to deteriorate even further, and when activity is resumed, the person is likely to injure the joint again because of a poor awareness of what position it is in.

It is now clear that proprioception plays an important role in preventing reinjury. This is especially evident in ankle sprains, but probably also in other joints. Exercises that stress proprioceptive awareness, such as balance boards and walking backward, help to improve joint recovery from injury. Other exercises might include rope skipping, toe or heel walking, walking with the eyes closed, or mini-trampoline jumping.

## Rehabilitation Progression

An approach that is sometimes helpful is to divide the rehabilitation of musculoskeletal disorders into four overlapping phases.

### Phase I

This is the initial period when inflammation and pain must be controlled for both a macrotraumatic injury or for overuse conditions. The RICE (rest, ice, compression, elevation) protocol is used after sports injuries and can be modified for just about any musculoskeletal condition. In addition, nonsteroidal antiinflammatory medications (NSAIDs) such as aspirin and ibuprofen may reduce inflammation. They are especially useful in overuse conditions such as tendonitis or bursitis. Ice is a helpful adjunct to treatment. It relieves pain and reduces edema. It is especially helpful in the acute postinjury period (or until swelling subsides). It is also useful for overuse conditions and both before and after exercise to avoid aggravating inflammation. Heat is generally used in the subacute postinjury period (after 1 to 2 days). It is also helpful in overuse syndromes. Modalities of heating and cooling are described further in Chapter 6.

Phase I usually lasts from 1 to 2 weeks. It is important not to neglect fitness of the rest of the body while the affected part is rested. In upper extremity injury, exercise bicycles may maintain cardiorespiratory and lower extremity fitness. In lower extremity injury, arm crank ergometry may be tried. Modified exercises such as kickboard swimming may be pursued if the patient wishes.

### Phase II

This may be the most important phase of rehabilitation, the mobilization phase. When a part of the body hurts, it is natural to try to not move it. Such "splinting" is helpful for a while, but if it is done for too long it will result in contracture, decreased strength and function, and ultimately even more pain. As soon as inflammation is controlled, the patient must work on restoring and maintaining normal range of motion. Inflexible muscles and joints are predisposed to further injury. Thus in conditions such as tennis elbow (lateral epicondylitis), one of the key points of treatment is to adequately stretch the muscles of the arm, shoulder, and forearm. The various parts of the body are interconnected in what is called the "kinetic linkage system." Abnormalities in one part, for instance in gait, may indirectly spread through the spine and into the neck and arms. Thus it is important to examine the whole patient, not just one part in isolation.

There are many reference tables for normal ranges of body motion. Hoppenfeld offers a particularly readable version.[9] While such tables are helpful, the patient often provides a normal control for range of motion in the opposite side of the body. Obviously, when joints are unstable or after supporting structures have been torn, for example, after ankle sprain or shoulder dislocation, flexibility exercises are not encouraged in the damaged structures. Slightly less flexibility in the defective areas compared with the normal side is sometimes allowable as long as flexibility in other planes is maintained.

Superficial or deep heat is often useful while working on flexibility. It is most effective if applied during stretching, while the connective tissue is still warm. Late in phase II isometric exercises may be started.

### *Phase III*

This is the strengthening phase. When starting this part of rehabilitation it is important first not to lose the gains made in phases I and II. Isometrics are continued, and added to this are isotonic and isokinetic strengthening exercises. These are described in more detail in Chapter 7, but as a general guideline one should start with relatively low weight and moderate-high repetitions and progress to higher weight, low-repetition exercises as tolerated.

### *Phase IV*

This phase is often neglected, and if not done properly will make your patient a repeat customer. Phase IV is that of functional restoration and corresponds to the principle of sports-specific training in sports medicine. It is not enough to achieve good flexibility and strength in the therapy department. Functional tasks similar to those that are to be resumed must be practiced before return to activity. For example after back injury to a laborer, a work hardening program consisting of limited and supervised shoveling and lifting may give him the strength, coordination, and confidence needed to return to work.

Injuries and overuse may of course occur in anyone, but most often they occur because of some faulty technique, whether while running, vacuuming, or doing assembly line work. Inadequate strength, poorly designed equipment, and improper motions are what cause a large proportion of musculoskeletal disorders.

To find and correct such predisposing factors is not always easy. It may take a visit to the patient's work site to see what is causing the problem. It may mean consulting with a coach or trainer about proper tennis strokes. When the necessary modifications have been identified, patients must learn to incorporate them into their routine. The changes should be simple at first to assure proper technique.

The following is an example of such a functional progression in an ankle sprain. First, the patient's playing technique and footwear must be assessed and if necessary modified. Then the patient may work through a progression of proprioceptive exercise: running forward and backward, running figure-of-eight's, running up stairs, etc. Each more complex exercise is added only when the previous ones are mastered. Patients successfully completing this process can return to their sports.

### Preventive Principles

From sports medicine we have learned that a proper screening evaluation is helpful in weeding out people most predisposed to injury. They can then be given the opportunity to make up for whatever deficiencies they may have. This principle is also useful for other activities and for pre-work evaluation. It does neither employer nor employee any good if the worker is not suited to the job. Such a screening evaluation may consist of a work simulation task, use of machines that measure lifting strength, or just a physical examination. It should not become an excuse to avoid employing someone, but rather a technique of identifying potential problem areas and correcting them before they result in disability.

Another part of the preventive approach is cross-training. Some people will argue that they work hard, walk a lot on the job, feel tired at the end of the day, and therefore do not need exercise. They are wrong. While they no doubt do work hard, it just is not the same as a regular exercise program. There are also zealots who are not happy unless they are competing in 100-mile runs, or for whom a regular marathon is not challenging enough unless preceded by a 1-mile swim and a 100-mile bike ride. For the average population, however, exercise in moderation is advisable. It is clear that active people feel better and perform better in their daily functions. A program of regular varied exercise, using strength and aerobic training in balance, optimizes health and well-being.

## Points of Summary

1. Prolonged immobility causes deterioration of the cardiorespiratory system, cartilage, muscles, bones, and impairs coordination.
2. Relative rest is preferred to immobilization when possible.
3. Ligament injury may impair proprioception.
4. The four phases of functional progression are phase I: control of inflammation; phase II: restore mobility; phase III: restore strength; and phase IV: functional progression to normal activity.
5. Cross-training may help prevent injury.

## References

1. Taylor HL, Henschel A, Brozek J, et al.: Effects of bed rest on cardiovascular function and work performance. *J Appl Physiol* 1949;2:223–239.
2. Akeson WH: The response of ligaments to stress modulation and overview of the ligament healing response. In Daniel D, Akeson W, O'Connor J (eds): *Knee Ligament Structure, Function, Injury, and Repair*. New York: Raven Press, 1990:315.
3. Noyes FR: Functional properties of knee ligaments and alterations induced by immobilization: A correlative biomechanical and histological study in primates. *Clin Orthop* 1977;123:210–242.
4. Akeson WH, Woo SLY, Amiel D, et al.: The connective tissue response to immobility: Biomechanical changes in periarticular connective tissue of the immobilized rabbit knee. *Clin Orthop* 1973;93:356–362.
5. Saltin B, Blomqvist G, Mitchell JH, et al.: Response to exercise after bedrest and after training: A longitudinal study of adaptive changes in oxygen transport and body composition. *Circulation* 1968;38 (Suppl 7):VII1–VII78.
6. Deitrick JE, Whedon GD, Shorr E: Effects of immobilization upon various metabolic and physiologic functions of normal men. *Am J Med* 1948;4:3–36.
7. Deyo RA, Diehl AK, Rosenthal M: How many days of bedrest for acute low back pain? A randomized clinical trial. *New Engl J Med* 1986;315:1064–1070.
8. Freeman MAR, Dean MRE, Hanham IWF: The etiology and prevention of functional instability of the foot. *J Bone Joint Surg* 1965;47B:678–685.
9. Hoppenfeld S: *Physical Examination of the Spine and Extremities*. East Norwalk, CT: Appleton-Century-Crofts, 1976.

## Suggested Readings

Saal JA (ed): Rehabilitation of Sports Injuries. *Physical Medicine and Rehabilitation: State of the Art Reviews* 1987;1(4).
Halar EM, Bell KR: Rehabilitation's relationship to inactivity. In Kottke FJ, Lehmann JR (eds), *Krusen's Handbook of Physical Medicine and Rehabilitation*, 4th ed. Philadelphia: WB Saunders, 1990:1113–1133.

# Chapter 5

# Medications Used in Musculoskeletal Rehabilitation

RALPH BUSCHBACHER
CHRISTINA DALMADY-ISRAEL

Patients often come to the physician or therapist looking for pain relief. All too often this translates into wanting a "pill" that will cure all their ills. Most musculoskeletal pain disorders are the result of an anatomic predisposition or something the patient is doing, such as overstressing a body part. In most instances, a pill will not cure the underlying problem. All that can really be expected of medications is temporary relief of symptoms so that the patient can better tolerate physical exercise, therapy, and rehabilitation to correct the root cause of the pain. Medications are usually an adjunct to care, rather than the prime focus. This must be made clear to every patient; otherwise, there is likely to be misunderstanding and frustration for all involved.

## Nonsteroidal Antiinflammatory Drugs

As a group nonsteroidal antiinflammatory drugs (NSAIDs) are the most widely used medications for treatment of musculoskeletal disorders, particularly for pain. As their name implies, they also reduce inflammation. The prototypical NSAID is aspirin (acetylsalicylic acid); however, there are numerous other salicylic acid derivatives as well as many other NSAIDs. Based on chemical structure, the NSAIDs can be divided into nine major groups as listed in Table 5-1. Usual dosages and costs are listed in Table 5-2.

The normal pathophysiologic pathway of pain production and inflammation involves the conversion of arachidonic acid to prostaglandins which then mediate the inflammatory process. Prostaglandins also sensitize the body's pain receptors to other pain generating compounds such as bradykinin. NSAIDs exert their analgesic and antiinflammatory effects by inhibiting cyclooxygenase, the enzyme that converts arachidonic acid to prostaglandin precursors (Figure 5-1).

NSAIDs are good analgesics for mild to moderate musculoskeletal pain. The onset of analgesia is relatively rapid, usually within minutes to hours. The antiinflammatory effects of the NSAIDs, on the other hand, usually take 2 to 3 weeks to take effect, and often require higher doses than used for analgesia (Table 5-2). Thus, when using an NSAID to reduce inflammation, it is important to obtain and maintain adequate blood concentrations of the drug for at least two weeks before assessing its efficacy. If an NSAID proves to be ineffective at relieving inflammation in a particular

**Table 5-1.** Commonly Utilized Nonsteroidal Antiinflammatory Drugs (NSAIDs)

| Chemical Class | Generic Name | Trade Name |
| --- | --- | --- |
| Acetylated Salicylates | Aspirin | Multiple products |
| Nonacetylated salicylates | Choline salicylate | Arthropan |
| | Magnesium and choline salicylate | Trilisate |
| | Magnesium salicylate | Magan, Mobidin, Doan's caplets |
| | Sodium salicylate | Multiple products |
| | Salsalate | Disalcid |
| | Diflunisal | Dolobid |
| Propionic acid derivatives | Ibuprofen | Motrin, Rufen, Advil and more |
| | Fenoprofen | Nalfon |
| | Naproxen | Naprosyn, Anaprox |
| | Ketoprofen | Orudis |
| | Flurbiprofen | Ansaid |
| | Ketorolac | Toradol |
| Pyrroleacetic acid derivatives | Sulindac | Clinoril |
| | Tolmetin | Tolectin |
| Indoleacetic acid derivatives | Indomethacin | Indocin |
| | Etodolac | Lodine |
| Anthranilic acid derivatives | Mefanamic acid | Ponstel |
| (Fenamates) | Meclofenamate | Meclomen |
| Phenylacetic acid derivatives | Diclonfenac | Voltaren |
| Oxicams | Piroxicam | Feldene |
| Pyrazolone derivatives | Phenylbutazone | Butazolidin, Azolid |

case, another NSAID may be tried instead. However, since NSAIDs within the same chemical classes have similar actions, it is recommended that a NSAID from a different group be substituted. Again a 2- to 3-week trial using an appropriate antiinflammatory dose is necessary before calling the trial a failure. Sometimes it may be necessary to try three or more agents before finding the drug that works. The agent that is ultimately successful cannot necessarily be predicted, as it is something of a "hit or miss" practice.

In the interest of the patient's pocketbook, it is generally advisable to use the least expensive agents first. Aspirin and ibuprofen are available without prescription and are generally effective and relatively inexpensive. One of their drawbacks is that they need to be given several times per day, so if compliance is an issue, a medication that can be scheduled once or twice a day may be preferred.

In most acute musculoskeletal conditions, NSAIDs are not given for long enough periods of time for medication side effects to be a major problem. These problems may be more evident when treating chronic arthritic or connective tissue dis-

orders, since long-term use for several years may be required. The main complications are gastrointestinal upset, gastrointestinal bleeding, liver or kidney damage, dizziness, headache, confusion, ringing in the ears, and allergy (Table 5-3).

Gastrointestinal upset can usually be avoided by administering the medication with meals. Gastrointestinal bleeding is more serious and may be a life threatening complication. When taken orally, all NSAIDs produce some damage to the gastric mucosa, the superficial layer of the stomach. By blocking prostaglandin synthesis, NSAIDs impair the formation of the mucus barrier that protects the gastrointestinal tract. Furthermore, all the NSAIDs except for Salsalate (Disalcid™) may prolong bleeding time by inhibiting platelets. Thus it is easy to see how prolonged use of NSAIDs may cause gastrointestinal bleeding.

Misoprostol, a prostaglandin-like substance that protects against mucosal ulceration, may be used to prevent the development of bleeding problems in high-risk patients. This agent is not without its own problems such as high cost, multiple daily dosing, and production of diarrhea; thus it is not

**Table 5-2.** Usual Dosages and Cost of Commonly Used Oral NSAIDs

| NSAID | Daily Analgesic Dose (mg) | Antiinflammatory Daily Dose | Daily Cost ($) |
|---|---|---|---|
| Aspirin | 650–975 q4h | 2.4–3.9 g* | 0.20 |
| Choline salicylate | 435–870 q4h | 4.8–7.2 g* | 2.20 |
| Dicolfenac | | 150–200 mg* in 2–4 divided doses | 3.34 |
| Diflunisal | 1 g load then 500 mg q8–12h | 250–500 mg* bid | 1.38 |
| Etodolac | 400 load then 200–400 q6–8h | 400 mg bid–tid or 300 mg tid–qid* | 3.85 |
| Fenoprofen | 200 q4–6h | 300–600 mg* tid or qid | 2.85 |
| Flurbiprofen | 50 mg qid | 200–300 mg* in 2–4 divided doses | 3.30 |
| Ibuprofen | 200–400 q4–6h | 1.2–3.2 g* in 3–4 divided doses | 1.39 |
| Indomethacin | 25–50 bid–qid | 25–50 mg bid–qid* | 3.16 |
| Ketoprofen | 50 q6–8h | 150–300 mg* in 3–4 divided doses | 3.89 |
| Magnesium and choline salicylate | 2–3 g salicylate in 2–3 divided doses | 1.5–4.5 g* salicylate in 2–3 divided doses | 3.31 |
| Magnesium salicylate | 300–600 q4h | 1.09–4.8 g* | 3.03 |
| Meclofenamate | 50 q4–6h | 200–400 mg* in 3–4 divided doses | 3.61 |
| Mefenamic acid | 500 load then 250 q6h* | | 3.22 |
| Naproxen | 500 load then 250 q6–8h | 250–500 mg* bid | 2.12 |
| Phenylbutazone | | Initial: 300–600 mg in 3–4 divided doses Maint: 100 mg qd–qid* | 0.62 |
| Piroxicam | | 10 mg bid or 20 mg* daily | 2.20 |
| Salsalate | 3000 in 2–3 divided doses | 3 g in 2–3 divided doses | 0.62 |
| Sodium salicylate | 325–650 q4h | 3.9–5.2 g* | 0.31 |
| Sulindac | 150–200 bid | 150–200 mg* bid | 2.12 |
| Tolmetin | | 600 mg–1.8 g* in 3–4 divided doses | 3.17 |

*Dosage used to calculate cost based on average wholesale price.
Source: *Redbook Drug Topics*. Oradell, NJ: Medical Economics Inc, 1992.

routinely prescribed for prophylaxis of bleeding events. NSAIDs are to be avoided in patients on anticoagulants, such as heparin or warfarin.

The hepatic effects of NSAIDs are usually seen as a reversible rise in liver function tests. Liver function should be checked with base laboratory values and periodic follow-up checks for the drugs most likely to cause damage, namely aspirin, ketoprofen, and diclofenac. True hepatitis is a rare complication.

Kidney effects are due to the inhibition of prostaglandins in the kidneys. This may result in glomerulonephritis, interstitial nephritis or nephrotic syndrome. In patients with compromised renal function, NSAIDs must be used with extreme caution, if at all, as they may induce frank renal failure. Sulindac is considered the safest NSAID for use in patients with poor kidney function since it is eliminated to a greater extent by nonrenal mechanisms. Care should also be exercised in using these agents in patients with congestive heart failure, as the tendency for sodium and water retention may adversely affect the underlying cardiac condition.

Allergies to NSAIDs are rare, but if a patient has a documented allergy to one agent, others,

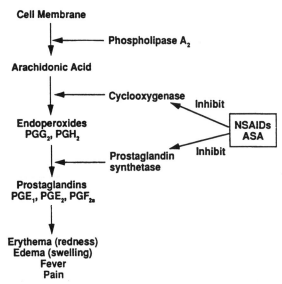

**Figure 5-1.** Mechanism of action of aspirin and NSAIDs in blocking the conversion of arachidonic acid into prostaglandins.

particularly within the same chemical class, should be avoided, as cross-sensitivity is a possibility.

Only one NSAID, ketorolac, can be administered by the intramuscular route. It is important to point out that it has no demonstrated antiinflammatory effect and should be used only for its analgesic properties. Ketorolac has been shown to be as effective as morphine at relieving pain and is often used postoperatively.

## Analgesics

In acute pain due to an injury, the first line of treatment is often pain control. Excessive pain leads to reflex muscle splinting and further pain. To provide comfort, analgesics are often used along with ice, proper position, and elevation of the injured area.

Analgesia is, of course, provided by the NSAIDs, but these agents are often avoided in the acute stage of injury since they may inhibit platelet aggregation necessary to halt bleeding. Instead, acetaminophen and narcotics, or combinations of the two, are often prescribed.

Acetaminophen is roughly equivalent to aspirin as an analgesic, but it has only weak antiinflammatory properties. It interrupts prostaglandin-mediated pain stimuli in the central nervous system. It is generally useful for treating mild to moderate pain. It potentiates the pain relieving properties of narcotic medications and is available in a number of combination preparations with various narcotics. Table 5-4 lists the frequently prescribed aspirin-narcotic and acetaminophen-narcotic products.

Narcotics are medications that activate or stimulate the body's own pain control mechanisms within the central nervous system. They do not diminish awareness of pain but do decrease the subjective distress of pain. The prototypical narcotic is morphine, and like morphine, the other narcotics generally have addictive qualities. The risk of addiction is very small when these medications are prescribed for acute pain and for short periods of time. More often than being overprescribed, these medications are usually underdosed by physicians afraid of causing addiction. When used appropriately this is rarely a problem. Narcotics are effective at reducing acute pain when there is an identifiable physiologic cause of the pain. They are notoriously ineffective at relieving chronic pain.

When prescribing a narcotic, a narcotic-acetaminophen, or a narcotic-aspirin combination it is important to use an adequate dose to provide true pain relief. All analgesics should be dosed on a scheduled basis, with the patient aware that they will be given for a short period of time and then discontinued in favor of another medication. Patients should not be allowed to get into the habit of requesting more and more narcotics as so often happens with emergency room visits or with phone calls to the doctor on call. Side effects of narcotic-containing medications include sedation, nausea, flushing, constipation, and rarely allergy. In addition, excessive doses of narcotics may cause respiratory depression (Table 5-5).

## Corticosteroids

Corticosteroids, or just "steroids" for short, are powerful antiinflammatory agents (Table 5-6). They may be administered by oral, intramuscular, intraarticular, epidural, or intravenous routes. They are not to be confused with the "anabolic steroids" used by some athletes to increase muscle mass. Technically, corticosteroids are of the catabolic type.

**Table 5-3.** Common Side Effects of NSAIDs

| Side Effect | DI | DF | FE | FL | IB | IN | E | K | MC | MF | N | PH | PI | S | T |
|---|---|---|---|---|---|---|---|---|---|---|---|---|---|---|---|
| **Gastrointestinal** | | | | | | | | | | | | | | | |
| Gastritis | – | 1 | 1 | 1 | 1 | – | 1 | 1 | – | – | – | 1 | – | 1 | 2 |
| Diarrhea | 3 | 3 | 2 | 3 | 2 | 2 | 3 | 3 | 4 | 3 | 2 | 1 | 2 | 3 | 3 |
| Nausea | 3 | 3 | 3 | 3 | 3 | 3 | 3 | 3 | 4 | 3 | 3 | 3 | 3 | 3 | 4 |
| Vomiting | 1 | 2 | 3 | 2 | 2 | 2 | 2 | 2 | – | – | 1 | 1 | 1 | 2 | 3 |
| **CNS Effects** | | | | | | | | | | | | | | | |
| Headache | 3 | 3 | 3 | 3 | 2 | 4 | 3 | 3 | 3 | – | 3 | 1 | 2 | 3 | 3 |
| Mood changes | 1 | 1 | 1 | 2 | 1 | 2 | – | 2 | 1 | – | 1 | 1 | 1 | 1 | 2 |
| Drowsiness | 1 | 2 | 3 | 2 | 1 | 1 | 2 | 2 | – | – | 3 | 1 | 2 | 1 | 2 |
| **Hepatic Effects** | | | | | | | | | | | | | | | |
| Hepatitis | 1 | 1 | 1 | 1 | 1 | 1 | – | 1 | – | 1 | 1 | 1 | 1 | 1 | 1 |
| ↑ LFTs* | 2 | 1 | 1 | – | 1 | 1 | – | 2 | 1 | 1 | 1 | 1 | 1 | 1 | 1 |
| **Dermatologic** | | | | | | | | | | | | | | | |
| Rash | 2 | 3 | 3 | 1 | 3 | 1 | 1 | 2 | 3 | – | 3 | 2 | 2 | 3 | 2 |
| Hives | 1 | 1 | 2 | 1 | 1 | 1 | 1 | 1 | 2 | – | 1 | 1 | 1 | – | 1 |
| Itching | 2 | 1 | 3 | 1 | 2 | 1 | 1 | 1 | 2 | – | 3 | 1 | 2 | 2 | 2 |
| **Renal Effects** | | | | | | | | | | | | | | | |
| Fluid retention | 3 | 1 | 2 | – | 2 | 2 | – | 3 | 2 | – | 3 | 3 | 2 | 2 | 3 |
| Renal impairment | 1 | 1 | 1 | 1 | 1 | 1 | – | 1 | 1 | 1 | 1 | 1 | 1 | 1 | 1 |
| **Cardiovascular†** | | | | | | | | | | | | | | | |
| Hypertension | 1 | – | – | 1 | 1 | 1 | – | 1 | – | – | – | 1 | 1 | 1 | 3 |
| Chest pain | 1 | 1 | – | 1 | – | 1 | – | – | – | – | – | – | – | – | 2 |
| ↑ CHF | 1 | – | – | 1 | 1 | 1 | – | 1 | – | – | 1 | 1 | 1 | 1 | 1 |
| Heartbeat change | 1 | 1 | 3 | 1 | 1 | 1 | 1 | 1 | 1 | 1 | 2 | – | 1 | 1 | – |
| **Hematologic** | | | | | | | | | | | | | | | |
| Leukopenia | 1 | – | – | 1 | 1 | 1 | – | 1 | 1 | 1 | 1 | 1 | 2 | 1 | – |
| Anemia | 1 | – | – | 1 | 1 | 1 | – | 1 | 1 | 2 | – | 1 | 2 | – | 2 |
| ↓ Platelets | 1 | 1 | 1 | 1 | 1 | 1 | – | 1 | 1 | 1 | 1 | 1 | 1 | 1 | 1 |
| **Ocular/Otic** | | | | | | | | | | | | | | | |
| Blurred vision | 1 | 1 | 2 | 1 | 1 | 1 | – | 2 | 1 | – | 2 | 1 | 1 | 1 | 2 |
| Ringing in ears | 2 | 2 | 2 | 2 | 2 | 2 | 1 | 2 | 2 | – | 3 | 1 | 2 | 2 | 2 |
| **Hypersensitivity** | | | | | | | | | | | | | | | |
| Anaphylaxis | 1 | 1 | 1 | 1 | 1 | 1 | 1 | 1 | – | – | 1 | 1 | 1 | 1 | 1 |

DI, diclofenac; DF, diflunisal; FE, fenoprofen; FL, flurbiprofen; IB, ibuprofen; IN, indomethacin; E, etodolac; K, ketoprofen; MC, meclofenamate; MF, mefenamic acid; N, naproxen; PH, phenylbutazone; PI, piroxicam; S, sulindac; T, tolmetin.

Incidence rates 4 = >10%; 3 = 3%-9%; 2 = 1%-3%; 1 = <1%; – = unknown.

*Greater than three times the upper limit of normal.

†Cardiovascular effects may be secondary to NSAID-induced renal impairment.

In conditions of systemic or multifocal inflammation, corticosteroids are usually administered orally. Examples of such use include patients with rheumatoid arthritis or other connective tissue disorders. They are also effective in the treatment of reflex sympathetic dystrophy and acute radiculopathy. In these conditions they are typically administered for 7 to 14 days at a high, but rapidly, tapered dose.

Intraarticular steroid injection is a common treatment for inflamed or arthritic joints. Care must be taken that the affected joint does not harbor any infection and that infection is not introduced into the joint by the injection. Joint injections with steroids provide excellent short-term relief of pain and inflammation but may hasten the ultimate demise of the articular cartilage. The use of intraarticular injections should be limited. The recommended frequency is not more than every 2 to 3 months, for a maximum of three to four injections per year. Intraarticular steroids can also be given in combination with a local anesthetic. The local anesthetic gives immediate pain relief, but since it wears off in a few hours, the symptoms may actually be worsened for a day or two before the steroid effect begins. The patient may need to apply ice to the joint to ease the pain.

**Table 5-4.** Frequently Used Analgesic-Narcotic Combination Products

| ASPIRIN/NARCOTIC COMBINATIONS | | |
| --- | --- | --- |
| **Trade Name** | **Amount ASA** | **Narcotic and (Other) Components** |
| Empirin 2 | 325 mg | 15 mg codeine |
| Empirin 3 | 325 mg | 30 mg codeine |
| Empirin 4 | 325 mg | 60 mg codeine |
| Synalgos-DC | 356.4 mg | 16 mg dihydrocodeine bitartrate (30 mg caffeine) |
| Azdone | 500 mg | 5 mg hydrocodone bitartrate |
| Percodan | 325 mg | 4.5 mg oxycodone hydrochloride + 0.38 mg oxycodone terephthalate |
| Talwin compound | 325 mg | 12.5 mg pentazocine |
| Darvon with ASA | 325 mg | 65 mg propoxyphene |
| Darvon compound | 389 mg | 32 mg propoxyphene (32.4 mg caffeine) |
| Darvon-N with ASA | 325 mg | 100 mg propoxyphene napsylate |
| Fiorinal | 325 mg | 50 mg butalbital (40 mg caffeine) |

| ACETAMINOPHEN/NARCOTIC COMBINATIONS | | |
| --- | --- | --- |
| **Trade Name** | **AMT APAP** | **Narcotic and (Other) Components** |
| Tylenol No. 1 | 300 mg | 7.5 mg codeine |
| Tylenol No. 2 | 300 mg | 15 mg codeine |
| Tylenol No. 3 | 300 mg | 30 mg codeine |
| Tylenol No. 4 | 300 mg | 60 mg codeine |
| Lortab 5/500 | 500 mg | 5 mg hydrocodone bitartrate |
| Vicodin | 500 mg | 5 mg hydrocodone bitartrate |
| Vicodin ES | 500 mg | 7.5 mg hydrocodone bitartrate |
| Hydrogesic | 500 mg | 5 mg hydrocodone bitartrate |
| Demerol-APAP | 300 mg | 50 mg meperidine |
| Percocet | 325 mg | 5 mg oxycodone |
| Tylox | 500 mg | 5 mg oxycodone |
| Talacen | 650 mg | 25 mg pentazocine |
| Darvocet-N 50 | 325 mg | 50 mg propoxyphene napsylate |
| Darvocet-N 100 | 650 mg | 100 mg propoxyphene napsylate |
| Fioricet | 325 mg | 50 mg butalbital (40 mg caffeine) |

APAP, acetaminophen; ASA, acetylsalicylic acid.

Steroids may also be injected into an inflamed bursa or tendon sheath for tendonitis. It is important to remember that the injection of steroid solution near tendons and ligaments may weaken those structures for periods of 2 to 6 weeks. Patients should be warned that relief of pain does not mean that the tendon should be overstressed, since tendon rupture may result.

The injection of steroid solution into the epidural space of the spinal canal may be useful in cases of radiculopathy or nerve root irritation, especially when it is due to disk herniation. This injection bathes the inflamed structures in the anti-inflammatory solution.

Steroids may also be administered systemically by the intramuscular route. From the injection

**Table 5-5.** Most Common Side Effects Associated with Narcotic Use

| *Gastrointestinal* | *Cardiovascular* |
| --- | --- |
| Constipation | Hypotension |
| Nausea/vomiting | *Respiratory* |
| *Central nervous system* | Respiratory depression |
| Dizziness | (high doses) |
| Drowsiness | *Allergic* (due to histamine |
| Confusion | release) |
| Seizures (rare) | Hypotension |
| Blurred or double vision | Flushing |
| False sense of well-being | Wheezing |
| | Tachycardia |

**Table 5-6.** Steroid Preparations Commonly Utilized in Musculoskeletal Disorders

| ORAL STEROID PREPARATIONS | | |
| --- | --- | --- |
| **Duration of Action** | **Generic Name** | **Trade Name** |
| Short acting | Cortisone | Cortone Acetate |
| | Hydrocortisone | Cortef, Hydrocortone |
| Intermediate acting | Methylprednisolone | Medrol |
| | Prednisolone | Delta-Cortel, Prelone |
| | Prednisone | Deltasone, Orasone |
| | Triamcinolone | Aristacort, Kenacort |
| Long acting | Betamethasone | Celestone |
| | Dexamethasone | Decadron, Dexone, Hexadrol |

| PARENTERAL STEROID PREPARATIONS | | | |
| --- | --- | --- | --- |
| | | **Parenteral Administration** | |
| **Generic Name** | **Trade Name** | **Systemic** | **Local** |
| Betamethasone | | | |
|   Sodium phosphate | Celestone Phosphate | IM, IV | IA, IL, ST |
|   Acetate/sodium phosphate | Celestone Soluspan | IM | IA, IL, IS, ST |
| Dexamethasone | | | |
|   Acetate | Decadron-LA | IM | IA, IL, ST |
|   Sodium phosphate | Decadrol, Decadron Phosphate | IM, IV | IA, IL, IS, ST |
| Hydrocortisone | | | |
|   Sterile suspension | – | IM | |
|   Acetate | Hydrocortone Acetate | | IA, IB, IL, IS, ST |
|   Sodium phosphate | Hydrocortone Phosphate | IM, IV, SC | |
|   Sodium succinate | Solu-Cortef, A-HydroCort | IM, IV | |
| Methylprednisolone | | | |
|   Acetate | Depo-Medrol | IM | IA, IL, ST |
|   Sodium succinate | Solu-Medrol, A-MethaPred | IM, IV | |
| Prednisolone | | | |
|   Acetate | Articulose-50, Predicort | IM | |
|   Acetate/sodium phosphate | – | IM | IA, IB, IS, ST |
|   Sodium phosphate | Hydeltrasol, Predicort RP | IM, IV | IA, IL, ST |
|   Tebutate | Hydeltra TBA | | IA, IL, ST |
| Triamcinolone | | | |
|   Acetonide | Kenalog | IM | IA, IB, IL |
|   Diacetate | Aristocort Forte, Triam-Forte | IM | IA, IL, IS, ST |
|   Hexacetonide | Aristospan Intra-articular | | IA, IL |

IA, Intraarticular; IB, intrabursal; IL, intralesional; IM, intramuscular; IS, intrasynovial; IV, intravenous; SC, subcutaneous; ST, soft tissue.

site, the medication is slowly released to provide systemic coverage. More commonly, however, the intramuscular route is used in myofascial pain conditions to inject trigger points. The rationale is that the local effect will relieve inflammation in these points. This is a common practice despite there being no good evidence to prove that these points are inflamed to begin with, nor that steroid injection by itself improves the symptoms.[1,2] Such injections of steroids are usually used in combination with a local anesthetic. Local administration of steroid reduces the risk of systemic side effects, and allows the administration of smaller doses of the medication.

Intravenous steroids are not used in musculoskeletal conditions and their use should be reserved for medical illnesses and acute spinal cord injury.

Steroids are generally safe when administered for short periods of time, but they can produce short- and long-term side effects. In the short term, oral steroids can unmask diabetes and weaken the body's defenses against infection. When used for longer periods of time, oral steroids may cause osteoporosis, hypertension, glucose intolerance, gastrointestinal bleeding, centripetal obesity, growth retardation in children, and a redistribution of body fat and water. Steroid use can also cause aseptic necrosis of joints and can cause flare-ups of latent infections such as tuberculosis (Table 5-7).

## Muscle Relaxants

The name "muscle relaxant" is, in essence, a misnomer as these medications do not truly relax the

**Table 5-7.** Side Effects Associated with Steroid Use

| Affected System | Side Effect |
| --- | --- |
| Endocrine/Metabolic | Glucose intolerance |
| | HPA axis suppression |
| | Altered lipid metabolism |
| | Negative nitrogen balance |
| | Hypokalemia |
| | Hypocalciuria |
| Cardiovascular | Hypertension |
| | Sodium and water retention |
| Central nervous system | Euphoria |
| | Disorientation, confusion |
| | Hallucinations |
| | Paranoia |
| Musculoskeletal system | Osteoporosis |
| | Growth suppression |
| | Aseptic necrosis of femoral head |
| | Myopathy |
| Gastrointestinal | Nausea/vomiting |
| | Peptic ulcer disease? |
| | Increased appetite |
| Hematologic | Leukocytosis |
| Immunologic | ↓ Function of white blood cells |
| | ↑ Risk of infections |
| | May mask infections |
| Dermatologic | Acne |
| | Striae |
| | Impaired wound healing |
| | Hypertrichosis |
| Ophthalmologic | Cataracts |
| Allergic reactions | Anaphylaxis |
| | Facial flushing |
| | Seizures |

muscles. A number of medications are marketed as such, but their effect is usually the indirect consequence of central nervous system sedation. These compounds cause drowsiness and should not be used when a patient must be alert, as in driving. Although these medications do not truly relax muscles, they are occasionally useful in musculoskeletal problems (Table 5-8). They may provide symptomatic relief of acute pain, perhaps by reducing secondary reflex muscle splinting. They are especially useful if given in a bedtime dose, as many of them increase the quantity of deep sleep (non-rapid eye movement or rest sleep) that helps some musculoskeletal symptoms. Nighttime use also minimizes daytime side effects.

## Antispasticity Medications

The three antispasticity medications include diazepam (Valium), baclofen (Lioresal), and dantrolene (Dantrium), which are usually used only in special musculoskeletal cases such as multiple sclerosis or after brain or spinal cord injury (Table 5-9). Diazepam reduces spasms by potentiating gamma-aminobutyric acid (GABA), an inhibitory neurotransmitter, within the central nervous system. Baclofen is thought to reduce spasticity by exerting GABA-like effects at the spinal cord level. Dantrolene is felt to reduce spasticity by inhibiting skeletal muscle directly. It blocks calcium release onto the myofilaments (see Chapter 2), thus preventing the muscle from contracting. Dantrolene may, in some cases, cause serious liver damage, and so liver function tests must be monitored. Since all three drugs produce systemic, rather than local effects, their side effects are also systemic. Often the weakness and drowsiness that they cause is more of a problem than the spasticity itself.

## Tricyclic Antidepressants and Anticonvulsants

In cases of chronic pain, tricyclic antidepressants (TCAs) and anticonvulsants may be helpful as adjuvant therapy (Table 5-10).[3] Although their mechanism of action in the treatment of pain is not entirely clear, they may be useful in treating neurogenic pain after nerve trauma, phantom limb

**Table 5-8.** Commonly Used Muscle Relaxants

| Generic Name (Trade Name) | Usual Doses | Side Effects |
|---|---|---|
| Cyclobenzaprine (Flexeril) | 20–40 mg/day in 2–4 divided doses | Anticholinergic effects Dizziness, drowsiness |
| Carisoprodol (Soma, Rela) | 350 mg qid | Drowsiness, dizziness Nausea/vomiting |
| Chlorphenesin (Maolate) | 400 mg qid | Drowsiness, dizziness |
| Chlorzoxazone (Parafon Forte) (Paraflex) | 250 mg tid–qid | Drowsiness, dizziness |
| Metaxalone (Skelaxin) | 800 mg tid–qid | Drowsiness, dizziness Rash ↑ in liver enzymes |
| Methocarbamol (Robaxin) | 1.5 g qid | Drowsiness, dizziness Blurred vision |
| Orphenadrine (Norflex) | 100 mg bid | Anticholinergic effects Drowsiness, dizziness Gastrointestinal upset |

pain after amputations, reflex sympathetic dystrophy, radiculopathy, low back pain, and chronic pain syndrome.

### Tricyclic Antidepressants

The TCAs work at nerve terminals by inhibiting the reuptake of neurotransmitters, thus potentiating the effect of the transmitters. One of these neurotransmitters, serotonin, is believed to play a role in inhibiting pain by a central nervous system mechanism.[4] The increase of serotonin concentration levels at the nerve terminals is felt to reduce pain transmission, especially the abnormal transmission seen in chronic and neurogenic pain states. The so-called tertiary amine TCAs and a related compound, trazodone, are generally the most effective in the treatment of pain.[5] The doses used in pain management are usually lower than those used for the treatment of depression. Patients should be made aware of the fact that these agents are also used for depression, and that this is not necessarily the reason for their treatment. Few

**Table 5-9.** Commonly Utilized Antispasticity Medications

| Generic Name (Trade Name) | Usual Dosage Range | Side Effects | Special Precautions |
|---|---|---|---|
| Baclofen (Lioresal) | Initial: 5 mg tid Max: 80 mg/day | CNS depression Muscle weakness Hypotension Constipation Insomnia | Elderly more likely to develop CNS effects Concurrent use with TCA antidepressants Concurrent use with antihypertensives Concurrent use with CNS depressants May ↑ blood glucose concentrations in diabetics |
| Dantrolene (Dantrium) | Initial: 25 mg qd Max: 100 mg qid | Hepatoxicity Diarrhea Dizziness Muscle weakness Insomnia Seizures | Rat studies show carcinogenicity with prolonged use Concurrent use with CNS depressants Concurrent use with hepatotoxins Females > 35 yr at higher risk for developing hepatotoxicity |
| Diazepam (Valium) | 2–10 mg tid–qid | Muscle weakness Ataxia Sedation Irritability | Geriatric and debilitated patients more sensitive to CNS side effects Concurrent use of CNS depressants |

**Table 5-10.** Adjunctive Pain Medications

| ANTIDEPRESSANTS | | | | |
| --- | --- | --- | --- | --- |
| Generic Name (Trade Name) | Usual Doses (mg/day) | Sedative Potential | Anticholinergic Effect | Orthostatic Hypotension |
| Amitriptyline (Elavil)* | 10-100 | ++++ | ++++ | ++++ |
| Desipramine (Norpramin)† | 10-100 | + | ++ | +++ |
| Doxepin (Sinequan)* | 10-100 | ++++ | +++ | ++++ |
| Imipramine (Tofranil)* | 10-100 | ++ | ++ | ++ |
| Nortriptyline (Aventyl)† | 10-100 | ++ | ++ | ++ |
| Trazodone (Desyrel) | 25-100 | +++ | + | +++‡ |

| ANTICONVULSANTS | | | |
| --- | --- | --- | --- |
| Generic Name (Trade Name) | Usual Doses | Side Effects | Special Precautions |
| Carbamazepine (Tegretol) | Initial: 100 mg bid Usual: 200 mg–1.2 g/day | Blurred vision Rash Hyponatremia Arrythmias Leukopenia Hepatotoxicity | Concurrent use of tricyclic antidepressants |
| Phenytoin (Dilantin) | 100–300 mg/day in divided doses | Gingival hyperplasia Nystagmus Ataxia Blood dyscrasias Hepatotoxicity Hypertrichosis | Monitor for possible drug interactions Teratogenicity |

*Is a tertiary amine.
†Is a secondary amine.
‡Orthostatic hypotension with trazodone can be eliminated by administering after meals.
+, Greater number of "+" indicates progressively greater potential effect.

things destroy a patient's trust as quickly as finding out from friends or the lay press that the drug the doctor prescribed is an antidepressant when he or she was told it was for pain.

Chronic pain states are almost invariably associated with abnormal sleep patterns. Serotonin is also associated with regulation of the sleep cycle, and this may be another mechanism by which TCAs help reduce pain. Due to their sedative potential, TCAs are usually given at bedtime or a few hours before retiring. The dose can be increased slowly to reduce side effects, which are usually only a problem with higher doses of TCAs.

When antidepressants are prescribed for pain or sleep disturbance the doses are generally less than those used for depression. The doses may be titrated upward as needed. If excessive daytime drowsiness occurs, the patient usually adjusts to it within a few days. If not, the dose may have to be decreased. At the low doses given for pain, side effects are rare and mainly include sedation and anticholinergic effects, such as dry mouth and orthostatic hypotension.

### Anticonvulsants

Carbamezepine (Tegretol), and phenytoin (Dilantin) are the two most commonly used anticonvulsants in chronic pain states. The mechanism by

**Table 5-11.** Commonly Used Local Anesthetics

| Generic Name (Trade Name) | Duration of Action | Indications |
|---|---|---|
| Bupivicaine (Marcaine) | Long | C, E, P, S |
| Chloroprocaine (Nesacaine) | Short | C, E, P |
| Etidocaine (Duranest) | Long | C, E, P |
| Lidocaine (Xylocaine) | Intermediate | C, E, P, S |
| Mepivicaine (Carbocaine) | Intermediate | C, E, P |
| Procaine (Novocain) | Short | P |
| Phenol† | Varies* | E, P, S |

*At low doses causes transient conduction blocks; at higher doses may cause irreversible conduction block by damaging nerves. Commonly used in motor point blocks.
†Phenol is primarily used for nerve or motor point blocks.
Short = 30–60 minutes; intermediate = 1–3 hours; long = 3–10 hours.
C, Caudal anesthesia; E, epidural anesthesia; P, peripheral nerve block; S, sympathetic block.

which they act is unknown but may be due to their membrane stabilizing effects.[3] Some of the more common side effects associated with these anticonvulsants are listed in Table 5-10.

## Injections

### Local Anesthetics

As described earlier, steroid injections into trigger points, bursae, or within joints are usually administered in a mixture with a local anesthetic. The commonly used anesthetics are listed in Table 5-11. When used for treating musculoskeletal pain they should not be combined with vasoconstrictors such as epinephrine since this may reduce blood flow to the painful area, possibly making it even more painful or causing tissue damage.

Local anesthetics work by inhibiting nerve transmission, and their effects usually wear off in a few hours. Sometimes they are used diagnostically, for instance in a facet joint injection. If the local anesthetic relieves the pain, it confirms the injection site as the locus of pain.

Often a local anesthetic is injected at trigger point sites without steroid. There is controversy regarding the efficacy of this practice, with some clinicians arguing that inserting a needle into a trigger point without injecting any medication, or injecting saline solution, is equally effective at giving long-term relief.[1,2]

Side effects of local anesthetics include cardiac and central nervous system depression, prolonged pain at the injection site, complications due to improperly placed injections, and in rare instances, allergic reactions.

### Nerve and Motor Point Blocks

In cases of extreme spasticity, it may sometimes be necessary to block the conduction of a nerve or a motor point (where the nerve enters the muscle). This procedure is usually performed with phenol, a long-acting local anesthetic that at high doses causes nerve damage. Such an injection may relieve spasticity for periods of time ranging from 3 months to 2 years. Side effects include reaction to the medication, weakness, and paresthesias, especially when sensory nerves are blocked.

### Sympathetic Ganglion Blocks

As described in Chapters 16 and 25, reflex sympathetic dystrophy (RSD) is a condition of increased sympathetic nervous system activity (see Chapter 2) to a limb. It can be excruciatingly painful, even incapacitating. Blocking the sympathetic outflow at the sympathetic ganglia (collection of nerve cell bodies) near the spinal cord can be both a diagnostic and a therapeutic procedure for RSD. This procedure should only be performed under fluoroscopic x-ray control by an experienced practitioner.

## Antianxiety Medications

Anxiety is often an integral part of pain syndromes, and antianxiety medications such as the benzodiazepines (Valium, Librium) are sometimes prescribed in pain conditions. While this is not recommended as a routine practice or in chronic pain syndromes,[5] it may find short-term utility in acute pain states in which anxiety has been identified as a major component. These agents have a potential for addiction and do not directly treat pain. Since they typically reduce serotonin levels, they may actually worsen the pain.

Antihistamines such as hydroxyzine (Vistaril) may also reduce anxiety by means of a sedative effect, and have been tried in combination with other medications, sometimes with good results.[5]

## Points of Summary

1. Nonsteroidal antiinflammatory agents reduce pain and inflammation by reducing prostaglandin production.
2. Acetaminophen is analgesic but only weakly antiinflammatory.
3. Corticosteroid injections weaken tendons and ligaments for 2 to 6 weeks.
4. "Muscle relaxants" do not really relax muscles, but cause central nervous system depression.
5. Tricyclic antidepressants increase serotonin levels at nerve synapses, help regulate the sleep cycle, and may be used to treat chronic or neurogenic pain.
6. The anticonvulsants carbamazepine and phenytoin may be used to treat chronic or neurogenic pain.

7. Benzodiazepines such as diazepam and chlordiazepoxide are not generally useful in treating pain. Antihistamines such as hydroxyzine may be helpful.

## References

1. Gunn CC, Milbrandt WE, Little AS, et al.: Dry needling of muscle motor points for chronic low-back pain: A randomized clinical trial with long term follow-up. *Spine* 1980;5:279–291.
2. Garvey TA, Marks MR, Wiesel SW: A prospective, randomized, double-blind evaluation of trigger-point injection therapy for low-back pain. *Spine* 1989;14:962–964.
3. Maciewicz R, Bouckoms A, Martin JB: Drug therapy of neuropathic pain. *Clin J Pain* 1985;1:39–49.
4. Basbaum AI, Fields HL: Endogenous pain control systems: Brainstem spinal pathways and endorphin circuitry. *Annu Rev Neurosci* 1984;7:309–338.
5. Hendler N: The anatomy and psychopharmacology of chronic pain. *J Clin Psychiatry* 1982;43(8):15–20.

## Suggested Readings

Kawahara NE, Spunt AL: Pharmacologic agents in musculoskeletal pain. *Physical Medicine and Rehabilitation: State of the Art Reviews* 1991;5(3):479–492.

# Chapter 6
# Therapeutic Modalities

RALPH BUSCHBACHER

Heat and cold have been known for some time to reduce pain. They appear to do so by equalizing the temperature gradient between injured and noninjured tissues.[1] In addition to relieving pain, these modalities have other actions, including effects on flexibility, joint stiffness, blood flow, and inflammation. To take advantage of these properties, both for treating pain and other conditions, numerous heating and cooling devices have been developed. This chapter describes the advantages and disadvantages of several such devices and also focuses on the use of electrical stimulation techniques and biofeedback in physical medicine.

## Heat

Heating modalities create both local and reflex effects. The local response is an increase in tissue temperature and metabolic rate. The reflex effects include both regional and generalized responses. The regional responses include increased blood flow to the treated area and muscle relaxation (Figure 6-1). The generalized responses include increased blood flow to the contralateral limb, sedation and relaxation, sweating, and body thermoregulation. The local responses are more vigorous as a rule.[2]

Heating modalities can be divided by their mechanism of heating, namely, conduction, con-

vection, or conversion. Table 6-1 lists the main modalities utilizing each of these mechanisms.

### Conduction

Conduction is the simplest heating modality (Figure 6-2). It occurs whenever two objects of differing temperatures come into contact with each other. Heat flows from the warmer to the cooler object. This occurs because the molecules in the warmer material vibrate faster and stimulate the cooler molecules to move faster as well. The temperature of the object being warmed rises most at the surface in contact with the heating source and drops off rapidly in a gradient from that point on. Similarly, the heating agent is warmest at its center and gets cooler closer to its surface of contact with the surroundings, also as a result of a temperature gradient. Because of this, heating by conduction is relatively inefficient. Unless the conducting material has a way of replenishing its own heat content, it quickly cools off and loses its effect.

### Convection

Convection is the exchange of heat from a moving liquid, such as a whirlpool (Figure 6-2). As described above, in conduction there is a temperature gradient such that the surface of the warming object is cooler than the rest of that object. This

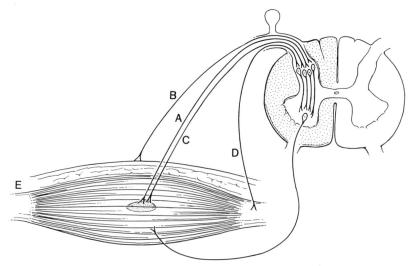

**Figure 6-1.** The effects of heat and cold on decreasing muscle tension. *A*, Heating certain afferent muscle spindle fibers causes them to have a decreased rate of firing, thus relaxing tonic muscle activity. *B*, Cooling the skin facilitates the alpha motor neurons, thus increasing spasticity and muscle stretch reflexes. *C*, Cooling the afferent muscle spindle fibers (deep cooling) causes the direct effect of inhibiting their firing, thus relaxing muscle spasticity. *D*, Heating the Golgi tendon organ increases its firing which inhibits the alpha motor neuron and decreases spasticity. *E*, Direct effect of heat increases collagen extensibility.

slows down effective heat transfer. Convection eliminates this gradient by constantly moving the fluid. Thus the heating fluid's temperature at the surface of the skin is constant and is not diluted by a temperature gradient. Convection is something we come into contact with often. When we are in a cool room with little air movement, there is a temperature gradient of the air closest to our skin and we may be comfortable. If we open the window or turn on a fan, the air is circulated and we lose the temperature gradient. Even though the ambient air temperature may be unchanged, we feel cooler because the temperature of the air next to our skin is no warmer than the rest of the air in the room; it loses its temperature gradient.

### Conversion

This type of heating involves the conversion of one type of energy, usually sound waves, electrical current, or electromagnetic radiation, into thermal energy. These modalities are described in detail under Superficial Heat Modalities and Deep Heat.

## Superficial Heat Modalities

Heating modalities are generally prescribed based on their ability to heat the body tissues either superficially or more deeply (see Deep Heat later in the chapter).

Superficial heating is created by all of the modalities except when deep heating conversion methods are used in conjunction with surface cooling systems. There is no method of conducting,

**Table 6-1.** Common Heating Modalities by Category

| | | |
|---|---|---|
| Conduction | Hot water bottle<br>Heating pad<br>Hydrocollator pack<br>Kenney pack<br>Paraffin bath | Superficial |
| Convection | Whirlpool<br>Hubbard tank<br>Fluidotherapy | |
| Conversion | Infrared lamp<br>Ultrasound<br>Shortwave<br>Microwave | Deep |

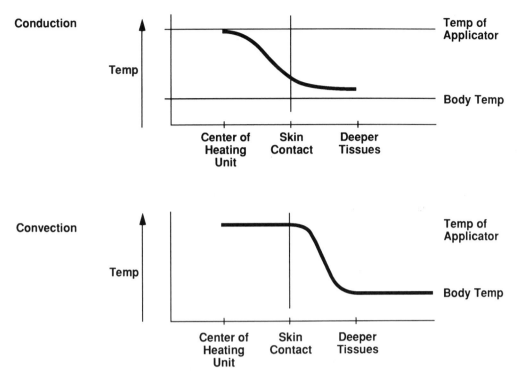

**Figure 6-2.** Temperature gradients for conductive and convective heating. In convection the temperature of the surface of the skin is the same as that of the rest of the heating element. This creates a more effective heating of the tissues.

convecting, or radiating heat into the deeper tissues without warming the superficial layers to some extent.

Superficial heating agents cause the greatest temperature rise to occur at the surface of the skin. The warming effect rapidly drops off, and is generally not appreciable deeper than 3 to 5 mm below the surface level of the skin. Deeper heating with such modalities is not practical because the temperature of the surface would have to be so high that it would burn the skin.

Superficial heat causes a reflex increase in blood flow to the skin and muscles below the heat as well as increasing blood flow in the skin of the limbs distal to the site of the heating. In conditions of painful muscle splinting, such as acute neck or back strain, superficial heat may provide significant relief of pain.

Superficial heat also causes a reflex generalized sedation and relaxation and a mild increase in blood flow to the contralateral limb in an area corresponding to the body part being heated. If applied over the abdomen it also decreases gastric acid production, gastrointestinal motility, and uterine menstrual cramping.

Because superficial heat increases the metabolic rate and oxygen requirements of the tissues being warmed, it should not be applied in patients with ischemic ulcers or arterial insufficiency. There are a number of different superficial heating devices.

### Hot Water Bottles

These are obviously simple and easy to use. They can be used in the home and have virtually no contraindications except that too high a water temperature in anesthetic areas may cause skin burns. The temperature in hot water bottles drops rapidly after a few minutes; thus their effect is relatively short-lived unless special water bottles are used that replenish the water to provide constant heat. Such water bottles are fairly complicated but may be found in some hospitals. Water bottles are used mainly to treat muscle strains.

### Electric Heating Pads and Blankets

These are also simple and easy to use sources of superficial heat. They provide a constant heat supply, but over the course of 30 to 60 minutes they actually become hotter. Therefore, care must be taken not to cause thermal burns (Figure 6-3), especially since the heat tends to reduce pain perception. Some special heating pads can be used to apply moist heat. This may be especially effective in conditions of muscle strain or in a stretching program. When used chronically, heating pads may cause a discoloration of the skin called erythema ab igne.

### Hydrocollator Packs

Silicate gel is sewn into a cloth cover. The gel holds a large amount of water so that when such a pack, known as a hydrocollator pack, is immersed in a

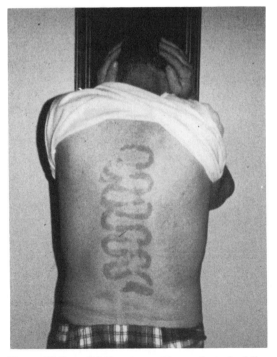

**Figure 6-3.** Superficial burn caused in a patient who fell asleep on a heating pad.

hot water bath it stores a large amount of heat energy. Water is especially effective at storing a high quantity of heat energy, known as specific heat. Hydrocollator packs are applied over a few layers of towels to prevent skin burns. They release heat slowly over the course of 20 to 30 minutes and are used in muscle strains and for relaxation and pain control.

### Kenney Packs

Developed originally for use in polio patients, these are pads of wool cloth which are steam heated and then spun to remove the water. They provide vigorous heating, but because of their low water content they cool rapidly. Effects are mainly due to reflex muscle relaxation. Kenney packs are somewhat cumbersome and are rarely used today.

### Paraffin Bath

Paraffin, a wax, is combined with oil in a 7:1 ratio. This combination turns liquid between 52 to 55°C (125 to 130°F). It is an effective vigorous superficial heating source, mainly used in painful conditions of the hand and wrist such as rheumatoid arthritis or scleroderma. There are two methods of paraffin bath technique: the immersion and the dipping techniques.

In the immersion method the hand is kept in the bath fluid. The paraffin next to the skin cools and solidifies around the skin to create an insulating layer which prevents the skin from being burned.

In the dipping technique the hand is dipped into the bath ten or so times. Each time a bit of the paraffin solidifies on the surface, much as in candle dipping. When the paraffin buildup is thick enough, the arm is wrapped in cellophane and covered by one or two towels to keep in the heat. This provides 10 to 15 minutes of heating effects. After the wrap is removed the solid paraffin is peeled from the skin and put back in the bath where it again melts. The exercise of removing the hardened wax is helpful in the patient with impaired hand function.

Because a paraffin bath set at too high a temperature could cause a burn, the liquid should always be inspected prior to use. At its proper temperature most of the paraffin will be liquid, but a few bits should have solidified around the edges. If all of the bath is in a liquid state it may well be too hot.

### Whirlpool Baths and Hubbard Tanks

So far all the superficial heating agents described have been heating methods by conduction. Whirlpool baths utilize agitated water to heat (or cool) by convection (Figure 6-4). One disadvantage of their use is that the limb being heated is necessarily placed in a dependent position, which may aggravate edema. Whirlpool baths heat a large body surface area. In order not to overheat the body they should not be used at temperatures greater than 46 °C (115 °F) when heating a limb or 41 °C (105 °F) when immersing the whole body.[2] Hubbard tanks are essentially just giant whirlpool baths. They have even more tendency to increase body temperature and should not be used above 41 °C (105 °F). This is especially important in the elderly and in patients with poor autonomic nervous system control or orthostatic hypotension. Also since the body is immersed in water, it cannot regulate temperature by sweating. The normal response to rising core body temperature, increased blood flow to the skin, only worsens hyperthermia in a heating tank. Thus when a water temperature

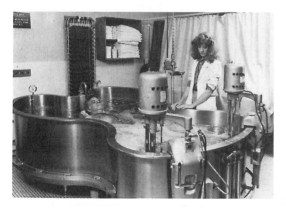

**Figure 6-4.** A Hubbard tank. (Basford JR: Physical agents and biofeedback. In DeLisa JA [ed]: *Rehabilitation Medicine: Principles and Practice* Philadelphia: JB Lippincott, 1988:257–275. Reproduced with permission.

above 38 °C (100 °F) is used, the patient's temperature should be monitored.[2] Both whirlpools and hubbard tanks are useful in patients with open sores or burns.

### Fluidotherapy

When hot air is blown through glass beads or small bits of corn cob, it creates a fluidlike medium that heats by convection. A limb can be inserted into a fluidotherapy box and heated as effectively as in a whirlpool. Advantages of such a system are that the skin can still sweat and the beads or corn cob particles can be sterilized by heat. Thus extensive cleaning and sterilization of the tank between patients is unnecessary.

### Infrared Heating Lamps or Cradles

Infrared radiation is emitted from all sources in proportion to their temperature. We radiate it to our surroundings and in turn receive it from our surroundings. It passes through the air. The net inflow (radiation from surroundings minus what we radiate) or outflow of infrared radiation helps determine whether we feel warm or cold. In two rooms with identical air temperatures the room with the warmer walls will feel warmer because those walls heat us more by radiation. Radiation increases the vibration of the molecules in our bodies and thus raises temperature. This principle is used mainly in heating lamps and is a form of heating by conversion.

Heating lamps or cradles utilize radiating energy to heat the skin. The energy does not penetrate deep tissues and may cause superficial skin burns. Such a modality has the advantage of being dry, inexpensive, easy to use, and it can be used at home. The bulb uses a reflector to spread the heat over a large surface area, especially in a heat cradle. This heating modality is especially useful in muscle strain, for producing relaxation, and can be used over areas of skin breakdown. Care must be taken not to overheat the patient, especially when multiple lamps or cradles are used. The lamps heat up over a period of 1 hour; thus care must be taken not to cause burn damage. As a rule, a maximum of 100 W at a minimum of 36 inches from the patient should be used for safety reasons.

## Deep Heating

When tissues deeper than 3 to 5mm need to be warmed, superficial heating agents cannot reach them. Deep heating modalities are used in conditions such as tendonitis or bursitis. They are used to help loosen contractures from tight joint capsules,[2] and may heat large joints of the body or just those joints, such as facet joints, that are hard to reach with other types of heat. There are three types of deep heating modalities. Only one, ultrasound, is used with any great frequency.

### Ultrasound Diathermy

Ultrasound machines create sound waves that are transmitted through the skin and deep into the tissues, down to the bone. The waves have a frequency of 0.8 to 1 MHz and cause the tissues to vibrate rapidly so that they generate heat. This effect is most evident at tissue interfaces, mainly muscle-bone, but also at fat-muscle, skin-fat, and applicator-skin.

To be effective, the ultrasound applicator must be pressed firmly to the skin. To reduce heat loss at the skin a "coupling agent" such as ultrasound gel or degassed water is placed between the applicator and the skin. This gel reduces the contrast in material at the surface of the skin and allows more heat to travel deeper. When the ultrasound waves hit bone they heat the surface of the bone and reflect back to the muscle. This creates the maximal heating effect right next to the bone, where joint capsules are often tight. At clinically used intensities ultrasound cannot pass through bone.

There are two techniques of ultrasound application: stroking and stationary. In the stationary technique, the applicator is not moved. This is usually discouraged because small variations in the ultrasound energy can create local "hot spots" which can burn the deep tissues. The stroking technique does not allow hot spots to form. When using the stroking technique it should be confined to a relatively small area so that the tissues do not cool down between passes.

Ultrasound, especially when used as a stationary technique, can cause "cavitation" of gases. This occurs when gases come out of solution and actually form small bubbles. These bubbles can cause tissue damage and are more likely to occur in fluid-filled organs.

Ultrasound is generally prescribed at a dosage of 0.5 to 4 $W/cm^2$ (2.5 $W/cm^2$ average) with the lower dose being used over small joints or with the stationary technique. The higher dose is rarely used except in deep structures such as the hip joint or in obese patients, and is always performed with the stroking technique. The average dose of 2.5 $W/cm^2$ is generally safe for most forms of tendonitis or contracture. Treatment is for 5 to 10 minutes once or twice a day followed by stretching. It is usually done for 5 to 10 days. When a large joint is treated it must be heated from multiple directions, since bone blocks the passage of the sound waves.

One advantage of ultrasound over the other deep heating modalities is that it can be applied to limbs with metallic implants as long as these implants are not secured with cement. It can also be applied to a limb immersed in a bucket of degassed water, for instance to heat the small joints of the hand.

Some clinicians prescribe a variant of ultrasound called phonophoresis. This (in theory) uses ultrasound to facilitate movement of surface creams or solutions into the tissues. Medications such as steroids or analgesics are commonly used. The problems with phonophoresis are that blood "washes out" the transmitted medications rapidly and that fairly small amounts, if any, of the solutions actually make it through the skin. It is a time-consuming procedure, and with other options such as oral medication or local injection available, there is almost never a good reason to use phonophoresis.

### Shortwave Diathermy

In this deep heating modality electrical currents are either passed directly through or are induced to pass through the tissues. It mainly heats superficial fat and muscle, and because the machine is expensive and cumbersome it is rarely used.

### Microwave Diathermy

Microwaves are a form of electromagnetic radiation which are preferentially absorbed in water-containing tissues. They mainly heat muscle. Microwave diathermy is relatively safe and easy to use. On the other hand, it does not usually offer a clear-cut advantage over ultrasound. If available, and if selective muscle heating is desired, it may be a good option to use.

## Guidelines for Use of Therapeutic Heat

The effects of and contraindications to using heat therapy are listed in Tables 6-2 and 6-3.[2] What follows are some general guidelines to help in using and prescribing heat.

1. When using superficial heating modalities, the patient should not lie on top of the heating source. This is more likely to cause skin burns because the pressure from the body weight masks the pain and prevents capillary blood flow from dissipating the heat.
2. When using heat to help increase flexibility, it should be accompanied and followed by prolonged gentle stretching. When collagen is warmed to a proper degree (42 to 45 °C) it will slowly elongate with this prolonged stretching.

**Table 6-2.** Effects of Therapeutic Heat

Increased collagen extensibility
Decreased joint stiffness
Increased inflammation
Reduced sensation of pain
General relaxation and sedation
Increased local blood flow
Mild consensual increase in blood flow (to the opposite limb)
Reduced spasticity
Increased core body temperature
Decreased gastrointestinal peristalsis and gastric acid production
Increased menstrual flow (deep heat)
Reduced menstrual cramping (superficial heat)

**Table 6-3.** Contraindications to the Use of Heat

Anesthetic area
Obtunded or uncommunicative patient
Impaired vascular flow to the limb
Acute injury
Acutely inflamed joints
Hemorrhagic conditions
Over the pregnant uterus
Over the testes
Over metallic implants (shortwave and microwave)
Over cemented metallic implants (ultrasound)
Over cancers
When used for multiple sessions over a child's epiphyseal growth plate
Over the eyes
Over the spinal column after laminectomy (deep heat)
Over the heart (deep heat)
Over sites of infection (except over some superficial skin infections)

Heat alone, without the stretching, will not increase flexibility. As a rule, the highest dose of heat that can be tolerated without producing tissue damage is required to have an effect on flexibility. This technique is mainly used to treat contractures.
3. Heat increases blood flow to the tissues being warmed. This increase in blood flow may help to resolve inflammation in some cases. In other instances it aggravates the inflammation. It may be followed by massage to reduce edema.
4. The increase in blood flow "washes out" the heat. Thus after a certain amount of time, prolonging the heating session is no longer useful. For most superficial heating sessions 20 to 30 minutes of heat application is useful. For deep heating 5 to 10 minutes per field is used.
5. Let the patient's sensation of warmth guide treatment. For ultrasound a useful technique to achieve optimal heating is to go right up to the point of pain and then back off on the intensity slightly. For superficial heat, pain to the patient is reduced by putting an extra towel or more distance between the skin and the heat source. This technique is reliable only if the patient is alert, mentally competent, and has normal sensation.
6. Heat can be used as a counterirritant to raise the pain threshold. This may be therapeutic in states of pain, but can also mask a skin burn by the heating source. Heat may also decrease

pain by increasing the blood flow to relatively ischemic muscles.[3,4] However, heat should not be used in peripheral vascular disease, since it increases the metabolic demands of the tissues even more than it increases the blood flow.

7. Vigorous heating is not generally indicated in acute injury or in inflamed joints. In these situations it may worsen the inflammation.

8. When possible, heat should be avoided in dependent limbs. The dependent (hanging down) position may generate edema worsened by heat application.

## Cryotherapy

Cold application is commonly used in musculoskeletal conditions, especially after acute injury. It helps decrease tissue inflammation and swelling. It also helps to decrease pain sensation, either by acting as a counterirritant or by blocking pain transmission directly.

Cold produces vasoconstriction, which decreases blood flow to the area being treated. Thus the cooling effect is not "washed out" as quickly as with heat, and the effects are more long-lasting. When the tissues are cooled enough to cause damage, there is an axonal-reflex mediated vasodilation that increases blood flow to prevent frostbite. This level of cooling should not be approached in a clinical setting.

Cryotherapy is usually used in the first 1 to 2 days after injury. It is commonly applied for 20 to 30 minutes every 1 to 2 hours as tolerated. It can also be used before or after exercise to decrease inflammation. In states of painful muscle splinting it can reduce pain and relax the muscle. It is also used to treat spasticity. Because of an effect on skin temperature receptors, cold may make spasticity slightly worse when it is first applied, but as the deeper muscles and muscle spindle are cooled, the spasticity decreases (see Figure 6-1).[5,6]

In deep burns, immediate cooling for 30 minutes may help to decrease injury. This is due to decreased edema formation which helps prevent secondary injury from the excess fluid. If the injured tissues are cooled 2 minutes or more after the burn it may actually worsen the outcome of the burn. With such delayed application edema is no

longer controlled, and by reflex vasoconstriction the healing process is impaired, at least in an animal study.[7]

In inflamed joints cold therapy may help decrease symptoms. There is some controversy over whether or not the superficially applied cold actually lowers or paradoxically raises intraarticular temperature, so the patient's subjective feelings should be used as a guide. Even though cooling a joint makes it more stiff, patients such as rheumatoid arthritics often have a significant improvement of function after such cooling. There are a number of methods of cold application.

### Ice Packs/Ice Slush/Ice Chips

This is an effective and easy way of achieving vigorous cooling. Care must be taken not to cause frostbite. If an ice pack is used, it can be wrapped around the skin with a moist towel to facilitate cooling. The water in the towel helps transfer heat out of the patient more effectively. Ice can be used along with compression in acute injuries to reduce swelling and inflammation. In arthritis and reflex sympathetic dystrophy it is sometimes used along with heat in a *contrast bath*. The limb is immersed in heat for 10 minutes (42 to 45 °C), then cold 1 minute (15 to 20 °C), then heat 4 minutes, cold 1 minute, and so on for 30 minutes. This creates an increase in blood flow and may help relieve pain in some patients.

### Vapocoolant Spray

Ethylene chloride and fluorimethane sprays evaporate when they hit the skin and thus cause superficial cooling. They are useful for myofascial pain conditions as a "spray and stretch" procedure when followed by a gentle prolonged stretching of the painful muscle. The liquid is sprayed onto the skin in a few passes in the direction of the muscle fibers. It may act as a counterirritant.

### Ice Massage

This technique allows cooling to be combined with a deep massage. Freezing water in a small paper cup and then peeling off the top is a simple way to form a piece of ice that is easier to handle than an ice cube. Alternatives include frozen drink containers that can be rolled over the muscle. The cold material is used to apply deep cooling massage in the direction of the muscle fibers for 15 to 30 minutes. This is followed by stretching.

### Cold Rooms or Pools

Patients with multiple sclerosis often do poorly in a warm environment or when exercising. A cool pool or room may allow them to reap the benefits of exercise without exacerbating their condition.

### Whirlpool

A cool whirlpool bath may be used in acute injury.

## Guidelines for Cryotherapy[2]

Tables 6-4 and 6-5 list the effects of and contraindications to cryotherapy. As a general rule, cold therapy should be used in conjunction with other therapies such as exercise and stretching. It is often not as well tolerated initially as heat, but once patients get accustomed to it they often experience significant relief of pain, splinting, spasticity, and inflammation. Cold is usually applied for 20 to 30 minutes two to three times a day or before and after exercise in conditions of tendonitis or overuse.

**Table 6-4.** Effects of Cryotherapy

Decreased pain
Decreased spasticity
Decreased blood flow
Decreased edema
Increased joint stiffness
Improved function in multiple sclerosis (cool pool or cold room)
Reduced damage from burns (if applied immediately)
Decreased joint inflammation
Decreased metabolic activity
Decreased nerve conduction velocity

**Table 6-5.** Contraindications to Cryotherapy

Anesthetic areas
Obtunded or unresponsive patient
Cold allergy
Cryoglobulinemia
Raynaud's phenomenon
Paroxysmal cold hemoglobinuria
Prolonged use over superficial nerves
Paramyotonia congenita
Delayed application after burns

## Electrical Stimulation

There are three main uses of electrical stimulation as therapeutic modalities. They are called transcutaneous electrical nerve stimulation (TENS), functional electrical stimulation (FES), and electrical stimulation (ES).

### Transcutaneous Electrical Nerve Stimulation

TENS units are small, battery powered sources of electrical current used to treat pain. By attaching wires and electrodes the current can be used to superficially stimulate the skin over various parts of the body. There are two types of TENS: high frequency, low intensity (conventional TENS), and low frequency, high intensity. The effects of low-frequency TENS are blocked by naloxone, an opiate antagonist, and therefore the stimulation is felt to be exerting its effect by increasing endogenous opiates in the brain and spinal cord. This is felt to be similar to the mechanism of action of acupuncture; thus low-frequency TENS is sometimes called acupuncture-like. Conventional TENS is not blocked by naloxone and is felt to act as a counterirritant (see Chapter 25).

TENS units are used to treat the symptom of pain. They do not affect the underlying disease. Which type of TENS to use and where to place the electrodes involve some educated guesswork. In general, for neurogenic or dermatomal pain the electrodes are placed in the painful skin distribution or over more proximal nerves supplying that area of skin. They are also sometimes placed over acupuncture points with good results.

TENS units are not for everyone, but in some patients they do result in significant pain relief. They require that the patient be taught to properly apply and adjust the unit. They should usually be prescribed initially for a trial period to see whether the particular patient in question will benefit from them.

TENS units are fairly safe; however, they should not be used over the pregnant uterus, over the neck, or over the chest of a patient with a pacemaker. Occasionally the stimulating pads cause superficial skin burns.

### Functional Electrical Stimulation

When electrical stimulation is used to produce functional movement it is called FES. While in principle FES could be used to create almost any motion in a patient with peripheral or central nervous system disorder, in practice it is not yet as useful.

One of the most successful uses of FES has been to decrease footdrop in patients with stroke or other dysfunction. Whenever the foot is lifted, the device stimulates nerves that supply the dorsiflexors. However, the same effect can be achieved more easily and reliably (and with less discomfort) with a good ankle-foot orthosis.

FES is also being used in patients with spinal cord injury for exercise purposes. The patient is placed on a special exercise bike while the muscles that cause a pedaling motion are stimulated in sequence over and over. This gives the patient good cardiovascular and psychological benefits of exercise. Another use of FES in spinal cord injury is to stimulate the phrenic nerve in "diaphragmatic pacing." This allows the paralyzed diaphragms in select quadriplegics to "breathe" independent of a ventilator.

### Electrical Stimulation

Electrical stimulation can also be applied directly to muscles to reduce pain, spasticity, or to retard atrophy. Unlike TENS in which the objective is to stimulate the skin, ES causes actual muscle movement. This can improve pain in myofascial pain states or can give prolonged relief of spasticity. In nerve damage which is expected to heal, ES can slow down muscle atrophy so that when the nerve heals, the muscle is more able to function and recover further.

### Biofeedback

While often discussed as a relaxation technique, biofeedback can actually be used for just about any bodily effect imagined. It involves bringing a bodily function which is not usually consciously perceived under voluntary control. For instance, we are not normally aware of our heart rate. By hooking a person up to a heart monitor he or she quickly learns to increase or decrease heart rate at will. The same can be done for muscle tension to reduce headaches or for motor learning after injury. Commonly used monitors are superficial electromyography electrodes (to measure muscle electrical activity), verbal feedback from therapists, or mirrors.

### Summary

The key to successful use of physical modalities is not to expect too much from them. Rarely do they cure any problems. Their real benefit comes in allowing the patient to move about better, feel better, and participate more fully in the rest of the rehabilitation exercise program.

### Points of Summary

1. Heat reduces pain, increases flexibility, reduces spasticity, increases blood flow, and reduces joint stiffness.
2. Cold reduces pain, reduces spasticity, decreases blood flow, and increases joint stiffness.
3. Heating can be applied superficially or deep. Care must be taken not to cause a skin burn.
4. Ultrasound diathermy is usually the preferred mode of deep heating.
5. Vapocoolant sprays are useful in myofascial pain syndromes.
6. In deep burns cold applied immediately may prevent secondary damage due to edema; if it is applied later it may impair healing.

7. TENS units treat pain, not the underlying condition.
8. ES may retard muscle atrophy and is used only if the damaged nerve is expected to recover.

## References

1. Wells HS: Temperature equalization for the relief of pain. *Arch Phys. Med* 1947;28:135–139.
2. Lehmann JF, deLateur BJ: Diathermy and superficial heat, laser, and cold therapy. In Kottke FJ, Lehmann JF (eds): *Krusen's Handbook of Physical Medicine and Rehabilitation*, 4th ed. Philadelphia: WB Saunders, 1990:285–367.
3. Lehmann JF, Brunner GD, Stow RW: Pain threshold measurements after therapeutic application of ultrasound, microwaves, and infrared. *Arch Phys Med Rehabil* 1958;39:560–565.
4. Gammon GD, Starr I: Studies on the relief of pain by counter-irritation. *J Clin Invest* 1941;20:13–20.
5. Miglietta O: Action of cold on spasticity. *Am J Phys Med* 1973;52:198–205.
6. Bell KR, Lehmann JF: Effects of cooling on H- and T-reflexes in normal subjects. *Arch Phys Med Rehabil* 1987;68:490–493.
7. Demling RH, Mazess RB, Wolberg W: The effect of immediate and delayed cold immersion on edema formation and resorption. *J Trauma* 1979;19:56–60.

## Suggested Readings

Lehmann JF, deLateur BJ: Diathermy and superficial heat, laser, and cold therapy. In Kottke FJ, Lehmann JF (eds): *Krusen's Handbook of Physical Medicine and Rehabilitation*, 4th ed. Philadelphia: WB Saunders, 1990:285–367.
Grabois M, Halstead LS: Physical modalities of treatment. In Halstead LS, Grabois M (eds): *Medical Rehabilitation*. New York: Raven Press, 1985:33–44.

# Chapter 7

# Exercise: Principles, Methods, and Prescription

MICHAEL D. ROBINSON
STEVEN E. BRAVERMAN

Exercise is defined as "bodily exertion for the sake of developing and maintaining physical fitness."[1] Not surprisingly, exercise is a necessary component of any fitness and conditioning program, whether for rehabilitation or increasing general fitness. This chapter summarizes the physiologic response to exercise, describes the several types of exercise used in rehabilitation and conditioning of the musculoskeletal system, and provides a rationale for prescribing particular exercises when rehabilitating musculoskeletal injuries.

## Physiologic Response to Exercise

The human body adapts to the demands placed on it. Muscles, bones, and ligaments all gain strength when they are regularly stressed. Similarly, cardiovascular and neural adaptations take place to provide for more efficient energy delivery and improved coordination. The body senses the demands placed upon it and within certain constraints, alters its structure and metabolism on a cellular level to meet those demands. This is explained as the overload principle: the body (or its component parts) must be stressed beyond its current level of activity or ability in order to adapt and enhance function.[2]

The ability to adapt is somewhat specific. Certain types, durations, intensities, and frequencies of exercise preferentially lead to certain results. Exercises that improve strength may not improve endurance and vice versa. However, recent research suggests that while specificity is important, exercise types may not be as mutually exclusive in achieving specific results as was once believed.[3-5] One should think of specificity as a continuum in which specific exercise types will maximally improve some tasks, with less improvement gained for other tasks.

### Strengthening Exercise

Strength gains from exercise stem from two components: the extent and synchrony of motor unit recruitment, and muscle hypertrophy. In the initial stages of strengthening (3 to 6 weeks), neural factors account for most of the increase in force capability.[6,7] Simply put, subjects learn to activate their muscles more completely and efficiently.

Then as repetitive overloads are imposed on the muscles, they develop hypertrophy, which

The opinions or assertions contained herein are the private views of the authors and are not to be construed as official or as reflecting the views of the Department of the Army or the Department of Defense.

leads to even greater strength gains. Hypertrophy is an increase in the size of the muscle fibers along with an increase in cellular components and enzyme activity. An increase in the actual number of muscle fibers, termed hyperplasia, has been documented by some researchers, but remains controversial.[8]

Both type I (slow twitch) and type II (fast twitch) muscle fibers develop hypertrophy with strengthening exercise, but type II fibers exhibit the greater degree of change (see Chapter 2).

### Endurance Exercise

**Fuel Utilization (Figure 7-1).** The immediate source of energy at the initiation of exercise is adenosine triphosphate (ATP). Primary ATP stores in the muscle are utilized within 3 to 4 seconds. Other local sources of ATP, that is, creatinine phosphate and adenosine diphosphate, are next converted to ATP. These sources are depleted within about 20 seconds of maximal exercise. By 20 to 30 seconds, carbohydrate stores (glycogen) are broken down into ATP and byproducts through anaerobic glycolysis. Two molecules of ATP are produced per molecule of glucose. This energy supply peaks at 40 to 50 seconds and then dissipates.

For high-intensity activity to continue, aerobic processes must then take over. Byproducts of the glycolytic pathway just described are routed to the mitochondria, and through the Krebs cycle 38 ATP molecules are produced for every molecule of glucose. This aerobic metabolism takes a minimum of 2 to 3 minutes to reach its maximum level of energy production. Later on, triglycerides (fats), and to a small extent proteins, are also broken down, netting 129 molecules of ATP per free fatty acid chain.

Regular endurance exercise increases the number of mitochondria and mitochondrial enzymes in the muscle fibers, thus raising the efficiency of oxidative metabolism.[9] Utilization of fat is enhanced and postpones glycogen depletion in prolonged exercise.

When energy requirements surpass the availability of oxygen, the byproducts of glycolysis can no longer be shunted into the oxidative pathways; anaerobic energy production once again becomes important. However, this mode of energy production cannot be sustained for long. Byproducts, such as lactate, accumulate and herald the onset of this "anaerobic threshold." Regular aerobic exercise raises the level of exertion at which this threshold is reached (primarily through the cardiovascular adaptations described next).

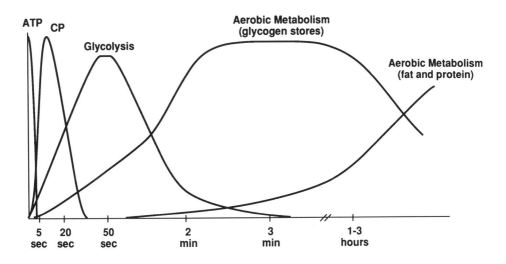

**ATP - Adenosine Triphosphate**
**CP - Creatine Phosphate**

**Figure 7-1.** Sources of energy during muscle contraction. ATP, adenosine triphosphate; CP, creatine phosphate.

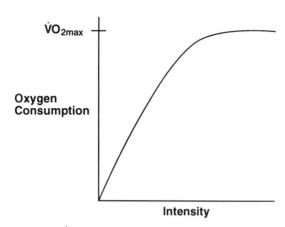

Figure 7-2. $\dot{V}O_2$max: As exercise intensity rises there is a nearly linear increase in oxygen consumption ($\dot{V}O_2$) up to a point, $\dot{V}O_2$max. Above this exercise intensity level, higher intensity no longer causes a rise in oxygen consumption, which is limited by the body's ability to distribute oxygen to the working tissues. Anaerobic exercise must generate any energy utilized above this level.

**Cardiovascular Response.**   During exercise the cardiovascular system must supply oxygen to and remove metabolic waste and heat from the active muscles. The rate of total body consumption of oxygen at peak exercise ($\dot{V}O_2$max) is a good correlate of work capacity. It is a measure of the maximal amount of oxygen that the body can possibly consume (Figure 7-2), and therefore gives an indication of one's maximal aerobic potential. It is limited by the amount of blood the heart can pump (cardiac output) and by the ability of the body to extract oxygen from this blood. Cardiac output (CO) is the product of the heart rate (HR) and the stroke volume (SV). During exercise HR increases, CO increases, and venous compliance decreases. Blood flow to the muscles is enhanced. The active muscles in turn help to push blood back to the heart, which increases SV and CO even further. Vasoconstriction of blood vessels feeding the internal organs also helps to shunt blood to the active muscles.

Over time and with regular exercise, SV may be improved by more efficient cardiac contractility, enhanced ejection fraction, and most importantly, by increased end-diastolic volume of the heart. Myocardial hypertrophy is variable and usually global, with little change in relative wall thickness versus end-diastolic volume. Enhanced parasympathetic tone at rest results in a resting bradycardia. The increased CO and peripheral extraction of oxygen allow for a smaller rise in HR with submaximal exercise. Maximal HR is not changed by endurance exercise.

### Flexibility

Flexibility is essential to allow for the greatest efficiency of the musculoskeletal system. It is a measure of the degree of normal motion surrounding a joint and is limited by the extensibility of the periarticular tissues. It must be differentiated from joint laxity, which is due to a failure of the joint supporting structures and which implies a degree of abnormal motion of the joint.

**Connective Tissue.**   Increased flexibility results primarily from stretching the connective tissues within and around the muscle and tendon rather than the contractile elements of muscle. Connective tissues are composed fundamentally of collagen enmeshed in a ground substance made of glycosaminoglycans.

Connective tissues progressively shorten when not opposed by a stretching force and elongate when challenged with a constant stress.[10] Stretching occurs when there is a linear deformation of the fibers that leads to an increase in length. There are two types of elongation. *Elastic stretch* occurs when the elongation produced by loading is followed by a recovery to resting length when the load is removed. *Plastic stretch* is produced when the elongation is maintained after removing the load.

Plastic elongation is the type necessary to improve the flexibility of connective tissue. It is maximized by applying a prolonged static stretch with the tissues warmed to 42 to 45 °C.[11] Bouncing stretch, heat without stretch, and short-duration stretching do not lead to increased flexibility (Table 7-1).

**Table 7-1.** Principles of Maintaining Flexibility

| |
|---|
| Prolonged stretch |
| Static stretch |
| Warming of the tissues to be stretched |
| Avoidance of bouncing |

**Neural Factors.** Neural factors may also play a role in muscle relaxation and flexibility. This involves a complex interaction between the muscle spindles, Golgi Tendon Organs, Central Nervous System, and muscles. It is unclear exactly how these elements interact, but it appears that a prolonged stretch (greater than 15 seconds) of moderate intensity will produce the greatest gains in flexibility.

## Exercise Methods (Table 7-2)

The theoretical basis for exercise has led to several methods to accomplish improvements in strength, flexibility, general conditioning, and endurance. Each method may be appropriate in a specific setting based on the goals of the exercise program.

Any exercise prescription is founded on four variables which can be manipulated: mode, intensity, frequency, and duration. Mode is the type of exercise to be undertaken. Intensity is the percent of the individual's maximum capacity, whether measured in weight lifted, % $\dot{V}O_2$ max, or % maximum HR achieved. Frequency refers to the number of workouts per unit of time (usually per week), and duration is the length of each workout.

### Strengthening Exercises

Techniques for building muscle strength employ high resistance loads against which a muscle must

**Table 7-2.** Types of Exercise Training

Strength
  Isometric
  Isotonic
    Concentric
    Eccentric
  Isokinetic
    Concentric
    Eccentric
  Plyometric
Endurance
Flexibility
  Static
  Passive
  Proprioceptive neuromuscular facilitation
Coordination
Activity specific

work. Resistance to motion can be applied manually by a therapist, by using weights, or through various types of equipment. Strengthening exercises take one of three forms: isometric, isotonic, or isokinetic. They can be varied in velocity of movement or contraction type: eccentric versus concentric.

### Force-Velocity Relationship

Fast, lengthening (eccentric) contractions develop the highest muscle tensions. Fast, shortening (concentric) contractions develop the lowest muscle tensions. Isometric contractions develop tension in between, at the inflection point shown in Figure 7-3.

### Isometric Exercises

An isometric contraction is a muscle contraction that does not produce movement of the joint. This exercise may be performed by exertion against an immovable object or by holding an object in a static position (such as holding a briefcase.) Peak isometric strength is the maximum force that can be exerted against an immovable object. Isometric contractions can generate a large amount of force, and daily isometric exercise at 50% of maximal strength may retard disuse atrophy. It may actually help build strength, especially in persons who are far removed from their peak strength potential.[12]

One drawback to isometric exercise is that strength gains are made primarily at the joint angle at which the muscle is exercised. It is also unclear how far the gains in strength can be further improved, and there may be little transference of strength to other activities. In addition, these exercises cause a rise in blood pressure and may therefore be contraindicated in persons with cardiac disease. On the other hand, isometrics have the advantage of being relatively easy to perform, and they require little or no equipment. Because of the lack of joint motion, they are useful in maintaining strength and muscle mass in the immobilized limb and when joint motion is painful or otherwise contraindicated (e.g., acute inflammatory phase of rheumatoid arthritis).

### Isotonic Exercises

Isotonic exercises involve moving a constant load through a full range of motion with or without

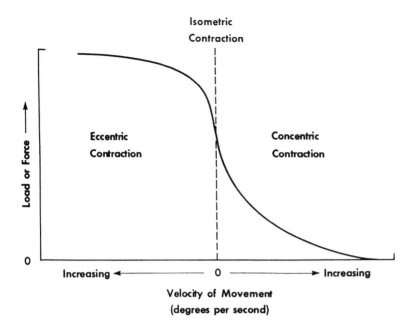

**Figure 7-3.** Relationship between velocity of movement and torque development capability. The highest torque can be developed by quickly lowering a heavy weight. The least torque is developed by quickly lifting a light weight. (Joynt RL: Therapeutic exercise. In DeLisa JA [ed]: *Rehabilitation Medicine: Principles and Practice.* Philadelphia: JB Lippincott, 1988:346–371. Reproduced with permission.)

changing the velocity of movement. Lighter weights can be lifted through more repetitions than can heavier weights (Figure 7-4). Lifting heavy weights is generally considered to be a

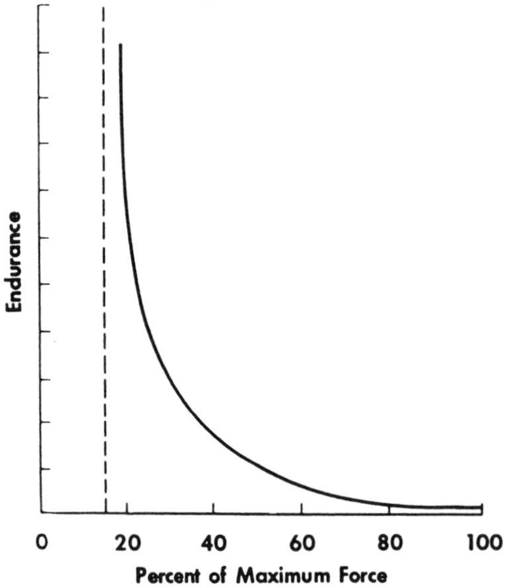

**Figure 7-4.** Relationship between strength and endurance. A lighter load can be lifted more often than a heavy one. (Joynt RL: Therapeutic exercise. In DeLisa JA [ed]: *Rehabilitation Medicine: Principles and Practice.* Philadelphia: JB Lippincott, 1988: 346–371. Reproduced with permission.)

strengthening exercise, while lifting lesser loads (or performing other activities that require relatively little strength) is called endurance exercise.

DeLorme is credited with establishing resistive exercises as a rehabilitative tool to increase strength.[13] His program involved the use of progressive resistance exercises with increasing loads. Each individual determined the maximal weight he or she could lift ten times with each muscle group to be strengthened. This was called the ten repetition maximum (10RM). Subjects would then perform three sets of 10 repetitions daily at 50%, 75%, and 100% of the 10RM with 2 minutes of rest between sets. Each week a new 10RM would be determined. The drawbacks to this exercise included difficulty in completing the final set of exercises due to fatigue and the fact that full motor unit recruitment was only accomplished during the last set.

The Oxford technique[14,15] reversed the DeLorme regimen by ordering the exercise sets with 100% 10RM first, followed by 75%, and then 50%. With this regimen, fatigue caused by the 100% 10RM set is offset by lower loads on the second and third sets.

Isotonic exercises can also be used for endurance training. DeLorme believed that high-repetition, low-resistance exercises only increase endurance, while low-repetition, high-resistance exercises only increase strength. While there is a tendency for DeLorme's belief to hold true at the extremes of exercise type, in practice there is much transferability of training; cross-training between the two exercise types does occur.[3] It is now generally believed that strength can be improved by many modes of exercise, as long as they are carried out to the point of muscle fatigue.

One problem with isotonic exercise is that maximal muscle torque varies with the length of the muscle. The muscle can contract at its maximum capacity at only one point in the full range of motion, at a point slightly longer than resting length (Figure 7-5). However, to lift a weight through a full range of motion requires that the muscle must be able to lift it even at its weakest point. Thus true isotonic exercise is inefficient, because it does not cause muscle overload throughout the whole contraction. The use of cams and pulleys, as in Nautilus exercise equipment, attempts to circumvent this problem by vary-

ing the resistance of the load to match the average torque curve for specific muscle groups.

Most isotonic exercises involve concentric and eccentric exercise. Unfortunately, eccentric contractions, while developing more tension, also produce more muscle soreness and more damage to type II muscle fibers than concentric contractions. When used judiciously, however, an eccentric strengthening program shows promise in some rehabilitation protocols.[16] The advantages of isotonic training are its effectiveness and its universal availability.

### Isokinetic Exercises

Isokinetic exercises employ special machines which have lever arms that rotate around fixed axes. The person pushes or pulls the lever arm through a set range of motion at a preset speed. The speed remains constant, no matter how hard the subject pushes. By maintaining the speed

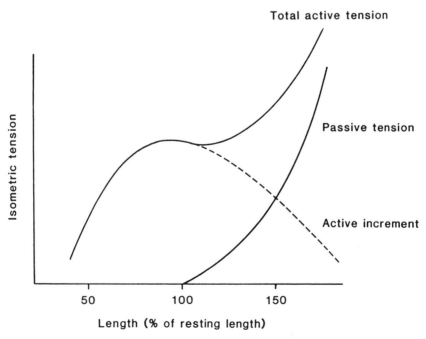

**Figure 7-5.** Muscle tension as a function of length. Passive tension increases as the connective tissues of the muscle are stretched. This is not related to active muscle contraction. By subtracting passive tension from total active tension which has been measured experimentally, the active increment can be calculated. The active increment is that portion of muscle tension that is due to muscle contraction. Maximal tension can be created at or slightly longer than the resting length of the muscle. (Rasch PJ: *Kinesiology and Applied Anatomy,* 7th ed. Philadelphia, Lea & Febiger, 1989. Reproduced with permission.)

(velocity), the person can generate maximal force (torque) at all angles of the range.

The chosen velocity of concentric isokinetic exercise may be important in strengthening.[17] Training at slow velocities generates the greatest torque, and strength gains are related to the maximal torque generated during training.[5] However, it must be stressed that activity or sport-specific training may require different training velocities than those designed just to build strength. Activities involving fast musculoskeletal movements may require training at fast velocities. Training at slower velocities leads to relatively larger strength gains, which, however, may not be completely transferable to the fast activities. The actual strengthening program can mimic the DeLorme or Oxford programs of progressive resistive exercises.

The biggest drawback to isokinetic exercise is the reliance on special equipment. These machines may be unavailable to the general public. The newer isokinetic machines allow training with eccentric as well as concentric resistance.

### Plyometric Exercise

Plyometric exercises are designed to increase power by linking sheer strength with speed of movement to produce an explosive-reactive movement.[18] These exercises train the neuromuscular system to react quickly and forcefully during stretch-shortening actions. Plyometrics are used primarily by the athlete to train in specific activities required of a sport (e.g., football linemen). Other individuals whose jobs may require these explosive types of movements may also benefit from this type of training.

These high-intensity bouncing/ballistic type drills are felt to utilize the muscle stretch reflex to augment normal muscle contraction to produce an explosive reaction (though possibly it is just the eccentric training which is helping to increase strength). The force of the concentric contraction is enhanced by the immediately preceding rapid eccentric contraction. The ability to rapidly switch from an eccentric to a concentric contraction determines the power. Squat jumps, drop pushups, catch and throws, and hops are examples of plyometrics. The action should try to duplicate any rapid movement with an intensity that is equal to or greater than that which is normally occurring.

Obviously, these rapid eccentric and concentric contractions may cause injury if the individual does not have adequate flexibility and agility. These exercises are only used after complete healing of any injury and after proper warm-up and flexibility exercises.

### Endurance Exercises

Endurance exercises may selectively cause hypertrophy of type I muscle fibers while increasing the oxidative capacity of some type II fibers. For cardiovascular fitness, the American College of Sports Medicine recommends aerobic exercise using large muscle groups which causes an elevation of training heart rate to 60% to 90% of the maximum HR or reaching 50% to 85% of $\dot{V}O_2$max for 20 to 60 minutes three to five times per week.[19] Training HR is calculated by taking 60% to 90% of predicted maximum HR, which is approximately 220 minus age (in years).

When starting an endurance training program one should start with low-intensity sessions to allow the exercise novice to maintain an appropriate training heart rate for the minimal length of time required to cause cardiovascular adaptation. Such a program results in improved cardiovascular fitness, aids in weight control, and improves the person's sense of well-being (see Chapter 26). Regular aerobic exercise is also an important adjunct to the treatment of myofascial pain and chronic pain states.

### Flexibility Training

A program to improve flexibility can be beneficial in a number of ways. It may lessen the likelihood of injury, minimize postexercise soreness, reduce contractures, decrease joint pain, and alleviate myofascial pain. Techniques for stretching include ballistic stretching, static stretching, passive stretching, and proprioceptive neuromuscular facilitation.[20]

Ballistic stretching involves repeated, rapid, forceful stretching maneuvers such as bouncing or twisting. This technique is no longer recommended for routine stretching due to the high risk of injury caused by the rapid generation of force.

The rapid movement creates a muscle stretch reflex response which actually makes it harder to achieve tissue lengthening. Athletes with good flexibility may utilize this technique after proper warm-up as part of plyometric exercises.

In static stretching, the body part is positioned to provide a gradual stretch over a duration of at least 15 seconds.[20,21] The stretch is usually repeated several times. It is the easiest stretch to perform and is widely used for preexercise stretching (after a warm-up). It also helps reduce muscular soreness following exercise. The best results are obtained when stretching is combined with an increase in tissue temperature into the therapeutic range (42 to 45 °C; 104 to 115 °F). This may be accomplished by using heating modalities or warm-up exercises.

Passive stretching is performed by a partner applying stretch to a relaxed muscle or extremity. Trainers and physical therapists commonly apply this method. Expertise and good communication between partners are essential to prevent injury from overstretching.

Proprioceptive neuromuscular facilitation (PNF) techniques were described by Knott and Voss.[22] They take advantage of the (theoretical) neural factors described earlier. Contract-relax or hold-relax techniques are the most commonly employed. For example, the gastrocnemius-soleus complex may be stretched by first isometrically contracting the muscle for 5 seconds followed by slow-duration passive or static stretching.[23] The initial contraction may decrease muscle activity by affecting the neural elements, or it may help stretch the fascia and tendons. Partners are often utilized for this technique. PNF techniques are especially helpful in reducing muscle splinting, decreasing tone, and stretching lower extremity muscles.

When stretching to correct connective tissue contractures, temperature elevation should be accomplished through heating modalities. The choice of modality depends on the depth of the tissue to be heated. Deep joint capsules with surrounding tendons, such as the hip or shoulder, require ultrasound diathermy. More superficial tissues such as the finger flexors or Achilles tendon are adequately heated by superficial modalities such as moist heat. Concomitant, gentle, prolonged stretching should be applied across the joint once elevated temperatures are attained.

Passive or static stretch is used depending on partner availability and the ability of the individual to participate in therapy.

When improving or maintaining flexibility in uninjured individuals, it is also important to elevate tissue temperature. Using therapeutic modalities, however, is impractical and unnecessary. Martin et al.[24] showed that a 15-minute light treadmill jog elevates peripheral muscle temperatures. Static stretching is done after the warm-up. Preactivity stretching without warm-up is of dubious benefit and may lead to injury. Postexercise static stretch is also efficacious. Holding the stretch until the muscle cools may help to maintain length deformation changes.[12,25]

### Coordination Exercise

While strength and endurance help prevent injury and reinjury, they cannot do so unless the body is coordinated. Coordination exercises, such as running in place, running backward, running in figure-of-eight patterns, running stairs, or various hand motion or ball catching exercises, help to develop coordination. The type of activity is limited only by the imagination of the clinician and the patient. In addition to improving coordination, such exercise helps to improve proprioception, which is often impaired after injury.

### Activity-Specific Training

While general coordination and strengthening exercises offer a great base on which to build, they cannot surpass activity-specific training to develop proper technique. In sports or work, the final coordination exercises need to at least resemble the activity being trained for. If the activity is complex, it can be broken down and practiced in component parts that are easier to master.

## Exercise Prescription

When prescribing an exercise program for the individual patient, some general guidelines are in order. They are described in Table 7-3. All of the types of exercise, for strengthening, endurance,

**Table 7-3.** Guidelines for Prescribing an Exercise Program

1. The needs, goals, and limitations of the individual must be addressed and defined prior to prescribing exercise.
2. The patient's introduction to exercise training should be at low to moderate intensity with slow to moderate progression to allow gradual adaptation.
3. Adequate medical information including medical history, physical examination, and when appropriate, laboratory and radiologic tests should be obtained prior to embarking on a rigorous exercise program. This allows for the prescription of a safe and effective program.
4. Realistic long- and short-term goals should be set.
5. The individual should be educated in the principles of exercise, including the prescription and methods of monitoring and recording progress.
6. Progress should be evaluated with timely follow-up visits.
7. When possible, exercise should approximate the specific movements or activities being trained for.
8. The exercise program should allow time for warm-up, and cool-down to prevent injuries.

flexibility, coordination, and activity-specific training, address specific deficits that may have occurred from disease or injury to the musculoskeletal system. Commonly, all of these exercises must be integrated into a rational, comprehensive, well managed, conservative rehabilitation program.

## Points of Summary

1. Exercises are activities used to develop and maintain physical fitness.
2. Strength, endurance, and flexibility may all be improved with specific exercises.
3. All exercise follows the overload principle of doing activity that stresses the body beyond its baseline, leading to adaptation and enhanced function.
4. Specificity of exercise is important. The exercise should simulate the activity being trained for.
5. All exercise prescriptions should include the mode, intensity, frequency, and duration of each exercise, as well as precautions.
6. Close monitoring is essential to prevent injury and to assure safe progression of training.

7. Exercise should be used in concert with other therapeutic interventions such as medications and modalities for a comprehensive integrated rehabilitation program.

## References

1. *Webster's New Collegiate Dictionary.* Springfield, MA: G & C Merriam, 1981.
2. Speilholz NI: Scientific basis of exercise programs. In Basmajian JV, Wolf SL (eds): *Therapeutic Exercise,* 5th ed. Baltimore: Williams & Wilkins, 1990:49–76.
3. DeLateur BJ, Lehmann JF, Fordyce WE: A test of the DeLorme axiom. *Arch Phys Med Rehabil* 1968;49:245–248.
4. Petersen S, Wessel J, Bagnall K, et al.: Influence of concentric resistance training on concentric and eccentric strength. *Arch Phys Med Rehabil* 1990;71:101–105.
5. Esselman PC, DeLateur BJ, Alquist AD, et al.: Torque development in isokinetic training. *Arch Phys Med Rehabil* 1991;72:723–728.
6. Milner-Brown HS, Stein RB, Lee RG: Synchronization of human motor units: Possible roles of exercise and supraspinal reflexes. *EEG Clin Neurophysiol* 1975; 38:245–254.
7. Moritani T, DeVries AH: Neural factors versus hypertrophy in the time course of muscle strength gain. *Am J Phys Med* 1979;58:115–130.
8. Gonyea WJ: Role of exercise in inducing increases in skeletal muscle fiber number. *J Appl Physiol* 1980; 48:421–426.
9. Barnard RJ, Edgerton VR, Peter JB: Effect of exercise on skeletal Muscle. I. Biochemical and histochemical properties. *J Appl Physiol* 1970;28:762–766.
10. Kottke FJ, Pauley DL, Ptak RA: The rationale for prolonged stretching for correction of shortening of connective tissue. *Arch Phys Med Rehabil* 1966;47:345–352.
11. Lehmann JF, Masock AJ, Warren CG, Koblanski JN: Effect of therapeutic temperatures on tendon extensibility. *Arch Phys Med Rehabil* 1970;51:481–487.
12. Muller EA: Influence of training and of inactivity on muscle strength. *Arch Phys Med Rehabil* 1970;51:449–462.
13. DeLorme TL, Watkins AL: Techniques of progressive resistance exercise. *Arch Phys Med Rehabil* 1948; 29:263–273.
14. Zinovieff AM: Heavy resistive exercise: The Oxford technique. *Br J Phys Med* 1951;14:6.
15. McGovern RE, Luscombe HB: Useful modifications of progressive resistive exercise technique. *Arch Phys Med Rehabil* 1953;34:475–477.
16. Stanish WD, Rubinovich RM, Curwin S: Eccentric exercise in chronic tendinitis. *Clin Orthop Rel Res* 1986; 208:65–68.

17. Moffroid MT,Whipple RH: Specificity of speed of exercise. *Phys Ther* 1970;50:1692–1700.
18. Gamble, JN: Strength and conditioning for the competitive athlete. In Kulund DN (ed): *The Injured Athlete,* 2nd ed. Philadelphia: JB Lippincott, 1988:132–135.
19. American College of Sports Medicine: *Guidelines for Exercise Testing and Prescription,* 4th ed. Philadelphia: Lea & Febiger, 1991.
20. Saal JS: Flexibility training. *Physical Medicine and Rehabilitation: State of the Art Reviews* 1987;1(4):537–554.
21. Medeiros J, Madding SW: Effect of duration of passive stretch on hip abduction range of motion. *Orthop Sports Phys Ther* 1987;8:409–411.
22. Knott M, Voss DE: *Proprioceptive Neuromuscular Facilitation.* New York: Harper & Row, 1968.
23. Moore MA, Hutton RS: Electromyographic investigation of muscle stretching techniques. *Med Sci Sports Exerc* 1980;12:322–329.
24. Martin BJ, Robinson S, Wiegman DL, et al.: Effect of warm-up on metabolic responses to strenuous exercise. *Med Sci Sports Exerc* 1975;7:146–152.
25. Sapega AA, Quedenfeld TC, Moyer RA, et al.: Biophysical factors in range of motion exercises. *Phys Sports Med* 1981;9(12):57–65.

## Suggested Readings

Speilholz NI: Scientific Basis of Exercise Programs. In Basmajian JV, Wolf SL (eds): *Therapeutic Exercise,* 5th ed. Baltimore: Williams & Wilkins, 1990.

Saal JS: Flexibility Training. *Physical Medicine and Rehabilitation: State of the Art Reviews* 1987; 1(4):537–554.

American College of Sports Medicine: *Guidelines for Exercise Testing and Prescription,* 4th ed. Philadelphia: Lea & Febiger, 1991.

Pollock M. (ed): *Exercise in Health and Disease: Evaluation and Prescription for Prevention and Rehabilitation,* 2nd ed. Philadelphia: WB Saunders, 1990.

# Chapter 8

# Electrodiagnostic, Imaging, and Laboratory Studies

RALPH BUSCHBACHER

## Electrodiagnostic Evaluation

When nerves conduct signals and muscles contract, their membranes undergo electrical changes. These changes can be detected by recording electrodes and are the basis for electrodiagnosis. It is primarily a method of detecting abnormalities of the peripheral nerves, of the neuromuscular junction, or of the muscles.

### Electromyographic Examinations

Electromyography (EMG) is the term used for two types of diagnostic examination: nerve conduction studies and electromyography proper, which is also known as the needle examination. There is also a variant of this technique called surface EMG, described later in the chapter.

### Nerve Conduction Studies

During normal voluntary muscle use motor nerves are stimulated in the spinal cord and pass an electrical wave or signal down the length of the axon to the muscle. At the muscle the signal is transmitted by a chemical messenger, acetylcholine, to the muscle, which then undergoes an electrical change

and contracts. In sensory nerves the principle is the same but the direction is reversed. Some stimulus at the nerve ending such as a pinprick or touch initiates an electrical impulse which passes up to the spinal cord and brain to let the central nervous system know what is going on in the body.

Normally, each nerve fires along its entire length whenever it is stimulated. The speed of conduction varies, depending on the nerve cell diameter, how much myelin it is surrounded by, and to some extent body temperature.

In nerve conduction studies (NCS) the nerve is stimulated at some point with a small electrical shock. This starts an electrical impulse which travels both up and down the nerve away from the stimulator. The nerves ordinarily transmit information in only one direction, but when fired with a stimulator they can pass an electrical wave in the opposite direction just as well. By placing a recording electrode over a nerve or muscle at a set distance from the electrical stimulator and measuring the time it takes for the impulse to travel between these two points, a conduction velocity of the nerve can be calculated (Figure 8-1). The electrical impulse can also be displayed on a television-like screen. It ordinarily has a characteristic speed, shape, and amplitude. Any deviations from the pattern guide the electromyographer to the appropriate diagnosis. For instance, if nerve

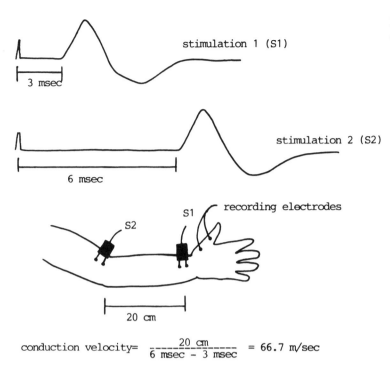

**Figure 8-1.** Calculation of nerve conduction velocity.

stimulation 1 (S1)

3 msec

stimulation 2 (S2)

6 msec

recording electrodes

S1

S2

20 cm

$$\text{conduction velocity} = \frac{20 \text{ cm}}{6 \text{ msec} - 3 \text{ msec}} = 66.7 \text{ m/sec}$$

conduction is diffusely slowed, it may be a sign that the myelin sheath insulation around the nerve is damaged, a condition called demyelination. If there is a localized slowing of the nerve impulse, it may be indicative of a nerve compression, such as carpal tunnel syndrome. If the amplitude of the wave is decreased, it may mean that some of the nerve fibers themselves are being blocked (neurapraxia) or are dead (axonopathy). In addition to standard NCSs there are special techniques to help diagnose myasthenia gravis, botulism, and numerous other conditions of the nerves, muscles, and neuromuscular junction.

*Electromyography (Needle Examination)*

While very valuable, the nerve conduction examination does not provide much information about the state of the muscles. It is also technically difficult to do and can be inadequate in proximal regions such as the back or a buttock. The EMG (needle examination) fills in these gaps.

The needle examination may be diagnostic when a muscle is damaged, when a nerve to a muscle is damaged, or if there is a loss of voluntary muscle control. It involves placing a small pin into various muscles of the body. This pin is an elec-

trode that is connected to the EMG machine in such a manner as to allow both seeing and hearing the muscle potentials. Denervated muscles display characteristic spontaneous activity such as fibrillation potentials (fibs) and positive sharp waves (Figure 8-2). They may also have characteristic firing patterns. This is extremely helpful in diagnosing radiculopathy, the recovery process from nerve trauma, and numerous other diseases of nerves and muscles. In radiculopathy, a sampling of muscles innervated by different myotomes helps diagnose the level of the lesion. It is almost always imperative that a full EMG/NCS be performed before making diagnoses of disorders of the nerves and muscles (Table 8-1).

Before referring patients for electrodiagnostic evaluation they should be well informed, so as not to create misunderstandings. They should be told that the procedure is moderately uncomfortable

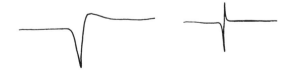

**Figure 8-2.** Positive sharp wave (*left*) and fibrillation potential (*right*) is indicative of muscle damage or denervation.

**Table 8-1.** Conditions Commonly Diagnosed with the Help of Electrodiagnosis

| |
| --- |
| Carpal tunnel syndrome |
| Ulnar neuropathy/Cubital tunnel syndrome |
| Radiculopathy |
| Peripheral neuropathy |
| Bell's palsy |
| Myasthenia gravis |
| Muscular dystrophies |
| Toxic/Metabolic neuropathies |

and in general very safe. When compared with the surgery and biopsies that EMG sometimes helps prevent it is clear that the minor discomfort is indeed a small price to pay for an accurate diagnosis. However, it must be appreciated that EMG is a complicated consultative diagnostic procedure, and the results of the examination are only as good as the examiner. EMG is by no means a simple "test" that anyone can interpret. The EMG examination itself is modified during the examination, depending on the results that are obtained.

*Surface Electromyography*

Surface electrodes can be applied to the skin to record gross information about underlying muscle activity. Such information is useful in biofeedback (described later) to help the patient perceive underlying muscle activity. It is also useful in analyzing muscle firing patterns in gait analysis and is often used as a research tool. The technique has also been abused as a substitute for true diagnostic EMG. It is not useful for this purpose.

*Somatosensory Evoked Potentials*

Whenever peripheral nerves or nerves in the skin are stimulated, they relay information to the brain. In the somatosensory evoked potential (SEP) test, the impulses are recorded with electrodes on the scalp and a general picture of nerve conduction from the periphery to the brain can be obtained. The waveforms that are recorded on the scalp are exceedingly small, and hundreds or thousands of stimuli are needed to obtain an accurate SEP. Variants of this procedure are used to test vision and hearing in the visual evoked potential and brain stem auditory evoked potential tests.

## Radiographic and Imaging Studies

### *Plain Radiographs (X-Rays)*

Ever since Wilhelm Konrad Roentgen discovered x-rays they have been a mainstay of musculoskeletal diagnosis. An energy beam (x-ray) is passed through the body onto a photographic plate to create an x-ray "picture." It is relatively inexpensive, safe, and easy to obtain. X-ray waves pass through soft tissues while largely being blocked by bone, thus creating a nice view of skeletal structures. Fractures, malalignment, arthritic changes, bony tumors, and congenital abnormalities may all be visualized. To a lesser extent the soft tissues can be assessed. Cartilage integrity can be indirectly evaluated by observing the bones of the joint. Also soft tissue swelling, abnormal calcification, and abnormal pockets of air can help in making a diagnosis (Figure 8-3). It must always be appreciated that x-rays (and the other radiographic diagnostic tests described in this section) detect anatomic defects. Not all such defects are clinically important. Often

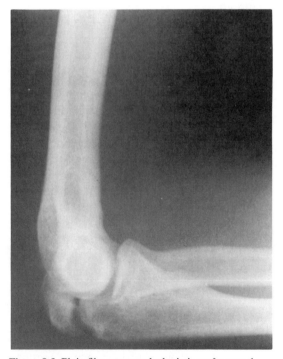

**Figure 8-3.** Plain film x-ray study depicting a fractured olecranon process of the ulna. (Nicholas JA, Hershman EB (eds): *The Upper Extremity in Sports Medicine*. St. Louis: CV Mosby, 1990:332. Reproduced with permission.)

a patient's symptoms are blamed on an x-ray abnormality, which may or may not reflect the true underlying pathology.

A variant of x-ray technique, the tomogram, is sometimes obtained. Here the x-ray source and the recording film are moved simultaneously in such a way as to visualize a "slice" of bone instead of the usual outline. It is much like using a camera to focus on a specified distance. Objects closer than or farther from this distance are blurry while the focused area is clear. This technique is sometimes helpful in detecting unusual fractures or vertebral column abnormalities (Figure 8-4).

### Computed Tomography

When x-ray beams are passed through the body in multiple directions and recorded by computer they can be used to generate a "slice" through the body (Figure 8-5) which is called a computed tomography (CT) scan. Multiple slices are used to detect abnormalities. CT gives a view that, prior to its advent, could only be obtained by surgery. Because it uses x-rays, it is much better at depicting bony structures than soft tissues. When used in conjunction with contrast dye injected into the veins it can

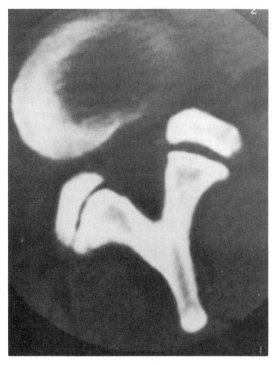

**Figure 8-5.** Computed tomography scan of the lumbar spine showing the facet joints. (Kirkaldy-Willis WH: *Managing Low Back Pain*, 2nd ed. New York: Churchill Livingstone, 1988:163. Reproduced with permission.)

sometimes be even more sensitive at detecting abnormalities. CT scanning is excellent at detecting fractures, bleeding strokes, and tumors. It is also often used to help make the diagnosis of herniated disk. It is somewhat limited in that it produces only cross-sectional images, but with newer computer programming, longitudinal reconstruction of fair quality is possible. Also, three-dimensional images can be produced, although this is still largely an experimental technique. One of the main drawbacks of CT is that the patient is exposed to fairly high doses of radiation.

### Magnetic Resonance Imaging

For magnetic resonance imaging (MRI) the body is placed in a strong magnetic field and is then subjected to radio waves which cause hydrogen atoms to enter a high energy state. When the atoms return to their lower energy state they produce a signal that is measured, and by computer

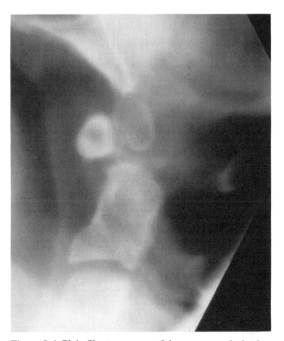

**Figure 8-4.** Plain film tomogram of the upper cervical spine.

program generates a cross-sectional or longitudinal "slice" picture through the body (Figure 8-6). Tissues such as water and fat which are rich in hydrogen are preferentially depicted. Thus while MRI is similar to CT scanning, it is much better at visualizing soft tissues than bones. Bones can be evaluated indirectly if they contain fatty marrow. MRI is good at diagnosing herniated disks, brain tumors, and many other soft tissue abnormalities. It has the advantage of not subjecting the patient to x-ray radiation.

There are two types of MRI pictures that can be produced, T1-weighted and T2-weighted. The technical differences between these two images are beyond the scope of this chapter; however, the reader should be aware that T1-weighted scans are best for evaluating structures containing fat, hemorrhage, or protein-containing fluid. T2-weighted scans are better at depicting areas of high water content such as cerebrospinal fluid, cysts, and intervertebral disks. Both are poor at imaging cortical bone.

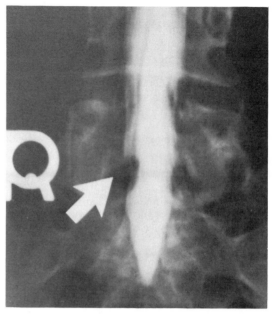

**Figure 8-7.** Myelogram of the lumbar spine depicting a radiopaque-dye filling defect due to single-level degenerative central stenosis (*arrow*). (Kirkaldy-Willis: *Managing Low Back Pain*, 2nd ed. New York: Churchill Livingstone, 1988:158. Reproduced with permission.)

*Myelogram*

Myelography involves the injection of a dye visible under x-ray into the space around the spinal cord to detect any compression of the spinal cord or nerve roots (Figure 8-7). This technique can be combined with either plain x-ray diagnosis or CT scanning to detect such compression. It is a time-consuming and uncomfortable procedure and is largely being supplanted by CT and MRI, but in some cases it still provides valuable information.

*Arthrogram*

In arthrography a radiopaque dye is injected into the joint and then viewed with x-ray or CT (Figure 8-8). It will sometimes detect joint pathology such as a ruptured ligament, torn rotator cuff, or joint capsule adhesions. It is largely being supplanted by newer techniques such as MRI and arthroscopic surgery, although it is still used, especially in the shoulder.

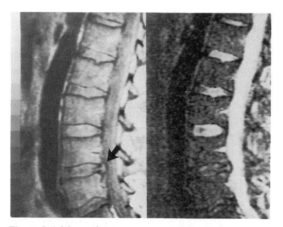

**Figure 8-6.** Magnetic resonance scan of the lumbar spine showing a disk herniation (*arrow* on the left). The Left scan depicts a T-1 weighted image. Right scan is a T-2 weighted image of the same scan. (Kirkaldy-Willis: *Managing Low Back Pain*, 2nd ed. New York: Churchill Livingstone, 1988:188. Reproduced with permission.)

*Ultrasound*

Diagnostic ultrasound uses sound waves that are directed into the body. By measuring the way the

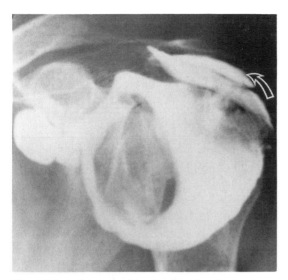

**Figure 8-8.** Arthrogram of the shoulder showing extravasation of contrast material (*arrow*) from the glenohumeral joint into the subdeltoid bursa, a sign of a rotator cuff tear. (Nicholas JA, Hershman EB (eds): *The Upper Extremity in Sports Medicine*. St. Louis: CV Mosby, 1990:114. Reproduced with permission.)

waves are reflected, a picture of deep body structures is created. This is commonly used in viewing fetuses and can also be used to detect soft tissue abnormalities such as torn ligaments and rotator cuff tears. Ultrasound is still in its infancy, and the images generated are not up to the standards of MRI and CT, but it holds a great deal of promise for the future.

### Thermography

Infrared cameras can create a thermal picture of the body surface by temperature gradients. Variations in temperature from side to side or from normal patterns have been advocated for use in diagnosing everything from carpal tunnel syndrome to fibromyalgia. However, because many factors, such as room temperature, season, and recent handwashing may affect the image, and because so many other good diagnostic tests are available, thermography is now rarely used. Its one major indication is in diagnosing or ruling out reflex sympathetic dystrophy.

### Bone Scan

A bone scan is performed by attaching a radioactive element to molecules that are preferentially drawn to regions of active bone turnover and injecting it into the bloodstream. A few hours later the patient is placed before a screen that measures radioactive emissions. Areas of abnormal concentration of the radioactive element may help diagnose osteomyelitis (bone infection), stress fractures, reflex sympathetic dystrophy, and may help differentiate old bony abnormalities from more recent ones. The radioactive element is washed out of the body by the kidneys and exposes the person to minimal radioactivity. Figure 8-9 depicts a bone scan.

## Laboratory Studies

Many laboratory studies of the body's fluids help to make musculoskeletal diagnoses, mainly of the rheumatic diseases (Table 8-2). Only a few of the more common laboratory tests ordered in musculoskeletal medicine are discussed here.

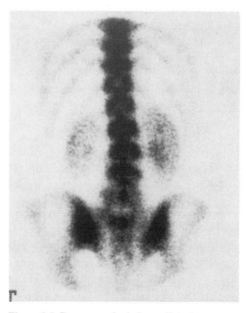

**Figure 8-9.** Bone scan depicting radioactive tracer uptake by the bones. (Courtesy of Eugene Jacobs, from *Medical Imaging: A Concise Textbook*. New York: Igaku-Shoin Medical Publishers, 1987.)

**Table 8-2.** Common Laboratory Studies in Musculoskeletal Medicine

Complete blood count
Thyroid function tests
Erythrocyte sedimentation rate/Rheumatoid
    factor/Antinuclear antibodies
Serum uric acid
Serum calcium, sodium, and potassium
Blood glucose
Liver function tests
Blood urea nitrogen/Serum creatinine
Stool hemoccult
Joint fluid analysis
Urinalysis

**Complete Blood Count (CBC).**    This is a simple blood test which gives information about possible anemia or infection.

**Thyroid Function Tests (TFT).**    Abnormal thyroid gland function can result in conditions of muscle pain, fatigue, impaired sleep, and can cause symptoms similar to fibromyalgia syndrome. TFTs should be obtained in such conditions.

**Erythrocyte Sedimentation Rate (ESR)/Rheumatoid Factor/Antinuclear Antibodies.**    These tests are abnormal in some of the connective tissue disorders. ESR is a nonspecific indicator of inflammation.

**Serum Uric Acid.**    This is usually elevated in gout.

**Serum Calcium, Sodium, and Potassium.**    The serum concentrations of these elements are abnormal in a number of mainly medical conditions. They may also be abnormal in conditions of muscular pain, weakness, and impaired muscular function.

**Blood Glucose.**    This is a screening test for diabetes, which of course may initially be diagnosed in a musculoskeletal clinic.

**Liver Function (LFTs).**    The liver may be damaged by a number of medications commonly prescribed. LFTs are often obtained to monitor the state of the liver when these medications are in use.

**Blood Urea Nitrogen (BUN)/Serum Creatinine.**    These tests are indicators of kidney function and are monitored when drugs that may affect the kidneys are used.

**Stool Hemoccult.**    Steroidal or nonsteroidal antiinflammatory drugs may cause gastrointestinal bleeding which can be detected by Hemoccult testing (guaiac test for occult blood) of the stool.

**Joint Fluid Analysis.**    Painful swollen joints should have their fluid aspirated to determine whether there is joint infection, bleeding, or gout or to ascertain if this is a connective tissue disease manifestation.

**Urinalysis.**    Urinary tract infection may cause back pain or fatigue. Routine urinalysis may help detect this. It also detects an elevated urine glucose level in the person with diabetes.

## Points of Summary

1. Electrodiagnostic evaluation, in particular electromyography, is the best diagnostic procedure for evaluating diseases of nerves and muscles.
2. CT scans are best at visualizing bone.
3. MRI scans are best at visualizing soft tissues.
4. Myelography involves x-ray dye injection into the spinal canal.
5. Arthrography involves x-ray dye injection into joints.

## Suggested Readings

Kirkaldy-Willis WH, Tchang S: Diagnostic techniques. In Kirkaldy-Willis WH (ed): *Managing Low Back Pain*, 2nd ed. New York: Churchill Livingstone, 1988:155–182.
Kraft GH: Electromyography: Doctor's questions answered. *Phys Med Rehabil Clin North Am* 1990;1:1–16.

# Chapter 9
# Manual Physiotherapy

PHILLIP R. BRYANT
SANDY TIMOK

Manual physiotherapy includes therapeutic massage, stretching and joint mobilization, traction, and manipulation. Details regarding these forms of therapy, including definitions, indications and contradications, and techniques are discussed in this chapter.

## Therapeutic Massage

Massage has been described as both an art and a science. One of the earliest works to document the role of massage is recorded in the *Yellow Emperor's Classic of Internal Medicine*.[1] In this ancient book, which dates back to about 1000 BC, there is a description of "breathing exercises, massage of the skin and flesh, and exercises of the hands and feet" used to address "complete paralysis and chills and fever." The Yoga cult in India reportedly used respiratory exercises for both religious and healing purposes, probably employing massage-like techniques, as early as 8000 BC.[2] The Greek physicians Hippocrates, Praxagoras, and especially Asclepiades reportedly acknowledged the therapeutic benefits of massage and frequently employed such techniques with success on their patients.[1,2] Per Henrik Ling of Sweden is credited with reviving massage in the West in 1813 after a period of relative obscurity during the Middle Ages. He established the Central Royal Institute of Gymnastics in Stockholm and formed a massage and therapeutic exercise system known as medical gymnastics.[3]

### Definition

Therapeutic massage refers to that set of techniques which mobilizes soft tissues either manually or mechanically to improve the health or well-being of a patient. The most popular techniques include effleurage, petrissage, tapotement, friction, and vibration. Effleurage uses a gliding stroke. Petrissage employs a kneading stroke. Tapotement requires a percussion or a repetitive striking technique. Friction involves mobilization of the deep soft tissues. Vibration can be employed alone, or in combination with the aforementioned stroke techniques.

### Effects

Massage is felt to have psychological, mechanical, physiologic, and reflexive effects. Potential psychological benefits include sedation, improved relaxation, and a higher pain threshold. Mechanical or physiologic effects include reduction or prevention of venous stasis and edema, mobilization of scar tissue, and improved removal of products of metabolism. Obligate edema, however, cannot be reduced with massage.[3] Additional physiologic effects may include a counterirritant phenomenon, sensory inhibition or excitation, a reflex increase in muscle tone, and arteriolar constriction or dilation (Table 9-1).

Manual manipulation of skin and underlying soft tissues may improve the movement of blood and lymph fluids.[4] This results in a reduction of swelling, a more rapid and complete oxygenation and reoxygenation of blood, an increased exchange of body fluids, improved availability of nutritive elements, and more complete and rapid elimination of wastes.[5] It cannot decrease obesity or increase strength.

### Indications and Contraindications

Indications for massage are to achieve relaxation, pain control, and to help reduce edema. It is a useful adjunct to other treatments to reduce soft tissue pain, especially after stretching and exercise. It is not typically used as a primary treatment by itself. Table 9-2 lists the major contraindications to massage therapy.[3,6,7]

### Techniques

**Effleurage.**    (Figure 9-1). This is a gliding massage stroke, usually applied with firm, even motion. It is typically used at the beginning and end of manual therapy. It can be applied with a light or deep stroke. Pressure is applied from distal to proximal with the intent of pushing tissue fluids in the direction of venous flow. The whole hand should be maintained in contact with the patient.

**Table 9-1.** Effects of Massage

**Effects**
 Relaxation (physical and emotional)
 Pain relief
 Reduction of edema
 Increase in range of motion
 Increase in superficial blood flow
 Prevention or breakup of adhesions

**Things massage cannot accomplish**
 Increase muscle mass or strength
 Decrease obligate edema
 Effect weight loss
 Improve sensation

**Table 9-2.** Contraindications to Massage[5,6]

Presence of skin disease, infection, or open wounds
Recently sutured or unhealed sites of surgical repair
Recently bruised sites
Patient on anticoagulation
Presence of thrombophlebitis
  (may cause breakup of the thrombus into emboli)
Near fracture sites
Over sites of active inflammation
Over calcified, atrophic, or grafted skin
Over malignant tumors (may facilitate metastasis)

**Petrissage.**    (Figure 9-2). This is a form of manual manipulation in which soft tissue, usually muscle, is lifted and compressed, or compressed against other soft tissue structures or against bone. Such strokes attempt to lift, wring, roll, shake, or squeeze the muscle mass. They are typically applied to assist in improving venous return, to stimulate removal of waste products from muscle tissue, and to break up adhesions.

**Friction Massage.**    Friction massage involves using deep pressure in small circular movements of the hands, fingers, or thumbs in an attempt to break up soft tissue adhesions. It is often followed by effleurage to induce relaxation.

Cross-fiber manipulation is a form of friction massage in which deep strokes are applied perpendicular to the direction of the muscle fibers. It is particularly useful for the erector spinae musculature. Deep short strokes with the thumb are performed to stretch or soften areas of tightness.

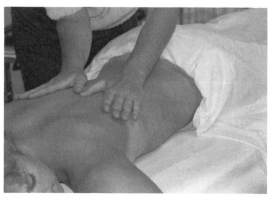

**Figure 9-1.** Effleurage (stroking) massage.

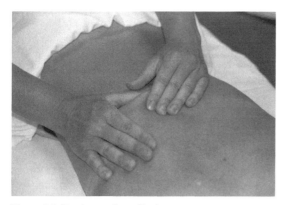

**Figure 9-2.** Petrissage (kneading) massage.

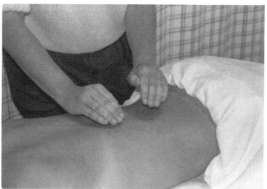

**Figure 9-4.** Tapotement massage, cupping technique.

**Tapotement.** This technique utilizes repetitive blows applied in a rapid, alternating fashion. Hacking (Figure 9-3), cupping (Figure 9-4), slapping, pincement, and tapping are forms of this massage technique.

## Stretching

### Definition

Stretching is a therapeutic maneuver designed to restore normal motion. It is used to lengthen pathologically shortened soft-tissue structures including muscles, ligaments, or joint capsules.

### Indications and Contraindications

Indications for prescribing a stretching program include any condition of limited range of motion

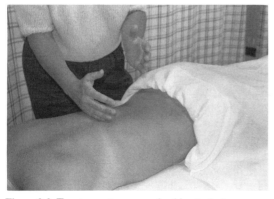

**Figure 9-3.** Tapotement massage, hacking technique.

which causes functional deficits. Such deficits may be caused by soft tissue contractures due to scar formation, muscle imbalance, or prolonged immobilization, among many other causes (Table 9-3).

Prevention is clearly the most important therapeutic intervention if contractures are to be avoided. Frequent daily attention to proper positioning must be included in any range of motion program. Positions such as lying in bed all day with a pillow under the knees or holding an amputated leg in flexion are to be avoided. Stretching is not usually performed when it appears that the contractures actually help to stabilize an impaired joint. Table 9-4 lists some of the contraindications to an aggressive range of motion program.

### Techniques

### Stretching

*Passive stretching* utilizes an extrinsic force applied in an appropriate direction and with sufficient magnitude to achieve optimal stretch without

**Table 9-3.** Causes of Soft Tissue Contracture

| | |
|---|---|
| Immobilization | Infection |
| Scar formation | Connective tissue disease |
| Muscle imbalance (especially | Bed rest |
| after amputation) | Burn |
| Contusion | Effusion |
| Frostbite | Hemorrhage |
| Radiation | Trauma |

**Table 9-4.** Contraindications to Stretching

Acute inflammation
Acute infection
Unhealed fracture
Recent surgery
Hematoma
Unstable joint
Weak connective tissue
Severe pain, or pain persisting more than 30 minutes
    after stretching

causing undue discomfort or injury. Close attention to the degree of soft tissue resistance and patient tolerance typically allows one to accomplish this goal. The patient does not contribute to this effort. Care must be taken in some joints, such as the knee, not to stretch too vigorously as this may cause ligamentous damage and joint subluxation. Flexion contractures at the elbow should not be aggressively stretched passively since this joint is easily damaged.

In *active assistive stretch*, the therapist and patient work together to achieve stretching. For example, in the case of heel cord tightness, the patient actively dorsiflexes the ankle while the therapist augments the patient's effort with additional force to further stretch the Achilles tendon. In *active stretch*, the patient is the sole participant in the stretching program.

It is important that the patient's affected limb or soft tissue be placed in a position of maximum relaxation prior to initiating the stretch. Heat application in the form of moist heat packs, infrared heating lamps, paraffin dip or immersion, and hydrotherapy prior to stretching have been effective in preparing the soft tissue for optimal stretch. It is also now recognized that a light calisthenic warm-up prior to active stretch may be useful in warming the tissues.

When spasticity is a cause of decreased mobility, ice application may be more effective than heat in aiding a stretching program. Similarly, patients with inflammatory conditions such as rheumatoid arthritis may be able to do their exercises better with cold application than with heat despite the fact that cold tends to stiffen joints. Ice offers an analgesic effect by raising the threshold of pain and reduces spasticity or spasm by decreasing the activity of the muscle spindles. By reducing the

individual's discomfort, greater stretch can be achieved. Although mild discomfort can occur, particularly early in treatment, stretching should be done in a gently progressive fashion to minimize pain and to avoid inflicting an injury.

### Serial Casting

Patients with severe contractures, or those who have not responded to manual stretching, may require serial casting to restore normal joint mobility. A cast is applied to the limb in a position of stretch and is changed at intervals (usually every 3 days) to a position of greater stretch. This allows a gradual elongation of the soft tissues to occur. Careful cast padding is necessary to prevent areas of pressure damage.

### Joint Mobilization Therapy

When decreased joint range of motion is due to joint capsule tightness it is often difficult to do stretching exercises. Pulling on the long lever arm of the limb may actually harm the joint by "prying" it apart. Joint mobilization techniques may help in such cases. The therapist manually applies a gliding motion to the joint in a direction perpendicular to the long axis of the joint or applies light longitudinal traction. Such techniques are very useful but must be performed gently to avoid causing injury.

## Manipulation

### Definition

The term *manipulation* is difficult to define because it is interpreted differently by the various professions employing such techniques. Chiropractors, osteopaths, some orthopedic surgeons and physiatrists, and physical therapists routinely perform spinal and extremity manipulation techniques. Some form of manipulation therapy is now taught to virtually all physical therapists in their undergraduate and/or basic Master's program curricula.[8] Sometimes it is referred to as soft tissue mobilization or spinal mobilization training by physical therapists.

*Effects*

It is unclear exactly what manipulation does to the spine or why it appears to relieve pain in some persons. Chapter 10 includes an in-depth review of the proposed mechanisms of action and possible effects of manipulation.

*Indications and Contraindications*

Manipulation is occasionally useful in a variety of musculoskeletal problems attributable to malalignment or dysfunction involving the neck, back, pelvis, and even the extremities. It should be viewed not as a cure for the dysfunction, but rather as an adjunct that may allow the patient to better perform exercises and return to normal function.

Spinal manipulation is fairly safe, and the incidence of serious complications attributable to manipulation therapy is apparently small. However, there have been cases of vascular insult to the vertebrobasilar system and/or spinal cord with cervical manipulation. The injury may not become manifest for some time after the manipulation, so the reported complication rate may be spuriously low. Most complications are due to poor technique or improper application in persons with contraindications to the procedure. Some of the contraindications to spinal manipulation are listed in Table 9-5.

*Techniques*

Manipulation is typically defined as a therapeutic modality designed to normalize joint alignment and motion. Various techniques of manipulation are available. Some are designed to address multiple spinal segments and therefore are classified as general spinal manipulation. Others attempt to identify and treat isolated segments of supposed spinal malalignment.

Manipulation techniques can be divided into a number of categories: direct versus indirect, contact versus noncontact, sustained pressure, thrust versus nonthrust, and surgical thrust.[8] *Direct manipulation* induces stretch in the direction of mo-

**Table 9-5.** Contraindications to Manipulation

| |
|---|
| Inexperienced or unskilled manipulator |
| Spine instability |
| Cauda equina syndrome |
| Spinal stenosis |
| Rheumatoid arthritis involvement of the neck |
| Unhealed fracture |
| Myelopathy |
| Malignancy |
| Vertebral artery insufficiency |
| Atherosclerosis of the arteries of the neck |
| Severe osteoarthritis |
| Radiculopathy (especially with objective neurologic signs) |
| Congenital joint laxity |
| Aneurysm |
| Osteomalacia/osteopenia |
| Aseptic necrosis |
| Pregnancy |
| "Hypermobile spine" |
| Vertigo |
| Vertebral inflammation |
| Anticoagulation |
| Severe diabetes mellitus |

tion restriction. *Indirect manipulation*, on the other hand, provides stretch in the opposite direction, that is, away from motion restriction.

In *contact manipulation*, a therapist or physician places a hand or finger on the segment concerned. This enables an isolation of the segment and helps in more accurately identifying the degree of restriction. It also provides a site to apply additional, focal force in a controlled fashion. The spinous and transverse processes are contact points in the thoracic and lumbar spine. *Noncontact manipulation*, as its name implies, does not involve focal contact with one's fingers or hand. It is usually used in those patients in whom greater force, sometimes achieved through greater leverage, is required to successfully mobilize and align a joint.

*Sustained pressure manipulation* utilizes a slow, gradual, continuous, and progressive force. Its proponents argue that this allows them to achieve improved sensitivity to tissue tension or spinal malalignment and provides them with the sensory feedback necessary to apply the appropriate force in the proper direction.

*Thrust techniques* use high-velocity, low-amplitude forces after placing the spinal segment concerned in its "end-range" position. The potential success of this technique is often improved when one takes time to adequately prepare the patient with relaxation procedures, such as moist heat application and gentle massage, prior to performing the maneuver. It can provide an appropriate patient with a dramatic sense of relief if done skillfully at the appropriate spinal level. On the other hand, if this technique is performed abruptly without an explanation and without an attempt to reassure and physically relax an apprehensive, tense patient, it is likely to result in less than favorable acceptance and little or no relief of the patient's discomfort.

*Surgical thrust manipulation* refers to the performance of manipulation under anesthesia. Although this technique eliminates the muscle guarding that can limit or block mobilization of the spine when the patient is alert, it also places the patient at risk for injury due to the potential for excessive or inappropriately directed manipulation.[8]

*Nonthrust techniques* are often called mobilization instead of manipulation and are generally more accepted by the medical community than the thrust techniques usually associated with chiropractic care. Nonthrust mobilization involves a number of techniques, all of which avoid the thrust action. Graded oscillation technique, progressive stretch mobilization, continuous stretch, muscle energy technique, functional technique, and counterstrain are all examples of nonthrust maneuvers. Two of these are commonly employed techniques and deserve additional attention.

The *muscle energy maneuver* uses the patient's muscle contraction force to normalize spinal mobility. An individual is placed in a specific position, usually toward the restriction. The therapist or physician then "takes up the slack" so an endpoint is reached. The patient is then asked to selectively contract those muscles that direct the spinal segment away from the restriction while the therapist or physician prevents actual movement in that direction. This creates an isometric muscle contraction. The force generated by the patient is carefully controlled and countered by the treating therapist or physician. The patient's muscle contraction is then followed by muscle relaxation. Further stretch is applied to the new "endpoint" and the cycle of contraction, relaxation, and stretch is repeated until optimal range is achieved without undue patient discomfort.

*Counterstrain* is a nonthrust technique that involves first localizing a myofascial trigger point. One then places the affected muscle and associated joint in a position of relaxation. Trigger point pressure is then applied for about 90 seconds. The latter maneuver, along with the proper positioning, is done with the intent of inhibiting the "muscle spasm" attributed to a pathologic reflex response. This technique is applied in those conditions in which joint dysfunction is felt to be caused by "self-perpetuating tonic-reflex" muscle spasms.[6,8]

## Traction

### Definition

Traction is a well-established mode of therapy for selected patients. It is a stretch force directed along a longitudinal axis. This pull can be performed manually with one's hands, with weights and a pulley system, or with a motorized device. It is generally limited to use in the neck and lumbar spine regions.

### Effects

The purpose of traction is to provide a separation of the vertebral elements, especially of the posterior spine, to relieve pain. It has been shown to cause such separation.[8] It may relieve pain due to compressed spinal nerves by decompressing them. It may also relieve pressure on painful facet joints or relax the neck muscles.

### Indications and Contraindications

Traction of the cervical and lumbar spine is generally prescribed for those individuals with radicular symptoms attributable to nerve root compression injury due to a herniated disk. It must always be preceded by x-ray evaluation to rule out bony instability or other abnormality that could be worsened by traction.

It is contraindicated in a number of cases. Relative contraindications include the elderly patient or overly anxious patient. In individuals with respiratory compromise, the use of a chest harness in lumbar traction may create further respiratory distress. Traction is unequivocally contraindicated when either the therapist or patient (if a home cervical traction unit is used) is inexperienced with regard to the proper angle of pull, optimal body position, and appropriate range of traction force. Other absolute contraindications include cervical ligamentous instability (may cause atlantoaxial subluxation and secondary spinal cord injury), existing vertebrobasilar artery disease, signs or symptoms of myelopathy, suspected or known spinal column tumors, significant osteoporosis, infection of the spine or paravertebral soft tissue, and diskitis. Lumbar traction is also contraindicated in pregnant patients. Some feel, and the authors of this chapter agree, that traction applied during acute neck or back injuries is more likely to exacerbate rather than to alleviate a patient's discomfort (see Table 9-6).[3]

### Techniques

When performing traction, it is imperative that one consider the position of the patient, the direction of pull, as well as the type, speed and duration of the force creating the traction. Regarding the patient's posture during traction, the supine position appears to be the most widely accepted and practiced. It is also felt to be the most effective posture for performing both cervical and lumbar traction. Crue is credited with being the first to

**Table 9-6.** Contraindications to Traction

| |
|---|
| Spinal instability |
| Spinal cord compromise |
| Vertebrobasilar artery disease |
| Myelopathy |
| Osteoporosis |
| Tumor |
| Spinal infection |
| Pregnancy (lumbar traction) |
| Acute soft tissue injury |

recognize that the maximal widening of the intervertebral foramina occurs between 20 to 30 degrees of neck flexion.[3]

When performing traction, it is important that one specify the appropriate amount of weight to prescribe. If cervical spine traction is done in the sitting position, at least 10 lb is necessary just to counter the weight of the heat. In the usual supine position, with the head at 24 degrees of flexion, a pull of 30 lb is most often adequate to achieve optimal vertebral distraction. In lumbar spine traction, it is necessary to overcome the friction produced by the weight of the body. It is established that one should produce a traction force equal to about one half of the weight of the body part being pulled to overcome this friction. This corresponds to about 26% of total body weight.[10] If one also hopes to cause vertebral separation at the lumbar level, then an additional 25% of the body weight is necessary.[3] In both cervical and lumbar spine areas, one should increase the force of traction progressively rather than abruptly while monitoring the patient's level of tolerance.

The issue of whether to perform traction continuously or intermittently remains controversial. There is no definite data which unequivocally supports one method in favor of the other. Nevertheless, it appears that most therapists use intermittent traction because it seems to be better tolerated by patients, particularly when heavier weights are employed in producing the traction force.

In general, it is recommended that one precede the traction with moist heat application to the posterior neck or low back area to induce greater muscle relaxation and patient comfort. This appears to be an effective means of preparing a patient to tolerate greater stretch. Soft tissue mobilization, including massage techniques, immediately following the traction also appears to add to the patient's relaxation and comfort.

### Summary

Manual physiotherapy, including therapeutic massage, stretching, traction, and manipulation, remains a valuable therapeutic option for many patients. Proper application of the various techniques and an awareness of the contraindications enable physicians and therapists to provide a broader spectrum of potentially effective therapies to their patients.

## Points of Summary

1. Massage is a useful adjunct to some therapy programs to effect relaxation, relief of pain, and decrease edema; it is a useless technique to treat obesity or to increase muscle mass.
2. Techniques of massage include effleurage, petrissage, tapotement, and friction massage.
3. Range of motion exercises should be instituted early in patients prone to contracture.
4. Traction may be useful in cases of radiculopathy; it causes vertebral body separation and intervertebral foraminal enlargement.

## References

1. Kamenetz HL: History of massage. In Basmajian JV (ed); *Manipulation, Traction, and Massage*, 3rd ed. Baltimore: Williams & Wilkins, 1985:214.
2. Tappan FM: *Healing Massage Techniques: Holistic, Classic, and Emerging Methods*, 2nd ed. Norwalk, CT: Appleton & Lange, 1988:5.
3. Geiringer SR, Kincaid CB, Rechtien JJ: Traction, manipulation, and massage. In DeLisa JA (ed): *Rehabilitation Medicine: Principles and Practice*. Philadelphia: JB Lippincott, 1988:276–294.
4. Elkins EC, Herrick JF, Grindlay JH, et al.: Effect of various procedures on the flow of lymph. *Arch Phys Med* 1953;34:31–39.
5. Wakim KG: In Licht S (ed): *Massage, Manipulation and Traction*. New Haven, CT: Elizabeth Licht Publisher, 1960:38–43.
6. Geiringer SR, deLateur BJ: Physiatric therapeutics: Traction, manipulation, and massage. *Arch Phys Med Rehabil* 1990;71:S264–S266.
7. Knapp ME: Massage. In Kottke FJ, Lehmann JF (eds): *Krusen's Handbook of Physical Medicine and Rehabilitation*, 4th ed. Philadelphia: WB Saunders, 1990:435.
8. Nyberg R: Role of physical therapists in spinal manipulation. In Basmajian JV (ed): *Manipulation, Traction and Massage*, 3rd ed. Baltimore: Williams & Wilkins, 1985:22–32.
9. Colachis SC, Strohm BR: Cervical traction: Relationship of traction time to varied tractive force with constant angle of pull. *Arch Phys Med Rehabil* 1965; 46:815–819.
10. Judovich BD: Lumbar traction therapy—elimination of physical factors that prevent lumbar stretch. *JAMA* 1955;159:549–550.

## Suggested Readings

Geiringer SR, Kincaid CB, Rechtien JJ: Traction, manipulation, and massage. In DeLisa JA (ed): *Rehabilitation Medicine: Principles and Practice*. Philadelphia: JB Lippincott, 1988:276–294.

Haldeman S: *Principles and Practice of Chiropractic*, 2nd ed. Norwalk, CT: Appleton & Lange, 1992.

Knapp ME: Massage. In Kottke FJ, Lehmann JF (eds): *Krusen's Handbook of Physical Medicine and Rehabilitation*, 4th ed. Philadelphia: WB Saunders, 1990:433–435.

Parry CBW: Stretching. In Basmajian JV (ed): *Manipulation, Traction and Massage*, 3rd ed. Baltimore: Williams & Wilkins, 1985:157–171.

# Chapter 10

# The Role of Manipulation in Disorders of the Spine

THOMAS FLORIAN

## Historical and Cultural Perspective

The role of manipulation in the management of spinal pain is controversial, partly because in the United States it is associated with the practice of chiropractic[1] and partly because of the perception among medical practitioners that there is little data to support its usefulness.

Manipulation has been practiced for thousands of years and in many cultures and countries. Hippocrates was the first clinician to clearly describe techniques of spinal manipulation in his book, *On Joints* (Figure 10-1).[2] In Iran, manipulation is practiced by unschooled common folk,[3] and in Mexico contemporary folk practitioners, called Sobadors, do spinal manipulation.[4] Traditional manipulators in England were called bonesetters, in a profession handed down from father to son in the time of the barber-surgeons.[5] Robert Anderson, MD, PhD, DC, a medical doctor and chiropractor who was also trained as an anthropologist, has written extensive reviews on the history and culture of spinal manipulation.[6,7]

## Contemporary Perspective

In the United States, two schools of manipulation, osteopathy and chiropractic, sprang from the independent-minded, frontier roots of this country almost simultaneously. Osteopathy, founded in the 1880s by a country doctor named A. T. Still, holds as a primary tenant that structure and function are intimately related and that function is adversely affected by structural asymmetry. Osteopaths further believe that in health, "the artery rules supreme." This means that an adequate blood supply is essential for healthy function. Structural imbalances are thought to adversely affect blood supply. The development of A. T. Still's thought is well outlined in *The Lengthening Shadow of Dr. Andrew Taylor Still*, written by Hildreth.[8] I. M. Korr has done significant research on osteopathic tenants and his work is often quoted in manipulation literature.[9,10]

Chiropractic was founded in 1895 by Daniel David Palmer, an itinerant grocer and magnetic healer. Palmer is reputed to have cured a janitor's deafness (Harvey Lillard) when he used the spinous process of a cervical vertebra as a lever to move the vertebra. Palmer held that spinal misalignments (subluxations) were the cause of disease. He felt that misalignments created pressure on nerves within the intervertebral canal and that this pressure was the cause of disease due to either too much or not enough "nerve energy." He felt that removing the misalignments would release the body's innate healing energy and that patients with various diseases would be cured.[11]

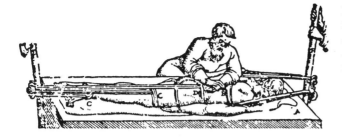

**Figure 10-1.** Hippocrates performing a spinal manipulation. (Haldeman S: *Principles and Practice of Chiropractic*, 2nd ed. Norwalk, CT: Appleton & Lange, 1992. Reproduced with permission.)

Today, few osteopaths or chiropractors accept the initial paradigms on which their professions were founded without major reservations. They are more likely to accept the more limited role of manipulation for musculoskeletal pain, and many in the chiropractic profession have argued eloquently for this position.[12,13] Several recent reviews have given manipulation tentative support for treatment of low back pain.[14–16] This is discussed later in the chapter.

Four persons within the medical community, Dr. John Mennell[17] and Dr. James Cyriax[18] (trained as orthopedists), and Stanley Paris[19] and G. D. Maitland[20] (trained as physical therapists), are prominent in the field of manipulation for musculoskeletal pain. Their work is most commonly practiced by physical therapists in the United States and by physiotherapists in commonwealth countries.

There is a great deal of overlap in the techniques practiced by osteopaths, chiropractors, and physical therapists. Physical therapists, grounded in traditional physical therapy (PT) techniques such as peripheral neuromuscular facilitation (PNF), are noted to do more soft tissue mobilization. Modern osteopaths generally tend to do more strain/counterstrain and muscle energy techniques, while those trained in the 1930s, 1940s, and 1950s do more osseous manipulation. Chiropractors are most noted for their osseous manipulation, often using mechanical devices such as drop-piece tables and spring loaded instruments to effect bone movement. These observations of the various schools are not scientific but are based on my personal interactions with practitioners from all three schools for the past 15 years.

## Active Versus Passive Therapy in the Management of Spinal Pain

Bed rest and surgery (both passive therapies) have been the mainstays of medical treatment for back pain. Surgery got its major impetus in 1934 when Mixter and Barr were able to show that a herniated disk can mechanically compress the spinal nerve root and that removal of the disk can relieve symptoms of nerve root pain.[21] By the 1970s a high incidence of failed back surgeries dampened enthusiasm for this modality. It became apparent that probably 99% of back pain patients would not benefit from surgery of any kind.[22]

Bed rest, measured in weeks, has been liberally recommended for low back pain since at least the turn of the century.[23] This approach has been called into question by the rehabilitation community because of the adverse effects of deconditioning[24] and shortening of connective tissue.[25] Klein and Sobel[26] showed in a patient survey that rehabilitation specialists were the most effective practitioners in giving patients relief from back pain. Their survey of 492 back pain sufferers who found relief included patients who had gone to all major practitioner groups: chiropractors, orthopedists, neurosurgeons, and neurologists, as well as many unorthodox practitioners such as acupuncturists and massage therapists. Doctors of rehabilitation (physiatrists) and physical therapists helped a much larger proportion of patients than the others. Perhaps the good results of physiatrists were due to the active non–bed rest therapy they tend to prescribe. More recent scientific evidence supporting active therapy for spinal pain includes a randomized controlled trial which showed that recommending 2 days of bed rest is just as good or better than 7 days for treatment of acute back pain.[27] Mayer[28] showed that patients undergoing "functional restoration," consisting of exercises, work hardening and education, did better in return-to-work status and need for subsequent surgeries than patients who underwent "usual" treatment. Finally, Saal[29] was able to show that 90% of patients with acute radiculopathy due to herniated disks had a favorable outcome with a program of lumbar stabilization. This active, non-surgical therapeutic paradigm was elegantly described by Waddell in an award-winning paper in 1987.[30]

### The Role of Manipulation in the New Patient-Active Paradigm of Spinal Pain Management

Spinal manipulation therapy has been justifiably criticized by third-party payers[31] and by the medical community[32] because it is a patient-passive therapy that requires the patient to keep coming back to get continued relief. In this context I favor manipulation not as a sole or primary modality for managing back pain, but as a supportive modality to help patients with back pain to become more active in therapy and in their daily lives, much as Saal has used epidural steroids to treat back pain.[29]

In defense of manipulative therapy, two points must be made. First, patients usually make more visits to the chiropractor for a given episode of back pain than to the medical doctor, but the final cost to society is lower because of less time off work.[15,33,34] Second, although it is not a patient-active therapy, it can be argued that manipulation does increase the patient's tissue mobility, which is the primary aim of treatment in the new patient-active paradigm for spinal pain treatment.[35]

## Spinal Manipulation Mechanisms of Action

The way spinal manipulation relieves pain remains speculative. Certainly, hands-on therapy is a powerful placebo, but there is likely also a specific biologic effect. Rahlmann[36] presented an excellent review on possible physiologic phenomena that cause back pain and prevent proper spinal motion which might be relieved by manipulation. He described four possible causes: (1) meniscoid entrapment in the facet joint; (2) displaced intervertebral disk fragments; (3) segmental or intersegmental muscle spasms; and (4) periarticular connective tissue adhesions. The last two explanations probably have the most evidence, clinically and in the laboratory, to support them.

Several investigators have shown that persistence of spinal muscle activity during terminal flexion is associated with back pain. Full forward flexion is normally accompanied by relaxation of the spinal muscles.[37-39] This is not so in the back pain patient. The persistent overactivity of spinal muscles is thought to be a contributor to pain; manipulation is held to decrease the muscle activity.

As alluded to previously, the breaking of periarticular connective tissue adhesions by manipulation certainly makes sense as a mechanism of action.[25] "Motion in joints and soft tissues is maintained by the normal movement of the parts of the body,"[25] but as described earlier, normal movement is limited in patients with spinal pain. The recognition that it is a normal reaction of connective tissue to be laid down and to shrink is the basis for manipulation to increase spinal mobility. Histological evidence of fibrosis after injury may occur in as short a time period as 4 days.[40] A short period of bed rest after spinal injury, as is often prescribed, may result in adhesions amenable to manipulative therapy.

The fact that manipulation does reduce paraspinal pain perception has been shown experimentally on normal persons without spinal pathology. Terret and associates[41] randomly assigned fifty persons to manipulation or sham manipulation after testing those persons to see how much electric current they could tolerate to the paraspinal muscles. The two groups were alike before spinal manipulation. After spinal manipulation the sham (soft tissue massage) treatment group showed no change in pain tolerance, but the manipulation group tolerated a significantly greater electric current.

Initially, many felt that manipulation may increase endorphin levels. This was supported experimentally in one study,[42] but independent investigators have not been able to confirm these findings.[43] It is possible that endorphin-release phenomenon is dose dependent. Perhaps a series of manipulations are necessary to increase plasma beta-endorphins, or perhaps only central endorphin levels are affected.

Despite some evidence supporting the theories outlined here, it is clear that experimental and laboratory evidence showing how manipulation works is inadequate at present.

## Brief Review of the Literature

A literature review was undertaken to evaluate the original research on manipulation. Only studies using randomized assignment and blinded outcome assessment were included in this review. Deyo's criteria were used to evaluate the quality of the studies (Table 10-1).[1,44] Deyo's criteria have been used previously to evaluate conservative treatment for back pain and neck pain.[45] An arbitrary scoring system giving one point for each criteria met was used (Table 10-2). (This is the quality number found in column 4 of Table 10-2.)

Twenty papers were evaluated (three on neck pain and seventeen on back pain).[34,46–64] Sixteen studies showed results favoring manipulation. The most convincing paper was the Meade Study,[34] published in the *British Medical Journal* in 1990. Meade and colleagues were able to show in a multicenter, 741-patient trial, that patients who underwent chiropractic manipulation had a better functional score on the Oswestry back pain questionnaire[65] after 2 years. They also missed less work. Meade and associates calculated that if all appropriate patients who presented to the hospital for back pain care were to be referred to chiropractors (about 72,000 of a total of 300,000 each year by Meade's estimate), then the British government would save £19.9 million in hospital costs, lost wages, and social security payments yearly. The Meade study has not been without its critics,[66] but taken in aggregate with the preponderance of other literature on manipulation, there is sufficient evidence to suggest that manipulation is sometimes helpful for acute and chronic low back pain.

## Conclusion

In 1988 it was estimated that 60,000 full-time practitioners of manipulation, primarily chiropractors,

**Table 10-1.** Criteria for Assessing the Validity and Applicability of Clinical Research on Conservative Treatments for Neck Pain

Validity

1. *Random Allocation:* The best way to achieve equal distribution of prognostic factors between active treatment and control groups and to eliminate biases that lead to false results.
2. *Minimal Patient Attrition:* Those who do very well or very poorly are most likely to drop out, biasing the remaining study sample. We require less than 15% attrition to meet this criterion.
3. *Blind Outcome Assessment:* The best way to reduce investigator bias in measuring outcomes. Though patient blinding is also desirable, a blinded observer is the minimum to meet this criterion.
4. *Equal Co-Interventions:* A wide variety of treatments for neck pain are readily available and may be obtained by subjects in the clinical trial. Some effort to describe or ensure equality of co-interventions is required.
5. *Compliance Measured:* Therapy cannot work if it is not received. Compliance with physical measures and lifestyle changes is often particularly poor. Inpatient studies are assumed to assure reasonable compliance.
6. *Minimal Contamination:* Unintended "crossovers" may occur if patients can obtain a study treatment elsewhere. A description of any contamination is judged adequate and inpatient trials are assumed to have little contamination.
7. *Both Statistical and Clinical Significance Considered:* A substantial clinical effect may fail to be statistically significant if the sample size is too small. For negative trials, some estimate of statistical power is required.

Applicability

1. *Good Demographic Description:* At least age, sex, and referral source of patients.
2. *Good Clinical Description:* Duration of pain, neurologic deficits, dermatomal pain, prior surgery, and other entry criteria are considered. A study is required to have four of these five items to judge the clinical description as adequate.
3. *Treatment Adequately Described:* Dose, duration, frequency, and reproducible description of technique are required.
4. *Reporting All Relevant Outcomes:* Four categories are considered: (1) symptoms and physiologic changes, (2) functional status, (3) cost of care, and (4) patient perceptions or psychological measures. Reporting is judged adequate if at least one measure is included from three of the four categories.

(Adapted from Deyo R: Clinical research methods in low back pain. *Spine: State of the Art Reviews* 1991;5(1):209–222.)

**Table 10-2.** Studies Evaluating Manipulation Using Randomized Allocation and Blinded Outcome Assessment

| Author | Journal | Year | Quality* | No. of Subjects/ No. Manipulated | Outcome Favorable to Manipulation |
|--------|---------|------|----------|----------------------------------|-----------------------------------|
| Glover et al.[46] | Br J of Ind Med | 1974 | 6/11 | 84/43 | Yes |
| Doran and Newell[47] | Br Med J | 1975 | 5/11 | 456/116 | Yes |
| Bergquist-Ullman[48] | Acta Orthop Scand | 1977 | 8/11 | 217/72 | Yes |
| Evans et al.[49] | Rheumatology Rehabil | 1978 | 7/11 | 32/32 (crossovers) | Yes |
| Sims-Williams et al.[50] | Br Med J | 1978 | 5/11 | 94/47 | Yes |
| Coxhead et al.[51] | Lancet | 1981 | 9/11 | 322/155 | Yes |
| Hoehler et al.[52] | JAMA | 1981 | 6/11 | 95/55 | Yes |
| Zybergold and Piper[53] | Arch Phys Med Rehabil | 1981 | 4/11 | 23/8 | No |
| Farrell and Twomey[54] | Med J Aust | 1982 | 7/11 | 48/26 | Yes |
| Sloop et al. (neck)[55] | Spine | 1982 | 8/11 | 39/21 | No |
| Howe et al. (neck)[56] | J Roy Coll Gen Pract | 1983 | 7/11 | 52/26 | Yes |
| Godfrey et al.[57] | Spine | 1984 | 6/11 | 81/22 | Yes |
| Gibson et al.[58] | Lancet | 1985 | 6/11 | 109/41 | No |
| Meade et al.[59] | J Epidemiol & Community Health | 1986 | 7/11 | 50/23 | Yes |
| Hadler et al.[60] | Spine | 1987 | 6/11 | 54/28 | Yes |
| Mathews et al.[61] | Br J Rheumatol | 1987 | 6/11 | 291/165 | No |
| Postacchini et al.[62] | Neuro-orthopedics | 1988 | 5/11 | 456/87 | Yes |
| MacDonald and Bell[63] | Spine | 1990 | 7/11 | 95/46 | Yes |
| Meade et al.[34] | Br Med J | 1990 | 7/11 | 741/357 | Yes |
| Vernon (neck) et al.[64] | J Manipulative Physiol Ther | 1990 | 7/11 | 9/5 | Yes |

*See text for explanation of quality score (out of a total of 11).

osteopathic physicians, and physical therapists, gave hundreds of millions of manipulation treatments a year for neck and back pain.[67] Low malpractice insurance rates to the chiropractor attest to the treatments' relative safety. For clinicians who want to give this service to their patients with musculoskeletal pain, there are only two options: learn to do the manipulations, or refer to a competent clinician who does. For those who decide to do manipulation themselves, the minimal initial learning time required is approximately 3 to 6 months.[17,68] This time commitment may not be practical for the busy practitioner of rehabilitative medicine. Isometric or muscle energy techniques sufficient for therapy initiation can usually be acquired in 1 to 2 weeks of formal course work.[69] The training time is short because the chances of injury to the patient using these techniques is low. For the clinician who wants to refer his patient to another practitioner for manipulation, the course is prob-

lematic. Medically trained osteopaths often do more traditional medicine than manipulation, and their skills may be rusty. Physical therapists most often limit themselves to nonosseous techniques, and chiropractors may espouse a health care model that is unacceptable to the medical practitioner. The most reasonable answer to this dilemma is to keep an open mind and ask persons in the community to whom they refer, or who they would go to personally, for musculoskeletal pain. The techniques of manipulation are described further in Chapter 9.

In the past few years there has been significantly more acceptance of the practice of manipulation for musculoskeletal pain in the medical community. The recent scientific studies reported on in the literature review are part of the reason. Another part of the reason is the publication in the *Journal of the American Medical Association* (JAMA) of the results of the Wilk trial in 1988.[70]

*Wilk et al.* alleged that the American Medical Association (AMA) had decided to eliminate chiropractic as a profession in the early 1960s. "One of the principal means used by the AMA to achieve its goal was to make it unethical for medical physicians to professionally associate with chiropractors."[70] Judge Getzendanner required the AMA to publish (in the JAMA) a permanent injunction order stating specifically that a medical practitioner can refer to and receive referrals from chiropractors when he or she "believe(s) the referral may benefit the patient."[70] The fallout of these developments was that at the 1991 meeting of the American Academy of Orthopedic Surgeons, a panel of physicians agreed that a short course of manipulation treatment is appropriate for some sufferers of back pain.[32] Scott Haldeman, MD, DC, PhD, Assistant Professor of Neurology at the University of California School of Medicine, was quoted as saying that these developments "seem to be spelling the end of the ostracism that manipulative therapy and its practitioners traditionally have received."[32] Manipulation has counted among its advocates many prominent clinicians from the past, including Hippocrates[2] and Paget,[6] and presently has begun to regain support in the scientific and medical communities as well. It is best viewed as an adjunctive treatment that allows patients to be more mobile and better able to perform their rehabilitative exercise program.

## Points of Summary

1. Manipulation is an ancient form of therapy found in many cultures.
2. Contemporary practitioners of manipulation are usually chiropractors, osteopaths, and physical therapists.
3. Patient-active therapy that increases patient mobility has scientific evidence to support it.
4. Spinal manipulation should play an adjunctive role in the management of back pain.
5. The way spinal manipulation relieves pain is not known.
6. A careful review of the scientific literature on spinal manipulation tends to support its use for musculoskeletal pain relief.
7. Spinal manipulation is gaining acceptance in the medical community partly because scientific evidence is accumulating that favors manipulation and partly because of political forces that favor manipulation.

## References

1. Deyo RA: Conservative treatment for low back pain: Distinguishing useful from useless therapy. *JAMA* 1983;250:1057–1062.
2. Withington ET: *Hippocrates* [with an English translation]. Cambridge, MA: Harvard University Press, 1928:285–301.
3. Bourdillon JF, Day EA: *Spinal Manipulation*, 4th ed. Norwalk, CT: Appleton & Lange, 1987.
4. Kay MA: Health and illness in a Mexican-American barrio. In Spicer EH (ed): *Ethnic Medicine in the Southwest*. Tucson: University of Arizona Press, 1977:96–168.
5. Moulton T: *The Compleat Bone-Setter*. Revised and enlarged by Robert Turner. London: Archives, Royal College of Surgeons, 1656.
6. Anderson R: Spinal manipulation before chiropractic. In Haldeman S (ed): *Principles and Practice of Chiropractic*, 2nd ed. Norwalk, CT: Appleton & Lange, 1992.
7. Anderson R: On doctors and bonesetters in the 16th and 17th centuries. *Chiropract Hist* 3(1):11–15, 1983.
8. Hildreth AG: *The Lengthening Shadow of Andrew Taylor Still*. Macon, MO: 1938.
9. Korr IM: *The Neurobiologic Mechanisms in Manipulation Therapy*. New York: Plenum Press, 1978.
10. Korr IM: Neural basis of osteopathic lesions. *J Am Osteopath Assoc* 1947;47:191.
11. Palmer DD: *The Chiropractor's Adjuster: The Science, Art and Philosophy of Chiropractic*. Portland, OR: Portland Printing House, 1910.
12. Homola S: Seeking a common denominator in the use of spinal manipulation. *Chiropract Technique* 1992;4:61–63.
13. Nimmo R: Receptor Tonus technique seminars given at Palmer College of Chiropractic, July 1977.
14. Shekelle PG, Adams AH, Chassin MR, et al.: The appropriateness of spinal manipulation for low back pain: Project overview and literature review, R-4025/1-CCR/FCER, Santa Monica, CA: Rand, 1991.
15. Ottenbacher K, Defabio RP: Efficacy of spinal manipulation/mobilization therapy: A meta-analysis. *Spine* 1985;10:833–837.
16. Koes BW, Assendelft WJJ, Van der Heijden GJMG, et al.: Spinal manipulation and mobilization for low back and neck pain: A blinded review. *Br Med J* 1991;303:1298–1303.
17. Mennell JM: *Back Pain*. Boston: Little Brown, 1960.
18. Cyriax J: *Textbook of Orthopedic Medicine*, Vol 2: *Diagnosis of Soft Tissue Lesions*. London, Ballière Tindall, 1982.

19. Paris SV: *The Spinal Lesion*. Christchurch, New Zealand, Pegasus Press, 1965.

20. Maitland GP: Vertebral manipulation, 2nd ed. London, Butterworth, 1968.

21. Mixter WJ, Barr JS: Rupture of the intervertebral disc with involvement of the spinal column. *New Eng J Med* 1934;211:210–215.

22. White AH: Introduction and purpose. In White AH, Rothman RH, Roy DC (eds): *Lumber Spine Surgery: Techniques and Complications*. St. Louis: CV Mosby, 1987.

23. Davenport HW: *Doctor Dock: Teaching and Learning Medicine at the Turn of the Century*. New Brunswick, NJ: Rutgers University Press, 1987.

24. Halar EM, Bell KR: Rehabilitation's relationship to inactivity. In Kottke FJ, Lehmann JF (eds): *Krusen's Handbook of Physical Medicine and Rehabilitation*, 4th ed. Philadelphia: WB Saunders, 1990:1113–1133.

25. Kottke FJ: Therapeutic exercise to maintain mobility. In Kottke FJ, Lehmann JF (eds): *Krusen's Handbook of Physical Medicine and Rehabilitation*, 4th ed. Philadelphia: 1990:452–479.

26. Sobel D, Klein AC: *Backache Relief*. New York: Random House, 1985.

27. Deyo RA, Diehl AK, Rosenthal M: How many days of bed rest for acute low back pain? A randomized clinical trial. *New Engl J Med* 1986;315:1064–1070.

28. Mayer TG, Gatchel RJ, Mayer H: A prospective 2-year study of functional restoration in industrial low back injury: An objective assessment procedure. *JAMA* 1987;258:1763–1767.

29. Saal JA, Saal JS: Non-operative treatment of herniated lumbar intervertebral disc with radiculopathy: An outcome study. *Spine* 1989;14:431–437.

30. Waddell G: A new clinical model for the treatment of low back pain. *Spine* 1987;12:632–644.

31. Simpson CA, Tilden RH: Standards of practice in third-party relationships. In Vear HF (ed): *Chiropractic Standards of Practice and Quality of Care*. Gaithersburg, MD: Aspen Publishers, 1992:257–258.

32. Newman A: Panel supports brief manipulative therapy for low back pain. *Intern Med News* 1991;24(9):3.

33. Jarvis KB, Phillips RB, Morris EK: Cost per case comparison of back injury claims of chiropractic versus medical management for conditions with identical diagnostic codes. *J Occup Med* 1991;33:847–852.

34. Meade TW, Dyer S, Browne W, et al.: Low back pain of mechanical origin: Randomized comparison of chiropractic and hospital outpatient treatment. *Br Med J* 1990;300:1431–1437.

35. Vernon AP: Chiropractic: A model on incorporating the illness behavior model in the management of low back pain patients. *J Manipulative Physiol Ther* 1991;14:379–389.

36. Rahlmann J: Mechanisms of intervertebral joint fixation. *J Manipulative Physiol Ther* 1987;10:177–187.

37. Hoyt W, Hunt H, DePauw M, et al. Electromyographic assessment of chronic low back pain syndrome. *J Am Osteopath Assoc* 1981;80:728–730.

38. Schultz A, Haderspeck-Grib K, Sinkora G, Warwick D: Quantitative studies of the flexion-relaxation phenomena in back muscles. *J Orthop Res* 1985;3:189–197.

39. Triano J, Shultz A: Correlation of objective measure of trunk motion and muscle function with low-back disability ratings. *Spine* 1987;12:561–565.

40. Jackson DS, Flickinger DB, Dumphy JE: Biochemical studies of connective tissue repair. *Ann NY Acad Sci* 1960;86:943–947.

41. Terret AC, Vernon H: Manipulation and pain tolerance. *Am J Phys Med* 1984;63:217–225.

42. Vernon HT, Dhami MSI, Howley TP, Annett R: Spinal manipulation and endorphin: A controlled study of the effect of spinal manipulation on plasma beta-endorphin levels in normal muscles. *J Manipulative Physiol Ther* 1986;9:115–123.

43. Christian GF, Stan GJ, Sissons D et al: Immunoreactive ACTH, B-endorphin and cortisol levels in plasma following spinal manipulative therapy. *Spine* 1988;13:1411–1417.

44. Deyo RA: Clinical research methods in low back pain. *Spine: State of the Art Reviews* 1991;5(1):209–222.

45. Florian, T: Conservative treatment for neck pain: Distinguishing useful from useless therapy. *J Back Musculoskel Rehabil* 1991;1:55–66.

46. Glover JL, Morris JG, Khosala T: Back pain: A randomized clinical trial of rotational manipulation of the trunk. *Br J Ind Med* 1974;31:59–64.

47. Doran DL, Newell JJ: Manipulation in the treatment of back pain: A multicentre study. *Br Med J* 1975;2:161–164.

48. Bergquist-Ullman M: Acute low back pain in industry. *Acta Orthop Scand Suppl* 1977;170:1–117.

49. Evans DP, Burke MS, Lloyd KN, et al.: Lumbar spinal manipulation on trial. Part 1. Clinical assessment. *Rheumatol Rehabil* 1978;17:46–53.

50. Sims-Williams H, Jayson M, Young S, et al.: Controlled trial of mobilization and manipulation for patients with low back pain in general practice. *Br Med J* 1978;2:1338–1340.

51. Coxhead CE, Inskip T, Meade W, et al.: Multicenter trial of physiotherapy in the management of sciatic symptoms. *Lancet* 1981;1:1065–1068.

52. Hoehler FK, Tobis JS, Buerger AA: Spinal manipulation for low back pain. *JAMA* 1981;245:1835–1838.

53. Zybergold RS, Piper MC: Lumbar disc disease: Comparative analysis of physical therapy treatments. *Arch Phys Med Rehabil* 1981;62:176–179.

54. Farrell JP, Twomey LT: Acute low back pain: Comparison of two conservative treatment approaches. *Med J Aust* 1982;1:160–164.

55. Sloop PR, Smith OS, Goldenberg E, et al.: Manipulation for chronic neck pain: A double blind controlled study. *Spine* 1982;7:532–535.

56. Howe DH, Newcombe RG, Wode MT: Manipulation of the cervical spine: A pilot study. *J Roy Coll Gen Pract* 1983;33:574–579.

57. Godfrey CM, Morgan PP, Schatzker J: A randomized trial of manipulation for low back pain in a medical setting. *Spine* 1984;9:301–304.

58. Gibson T, Grahame R, Harkness J, et al.: Controlled comparison of short wave diathermy with osteopathic treatment in non-specific low back pain. *Lancet* 1985;2:1258–1261.

59. Meade TW, Browne W, Mellows S, et al.: Comparison of chiropractic and hospital outpatient management of low back pain: A feasibility study. *J Epidemiol Community Health* 1986;40:12–17.

60. Hadler NM, Curtis P, Gillings DB, Stinnett S: A benefit of spinal manipulation as adjunctive therapy for acute low back pain: A stratified controlled trial. *Spine* 1987;12:703–706.

61. Mathews JA, Mills SB, Jenkins VM, et al.: Back pain and sciatica: Controlled trials of manipulation, traction, sclerosant, and epidural injections. *Br J Rheumatol* 1987;26:416–423.

62. Postacchini F, Faccini M, Palieri P: Efficacy of various forms of conservative treatment in low back pain: A comparative study. *Neuro-orthopedics* 1988;6:28–35.

63. MacDonald RS, Bell CJ: An open controlled assessment of osteopathic manipulation in nonspecific low back pain. *Spine* 1990;15:364–370.

64. Vernon HT, Aker P, Burns S: Pressure pain threshold evaluation of the effect of spinal manipulation in the treatment of chronic neck pain: A pilot study. *J Manipulative Physiol Ther* 1990;13:13–16.

65. Fairbank J, Davis J, Cougar J, O'Brien JP: The Oswestry low back pain disability questionnaire. *Physio Therapy* 1980;66:271–273.

66. Assendelft WJ, Boulter LM, Kessels AG: Effectiveness of chiropractic and physiotherapy in the treatment of low back pain: A critical discussion of the British randomized clinical trial. *J Manipulative Physiol Ther* 1991;14:281–286.

67. Henderson DJ: Vertebral basilar vascular accidents associated with cervical manipulation. In Vernon H (ed): *Upper Cervical Syndrome: Chiropractic Diagnosis and Treatment*. Baltimore: Williams & Wilkins, 1988:194–206.

68. Lewitt K: *Manipulation Therapy in the Rehabilitation of the Motor System*. London: Butterworths, 1985.

69. Geiringer SR, Kincaid CB, Rechtien JJ: Traction manipulation and massage. In DeLisa J (ed): *Rehabilitation Medicine: Principles and Practice*. Philadelphia, JB Lippincott, 1988:281.

70. Getzendanner S: Permanent injunction order against AMA. *JAMA* 1987;259:81-82.

## Suggested Readings

Bourdillon JF, Day EA: *Spinal Manipulation*, 4th ed. Norwalk, CT: Appleton & Lange, 1992.

Haldeman S (ed): *The Principles and Practice of Chiropractic*, 2nd ed. Norwalk, CT: Appleton & Lange, 1992.

# Chapter 11

# The Musculoskeletal Examination

RALPH BUSCHBACHER

The complete musculoskeletal examination must be studied in relation to the body part in question, and such a detailed account is beyond the scope of this chapter. There are, however, a number of general principles that should be adhered to in the examination process. The total process can be divided into three overlapping stages: history, physical examination, and ancillary testing. This chapter deals with each of these stages, as well as presents select items within those stages.

## History

A detailed history often suggests the most likely diagnosis and in some conditions is more valuable than any other part of the examination. It should include the obvious questions of what the major and secondary complaints are, how they started, what aggravates or alleviates them, and how much they bother the patient in daily activities.

In addition, the patient should always be asked whether or not the same or similar symptoms have been present at some time in the past. It is surprising how few patients volunteer this information on their own, even if the identical condition occurred in the past.

Patients should be asked about the onset of their problem. Was it due to trauma? Did it start all of a sudden or creep up on them gradually? Have they received any treatment to date (both medical and home remedy)? When possible, open-ended questions such as "Tell me when your pain began" are preferred over yes/no inquiries. Also, the questions should be asked in a way that a nonmedical person can understand. If too many jargon-filled yes or no questions are rattled off by the examiner, the patient may simply be answering without really understanding the questions.

Past medical or surgical illness, current and past medications, drug use and abuse, and family history are important areas that should be addressed. The patient's age should be noted as it may make some problems more likely than others. Occupation should be explored. Many work-related hazards predispose workers to one musculoskeletal disorder or another. The same holds true for sports activity or hobbies.

Patients commonly complain of "pain or numbness" without adequately defining these terms. One person's weakness may be another's joint instability. The examiner must understand exactly what is meant by the patient.

Sleeping patterns are an often overlooked aspect of a patient's history. Sleep disorders may cause or be caused by musculoskeletal pain conditions. Often treating the sleep pattern will help to restore the patient to health. Similarly, changes in mood and social habits may be associated with pain disorders and should be investigated.

A final point about the history is that it should relate to the patient's functional level. An elderly sedentary man may be found to have a rotator cuff tear, but if it is not causing him any pain or dysfunction, it really cannot be called a problem. Finding out what the dysfunction is will lead the examiner to the musculoskeletal abnormalities underlying the dysfunction. Once identified and treated, it will lead to a more satisfactory outcome than if every nonsignificant physical finding is addressed while ignoring the patient's overall function. Of course, it must also be recognized that different body parts interact. A painless rotator cuff weakness, for instance, may lead to painful tennis elbow. Until the weakness is corrected the elbow pain will not improve.

## Physical Examination

### Inspection

Inspection of the patient is done throughout the examination, from the time of arrival at the office until departure. It yields information about function, mood, and the reaction to the examination. Specific areas that should be assessed are signs of muscle atrophy, skin changes, posture, and scars. Most textbooks recommend observing the patient undressing to get an idea of dressing/undressing function; however, in practice this is rarely done. It is, however, a very good practice to observe the patient performing some common activities such as standing up and walking.

### Palpation

Palpation techniques vary according to the body part being examined. In general, both the soft tissues and the bones should be assessed. Joints are checked for effusion (excess fluid), muscles are checked for hematoma or disruption, and tendons and ligaments are palpated to detect signs of partial or complete rupture. Palpating the origins and insertions of muscles and ligaments often helps make diagnoses of sprains and overuse.

### Strength Testing

Muscle strength testing is commonly graded on a scale of 1 to 5 (Table 11-1). While this system is useful in some conditions, and it does help to standardize strength testing, it does have the drawback of not being very functional. Patients often have a poor understanding of what is being asked of them in isolating the various muscles. Additionally, some muscle groups, such as those in the back, are hard to isolate from each other. When possible, strength should be compared in the comparable muscles from side to side. Some allowance for slight differences needs to be made because the dominant side is usually stronger. Allowances also need to be made for the general size and physique of the patient and the examiner.

Substitution movements are used by patients with specific muscle weakness. For instance, a patient with weakness in initiating shoulder abduction may be able to hold the arm up once it is raised. He or she may substitute for a weak supraspinatus by swinging the arm up with the trunk or bending to the side. Such substitutions may hide a more profound weakness and should be eliminated in the examination.

Muscles are reproducibly innervated in most people by the same spinal cord levels (within one or two levels). The nerve fibers travel through a characteristic pattern of peripheral nerves to reach their appointed muscles (see Chapter 2). Therefore, when several muscles are weak, the site of pathology may sometimes be traced to a specific

**Table 11-1.** Muscle Strength Grading*

|  | Grade (Number) | Grade (Name) |
|---|---|---|
| No motion | 0 | Zero |
| Palpable muscle twitch with no joint motion | 1 | Trace |
| Joint movement normal with gravity eliminated | 2 | Poor |
| Joint movement normal against gravity with no other resistance | 3 | Fair |
| Joint movement against gravity with some resistance | 4 | Good |
| Normal strength | 5 | Normal |

*In addition each individual grade is sometimes split into three subgrades; for instance 4 −, 4, and 4+.

spinal cord or peripheral nerve level. Some of the main muscle groups along with their innervation are listed in Table 11-2. A patient who has weakness of foot dorsiflexion as well as hip abduction is likely to have lumbar level 5 (L5) spinal nerve injury, since these actions share the L5 spinal cord level but not the same peripheral nerve innervation. A patient with isolated weakness of foot dorsiflexion is more likely to have peripheral nerve damage, possibly of the deep peroneal nerve. The muscle distribution that belongs to a spinal nerve is called a myotome. Care must be taken not to overreact to muscular weakness by forcing it into a myotomal or peripheral nerve pattern. Such problems are actually relatively rare, and should only be diagnosed by an experienced clinician.

**Table 11-2.** Myotomal* and Peripheral Nerve Innervation of the Major Muscle Groups

| | Major Cranial or Spinal Nerve Level | Peripheral Nerve |
|---|---|---|
| **Upper Extremity** | | |
| Shoulder Muscles | | |
|    Elevators | CN XI, $C_4$, $C_5$ | Spinal accessory nerve; posterior branches of spinal nerves |
|    Protractors | $C_5$, $C_6$, $C_7$ | Long thoracic nerve; pectoral nerves |
|    Retractors | $C_5$, $C_6$, $C_7$, $C_8$ | Dorsal scapular nerve; spinal accessory nerve; thoracodorsal nerve |
|    Upward rotators | CN XI, $C_5$, $C_6$ | Long thoracic nerve; spinal accessory nerve |
|    Downward rotators | $C_6$, $C_7$, $C_8$ | Thoracodorsal nerve; pectoral nerves |
|    Abductors | $C_5$, $C_6$ | Axillary and suprascapular nerves |
|    Extensors | $C_6$, $C_7$, $C_8$ | Thoracodorsal, axillary, and pectoral nerves |
|    Flexors | $C_5$, $C_6$ | Axillary, musculocutaneous, and pectoral nerves |
|    Internal rotators | $C_5$, $C_6$ | Pectoral nerves; thoracodorsal and subscapular nerves |
|    External rotators | $C_5$, $C_6$ | Axillary and suprascapular nerves |
| Elbow flexors | $C_5$, $C_6$ | Musculocutaneous nerve |
| Elbow extensors | $C_7$ | Radial nerve |
| Wrist extensors | $C_6$, $C_7$ | Radial nerve |
| Wrist flexors | $C_7$, $C_8$ | Median and ulnar nerves |
| Finger extensors | $C_7$ | Radial nerve |
| Finger flexors | $C_7$, $C_8$ | Median and ulnar nerves |
| Intrinsic hand muscles | $T_1$ | Ulnar and median (thumb) nerves |
| **Trunk and Back** | | |
| Abdominal muscles | $T_7$–$T_{12}$ | Segmental innervation |
| Back muscles | $C_2$–$L_5$ | Segmental innervation |
| **Lower Extremity** | | |
| Hip flexors | $T_{12}$, $L_1$, $L_2$ | Lumbosacral plexus |
| Hip extensors | $L_5$, $S_1$, $S_2$ | Inferior gluteal nerve |
| Hip abductors | $L_4$, $L_5$, $S_1$ | Superior gluteal nerve |
| Hip adductors | $L_2$–$L_4$ | Obturator nerve |
| Knee flexors | $L_5$, $S_1$ | Sciatic nerve |
| Knee extensors | $L_2$–$L_4$ | Femoral nerve |
| Foot dorsiflexors | $L_4$, $L_5$ | Deep peroneal nerve |
| Foot plantarflexors | $S_1$ | Tibial nerve |
| Foot inverters | $L_4$ | Deep peroneal and tibial nerve |
| Foot everters | $L_5$, $S_1$ | Superficial peroneal nerve |

*C, Cervical level; T, thoracic level; L, lumbar level; S, sacral level; CN, cranial nerve.

### Neurologic Examination

Since neurologic conditions often lead to musculoskeletal symptoms, a good neurologic examination is usually necessary. It should include testing of light touch and pinprick sensation, temperature sensation, proprioception, balance and coordination, and deep tendon (muscle stretch) reflexes (DTRs).

DTRs are graded from 1 to 4 as shown in Table 11-3. They are caused by a stretching of the muscle spindle (see Chapter 2), usually elicited by a tapping with a reflex hammer. This sends an impulse to the spinal cord where it immediately stimulates the motor neuron to send a message for the muscle to contract.

Pain is sometimes felt at sites distant to the site of disorder. For instance, irritation of a spinal nerve by a herniated disk may cause pain down the leg and into the foot. When this follows a dermatomal pattern it is called *radicular pain*.

Other types of distantly felt pain are "referred" and "radiating" pain. *Referred pain* occurs because nerve cells that are close together in the spinal cord may correspond to widely separate parts of the body. When pain signals come in from one part it often "spills over" to the nerves related to the other part, and so the person perceives pain to be coming from a wholly unrelated area. For instance, gallbladder pain may be referred to the shoulder and heart pain may be referred to the left arm. This type of pain is usually due to internal organ problems.

*Radiating pain* occurs when a proximal musculoskeletal disorder causes pain to spread down the limb. For instance, palpation of tender spots in the neck muscles may cause pain to be felt down the arm into the fingertips. This type of pain is often confused with radicular or neurogenic pain.

Sensory testing is similar to muscle strength testing in that patches of skin are innervated both by a distinct pattern of spinal nerves and by distinct peripheral nerves. The spinal nerve innervation pattern is called a dermatome and is depicted in Figure 11-1. The sensory nerve distributions and dermatomes, however, are not really as clear-cut as depicted in this diagram. There is overlap among the nerves, which makes localization of any problem difficult.

### Joint Examination

Joints should be examined for swelling, erythema, excessive warmth, and for range of motion. The range of motion should be compared from left to right body sides and also with active and passive movement. It is often measured with devices called goniometers (Figure 11-2) (or in the back with an inclinometer). If a patient has restriction of active but not passive movement it is likely due to muscle weakness. If both are restricted then there

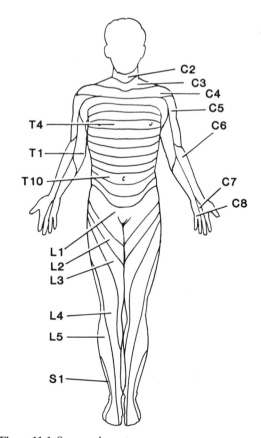

**Figure 11-1.** Sensory dermatomes.

**Table 11-3.** Deep Tendon Reflex Grades

| | |
|---|---|
| 0 | No response |
| 1+ | Low normal |
| 2+ | Average normal |
| 3+ | Brisker than normal, but not necessarily pathologic |
| 4+ | Hyperactive, usually with clonus |

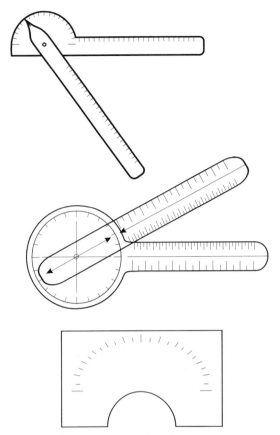

**Figure 11-2.** Common types of goniometers.

may be joint contracture or a bony block. The end-point of range should always be assessed when testing range of motion. A hard, rigid endpoint may be indicative of a bony block. Firm endpoints are normal, while pain on a firm endpoint may be indicative of a ligamentous sprain. Softer than usual endpoints are signs of partial ligamentous rupture, and lack of an endpoint is a sign of a complete ligamentous tear.

*Gait*

Since gait abnormalities can be manifestations of a large variety of disorders, the normal gait cycle must be understood. The normal gait pattern is presented in Figure 11-3. As depicted, a full cycle, or stride, goes from heel strike of one foot to the next heel strike of that same foot. Step length is the distance from heel strike of one foot to heel strike of the opposite side. Ordinarily 60% of the gait

cycle is in stance phase while 40% is in swing phase. About 25% of the time both feet are in contact with the ground. The purpose of normal gait is to propel the body's center of mass along a smooth sinusoidal wave to minimize energy consumption. Any deviations from this pattern increases the energy requirements of ambulation.

There are six *determinants of gait* that help to propel the body along the path of least energy consumption.[1] They are listed in Table 11-4. Gait must be analyzed by observing the patient from the sides, front, and from the rear. From the side the stride length, knee and ankle motions, and foot clearance can be assessed. Common abnormalities seen here are a footdrop or backbending (hyperextension) of the knee, called genu recurvatum. The tilt of the pelvis and the ankle are best viewed from the rear. Weakness of the hip abductors causes the pelvis to drop during stance in what is called an uncompensated Trendelenburg gait. In more severe weakness of the abductors, the patient lists to the side of weakness during stance to compensate for excessive pelvic drop in what is called the compensated Trendelenburg gait (Figure 11-4). The ankle is assessed for excessive varus or valgus position and the foot is checked for excess pronation. The centers of the heels should normally hit the ground within a side to side distance of 5 to 10 cm (2 to 4 inches).

Gait should be assessed both with shoes on and off. In addition, the shoes should be examined for abnormal wear patterns. Table 11-5 lists the major muscle groups in the leg along with what points of the gait cycle they are normally active in and what happens if they are weak.

**Table 11-4.** The Six Determinants of Gait

|  |  | **Effect on Gait** |
|---|---|---|
| 1. | Pelvic rotation | Raises low point in gait |
| 2. | Pelvic tilt in stance | Lowers high point in gait |
| 3. | Knee flexion in stance | Lowers high point in gait |
| 4&5. | Knee and ankle motion | Smoothes gait cycle |
| 6. | Lateral displacement of hips | Decreases side to side displacement |

*Source:* Lehmann JF, deLatour BJ: Gait analysis: Diagnosis and management. In Kottke FJ, Lehmann JF (eds): *Krusen's Handbook of Physical Medicine and Rehabilitation*, 4th ed. Philadelphia, WB Saunders, 1990.

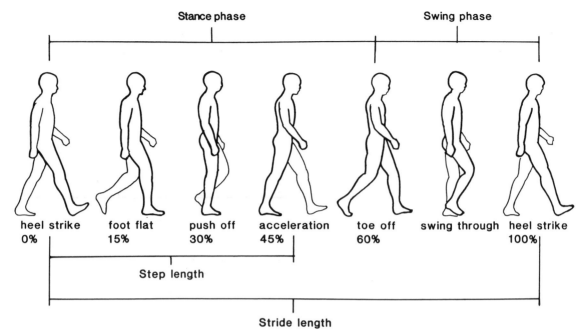

**Figure 11-3.** The normal gait cycle: Stride length is defined as the distance from one heel strike to the next heel strike on the same foot (the right heel is depicted in this figure). Step length is from heel strike of one foot to heel strike of the other. Ordinarily the gait cycle is viewed from the perspective of one foot or the other. The cycle consists of 60% stance phase and 40% swing phase. The stance phase is divided into stages by increments of 15% of the total stride as depicted in the figure.

## Ancillary Testing: Radiographic Tests, Laboratory Studies, and Other Diagnostic Procedures

When the history and physical examination are complete but the diagnosis is still in question, it is often time to turn to laboratory and other studies to help make the diagnosis. This is an integral part of the examination process but should not take the place of the hands-on examination.

## Points of Summary

1. Sleeping patterns are an often overlooked but important part of the history.
2. History taking should concentrate on function.
3. Strength testing is most reliable when comparing the two sides of the body for differences.
4. Radicular pain is due to nerve root irritation and follows a dermatomal pattern.

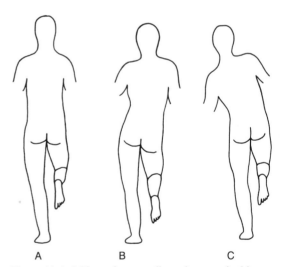

**Figure 11-4.** *A,* Normal stance allows the opposite hip to drop slightly. This drop is controlled by the hip abductors on the stance side, which keeps the pelvis from dropping too much. *B,* An uncompensated Trendelenburg gait results when the hip abductors are weak and allow the opposite pelvis to drop. *C,* When the hip abductors are even weaker, the person resorts to a compensated Trendelenburg gait. Weight is shifted to the side of the weak abductors to keep the pelvis from dropping excessively.

**Table 11-5.** Major Muscle Groups Involved in Ambulation, the Time of the Gait Cycle They Are Active in, and the Gait Abnormalities That Occur When They Are Weak

| Muscle Groups | Active During | Weakness Results in |
|---|---|---|
| Hip flexors | Acceleration | Abnormal acceleration and swing (patient compensates by thrusting trunk backward to passively swing the leg) |
| Hip extensors | Heel strike | Forward lurch of trunk on heel strike (patient compensates by excessive lordosis) |
| Hip abductors | Stance phase | Trendelenburg gait (see Figure 11-4) |
| Hip adductors | Heel strike, toe-off | Abnormal rotation of leg and pelvis |
| Knee extensors | Heel strike, acceleration | Knee buckling, especially when walking downhill |
| Knee flexors | Deceleration, heel strike | Knee snaps out too hard at end of swing; knee buckling at heel strike |
| Foot dorsiflexors | Swing phase, heel strike | Footdrop; steppage gait; foot slap at heel strike |
| Foot plantar flexors | Push-off | Short step on unaffected side; poor push-off |

5. Referred pain is due to "spill over," when pain from a body organ is transmitted to the spinal cord to the vicinity of other sensory fibers. The body misinterprets the pain signals as coming from another area, such as arm pain during a heart attack.

6. Radiating pain occurs when stimulation of an area causes pain to be felt distally.

# References

1. Lehmann JF, deLateur BJ: Gait analysis: Diagnosis and management. In Kottke FJ, Lehmann JF (eds): *Krusen's Handbook of Physical Medicine and Rehabilitation*, 4th ed. Philadelphia: WB Saunders, 1990:108–125.

# Suggested Readings

*Aids to the Examination of the Peripheral Nervous System*, London, Baillière Tindall, 1986.

Hoppenfeld S: *Physical Examination of the Spine and Extremities*. Norwalk, CT: Appleton-Century-Crofts, 1976.

Hoppenfeld S: *Orthopedic Neurology: A Diagnostic Guide to Neurologic Levels*. Philadelphia: JB Lippincott, 1977.

# PART TWO

## Management of Specific Anatomic Regions

# Chapter 12
# Head and Neck

RALPH BUSCHBACHER

The neck, perhaps more than any other body structure, reflects who we are and how we feel. When we are happy we hold our heads high. When sad, we allow our necks to droop. Neck posture is affected by occupation and by habit. When the posture is poor it can set off a series of events leading to pain, continued poor posture, degeneration, and continued pain.

This chapter covers the most common neck disorders that are encountered in a musculoskeletal practice, and its main focus is on the basic principles needed to assess and treat the neck. For completeness, some of the less common problems are also mentioned.

## Anatomy

### Bones, Joints and Ligaments

There are seven cervical vertebrae: C1–C7 (Figure 12-1). The upper two differ from the rest in form and function. They are called the atlas (C1) and axis (C2) (Figure 12-2). The atlas holds the head on two concave surfaces. The occipital condyles of the base of the skull rest on these somewhat shallow planes and are held in place to a large extent by ligamentous support.

The atlas and axis articulate through a pivot joint, with the dens of the axis, a fingerlike upward projection, providing a point around which the atlas can turn. The atlas and axis are both bony rings.

The atlas has no vertebral body like the rest of the vertebrae, and the space the body would usually occupy is taken up by the dens. The dens is kept from slipping out of place by the transverse ligament.

The axis attaches to the C3 vertebra by way of an intervertebral disk and two posterior facet joints (Figure 12-3). There are disks between all the cervical vertebrae including and below this level, but none between the occiput and atlas or the atlas and axis. The C3–C7 vertebrae are all basically similar. They consist of a body to which is attached a ring consisting of two laminae and two pedicles. At the laminopedicular junction bony processes articulate with the corresponding processes above and below them to form the facet joints (zygapophyseal joints). The facet joints are synovial plane joints lined with hyaline cartilage and surrounded by a synovial membrane and capsule. They face posteriorly at about a 45-degree angle and allow a relatively large amount of motion in all directions. The rings of the vertebrae are stacked on top of each other to form the spinal canal, through which passes the spinal cord and its associated structures. The bodies of the cervical vertebrae have an upper and lower vertebral endplate lined by hyaline cartilage. They are curved to allow them to glide upon one another.

There are lateral and posterior projections of the rings of the vertebrae called the transverse and spinous processes, respectively. These are sites of muscular and ligamentous attachments. The spinous process of C7 (or sometimes T1) is particularly

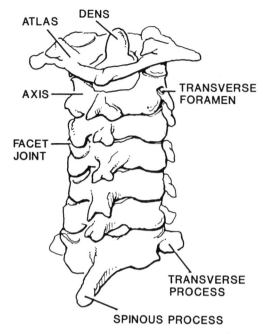

**Figure 12-1.** The cervical vertebrae viewed from a posterolateral angle.

prominent on physical examination and is used as a bony landmark, the "vertebra prominens."

The disks between the vertebral bodies are composed of an inner nucleus pulposus and an outer annulus fibrosus. The nucleus is made up of a gelatinous connective tissue with a high water content. It is connected to the vertebrae on its top and bottom at the vertebral end-plates, which are lined with cartilage. The nucleus has no direct innervation or blood supply. It receives its nutrition through a regular loading and unloading of weight (or force), which pushes water in and pulls it out of the disk by hydraulic pressure. This seems like a somewhat tenuous way to receive nutrition, but it works fairly well most of the time. During a day of standing the disk gradually loses water, which leads to a shortening in body height of about ¾ inch per day. The fluid returns and restores height during sleep.

The annulus fibrosus is composed of collagenous fibers that encircle the nucleus in an angular manner. The structure somewhat resembles a radial tire.

There are several ligaments which help hold the vertebral column together (Figure 12-4). The anterior longitudinal ligament runs along the anterior surfaces of the vertebral bodies and disks. The posterior longitudinal ligament runs along the posterior vertebral bodies and disks. In the neck this posterior ligament is broader than in the low back; thus it helps protect the vertebral canal to a greater extent. The ligamentum flavum (yellow ligament), which starts at C2, has a high elastin content. It runs along the posterior part of the spinal canal. Its elasticity allows it to stretch to accommodate neck flexion and to retract without buckling during extension.

On the posterolateral vertebral bodies there are rims of bone, the uncinate processes, which project upward and downward.[1] They interact with the corresponding projections above and below them in a pseudarthrosis (false joint), not a true joint, known as the uncovertebral joint of von Luschka. This pseudarthrosis, which is not present at birth, protects the vertebral canal.

Behind the joints of von Luschka and in front of the facet joints is a hole, the intervertebral foramen, through which passes the spinal nerve. Both afferent and efferent nerve fibers pass through this tunnel.

### Muscles

The muscles of the neck are numerous and complex, and a complete discussion of them is not

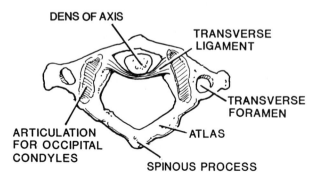

**Figure 12-2.** The atlas and axis viewed from above.

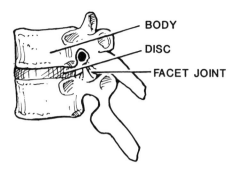

**Figure 12-3.** The functional spinal unit includes two vertebrae and the disk between them, viewed from the side.

important to the focus of this chapter. They are depicted in Figure 12-5.

### Nerves

The spinal cord passes through the vertebral canal giving off segmental spinal nerves. There are eight cervical spinal nerves. The first exits above the atlas. The last exits below C7. They pass out of the vertebral canal through the intervertebral foramina. After exiting the foramina, they give off small recurrent branches called the sinuvertebral nerves (of von Luschka) which innervate some of the structures within the spinal canal.[2] The upper cervical nerves also give rise to the sensory nerves of the scalp, including the greater occipital nerve which passes from the neck into the scalp a few centimeters lateral to the midline of the base of the skull.

### Pain-Sensitive Structures

When discussing the spine it is probably easier to focus on the structures that do not cause pain rather than those that do. The intervertebral disk is commonly felt not to contain pain-sensitive nerve fibers, although there may be pain receptors in the very outer layers of the annulus fibrosus. Also, with tears of the annulus fibrosus there may be an ingrowth of nerves into the disk. This may be a cause of pain in disk degeneration.

Another structure which does not have pain innervation is the interior of the vertebral body. The exterior, or periosteum, does contain pain innervation; thus vertebral fractures cause pain.

Lastly, the ligamentum flavum and the interspinous ligaments are not felt to be pain sensitive.[3] All other structures, including the anterior and posterior longitudinal ligaments, the facet joints, muscles, dura, and spinal nerves can be the source of neck pain. In addition, pain can be referred to the neck from distant sites.

### Head and Neck Motion

Motion of the head and neck consists of flexion, extension, lateral bending, and rotation. Aside from a few segmental exceptions, the motion at each functional unit (two vertebrae and the disk between them) is small. Overall, however, the motion of the head and neck is quite remarkable.

About 50% of total flexion/extension occurs at the atlanto-occipital joint with the base of the skull essentially rocking on the atlas. The rest of the flexion/extension motion is spread throughout the rest of the vertebrae, being concentrated preferentially at the C4–C6 level. Because of the slight concave/convex interface of the vertebral bodies, flexion involves not just a "bending" of the spine, but also a slight gliding of the upper vertebrae forward on the ones below. Extension involves a reversal of this glide. The facet joints, which face posteriorly at about a 45-degree angle, allow both

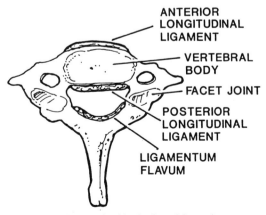

**Figure 12-4.** The vertebral body viewed from above to depict the longitudinal ligaments of the spine.

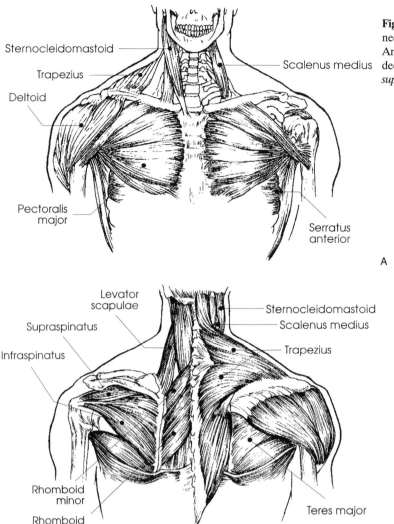

**Figure 12-5.** The muscles of the neck and shoulder girdle. *A,* Anterior view (*left:* superficial; *right:* deep). B *Posterior view (*right: *superficial;* left: *deep).*

Sternocleidomastoid

Trapezius

Deltoid

Pectoralis major

Scalenus medius

Serratus anterior

A

Levator scapulae

Supraspinatus

Infraspinatus

Sternocleidomastoid

Scalenus medius

Trapezius

Rhomboid minor

Rhomboid major

Teres major

B

flexion and extension to occur. Ordinarily, flexion is limited by the chin hitting the sternum. Extension is limited by the stretch of the anterior longitudinal ligament. During flexion the anterior disk is compressed, while the posterior edge widens. Extension reverses this deformation. Thus flexion opens up the intervertebral foramina, while extension causes their narrowing. Extreme flexion stretches the spinal nerve roots.

Pure rotation is possible only at the atlantoaxial joint, which contributes about 50% of total rotation. The remainder of the rotatory movement is intertwined with lateral bending. It is nearly impossible to laterally bend without also rotating the spine, or to rotate the spine without bending.

When rotating or bending, the disks deform and the intervertebral foramina narrows on the side being turned or bent toward. The foramina on the opposite side widen.

## Rehabilitative Approach

When approaching the treatment of disorders of the neck it is helpful to follow a few general guiding principles. This section deals with some of these principles as well as the specific therapeutic modalities and other interventions which can be used in treatment.

### Early Rest

In acute soft tissue injury, such as a flexion-extension sprain (whiplash), a period of relative rest is often prescribed. This can help reduce pain, anxiety, and painful muscle splinting.

Obviously patients with fractures, subluxations, or spinal cord injury must be treated by the appropriate specialist. In individuals with a stable spine, soft tissue injury treatment should be conservative. Following such injury the muscles contract to splint the neck. Prolonged neck muscle contraction leads to further pain and fatigue of the neck muscles. A soft collar can provide a comfortable place to rest the head so that the muscles can relax. It does very little by way of immobilization, although it does moderately reduce flexion range of motion. More importantly it provides tactile and proprioceptive feedback to the patient to refrain from moving to the extremes of mobility. It should hold the neck in a position of slight flexion to open up the posterior neck structures. It may be taken off at night for comfort, and a cervical pillow may be used instead (or nothing at all). A collar should be worn for a maximum of 1 to 2 weeks; longer periods of time lead to disuse atrophy. The collar is gradually removed, as tolerated, for ordinary activity and is finally used only for exacerbating activity such as driving. It should never be used as a substitute for other treatment.

### Early Mobilization for Proper Motion

Before expounding on the virtues of early mobilization, I must warn against too early and too vigorous mobilization. After soft tissue injury there must be adequate time to allow healing to take place. If there was a flexion-extension injury then early work on flexion and extension range of motion is contraindicated. Instead, rotation and lateral bending can be done, with more flexion and extension added, as tolerated, within a few weeks. In more chronic or overuse conditions range of motion exercises in all planes is indicated, with a goal of restoring proper mobility. In general the extremes of flexion and extension are avoided. A moderate degree of flexion opens up the posterior spine and may improve symptoms related to this area. More extreme flexion stretches the nerves and may worsen symptoms. Extreme extension, of course, compresses the posterior spine elements.

When one segment of the spine is injured or becomes dysfunctional it is splinted by muscular action. In acute injury this may be helpful, but later on it can be a problem. The patient may be performing a home stretching program and regaining flexibility but not improving as far as pain goes. What may be occurring is that the already hypermobile or normal segments are being stretched, while the tight segments remain tight. It is nearly impossible for persons to mobilize individual segments of their own necks properly. Thus it is cost-effective, in such cases, to get help from a physical spine therapist early on. Such a therapist must be well versed in evaluating and treating individual spine segments. After restoring proper mobility to the proper spinal segments the patient must be instructed in proper neck mechanics and posture. If such intervention is not made, the problem is likely to become chronic or recurrent. Ultimately the patient is taught a maintenance stretching and range of motion program as well as isometric exercises to restore and maintain strength.

### Maintaining (or Attaining) Conditioning

Neck pain, as does low back pain, affects the entire mood and outlook of the person. Maintaining, regaining, or attaining general conditioning is an important part of treating any pain condition. Obviously this is not important in the first days after injury, but in overuse conditions, myofascial pain, or chronic pain states it becomes an important part of treatment. As tolerated, the patient should recondition the neck. This is done with isometric exercise, often with the help of a physical therapist. A technique known as rhythmic stabilization is performed by the patient resisting various forces applied by the therapist. The contractions are isometric and alternate. This strengthens the muscles needed for posture, aids in blood flow to the area, and loosens the connective tissues.

### Therapeutic Interventions

In acute injury, modalities are selected to reduce pain, inflammation, and secondary muscle splinting. In subacute and chronic conditions, pain control is still a goal but is more likely achieved by restoring proper mobility and strength and by modifying behavior. What follows is a short list of interventions that may be useful in treating neck pain.

**Heat and Cold.** As a rule, either heat or cold can be used for soft tissue pain depending on patient preference. In the acute stage of an injury cold application may be preferable, but later on either can be used. In conditions of myofascial pain a useful technique to use is ice massage. This is performed by a helper massaging in the direction of the muscle fibers until deep cooling, pain relief, and muscle relaxation are achieved. This can either precede or follow an exercise or stretching session, depending on patient preference.

One helpful hint for applying ice massage is to put a small paper cup filled with water in the freezer. When it is frozen, the lip of the cup is torn off and the helper has a nice comfortable way to hold the ice for the massage.

**Massage.** This technique helps reduce anxiety by relaxing the patient. Often such relaxation helps to break the cycle of muscle tension and pain, and massage can definitely be helpful as part of an overall treatment program.

One technique that the patient can be taught to do at home is ischemic compression massage. The theory behind this is that sustained pressure, enough to cause muscle ischemia, causes the fibers within tender or trigger points in muscle to relax. This can be done several times a day as needed. To select patients who will respond to such treatment the clinician may do a trial of compression for 30 seconds to 2 minutes in the office. Posture is adjusted to a position in which pain is minimized. If the muscle relaxes and pain lessens the patient should be taught the technique for home use. It can be performed by leaning against a tennis ball (either on the wall or on the floor) to apply pressure to the tender area. It should be a sustained pressure, not a deep massage. Such deep massage, while useful if done once a day or every other day, is not tolerated well if done several times a day. It may actually make the symptoms worse.

**Manipulation.** A large proportion of the population quickly seeks manipulation when neck pain arises. Many report good results, but then again most patients recover no matter what the treatment is. It is unclear exactly why manipulation works, if in fact it does. The literature is inadequate, although Florian recently performed an excellent review of articles dealing in treatment for neck pain and found some evidence supporting a role for manipulation.[4] It must not be viewed as a cure in itself, but rather as one more modality to help patients better cure themselves.

**Electrotherapy.** Transcutaneous electrical nerve stimulation (TENS) units can be used in treating acute neck pain for temporary relief. Other forms of electrotherapy include electrical stimulation of muscles to relieve tightness and pain, and pulsed electromagnetic therapy (PEMT). PEMT is sometimes used to accelerate fracture healing. It has also been advocated for use in treating neck pain,[4] although its use is not widely accepted for such treatment.

**Traction.** This is commonly used for the treatment of neck disorders, although in Florian's review its use was not well supported.[4] It is probably best reserved for patients with signs of nerve root irritation, since the traction helps to open up the intervertebral foramina through which the nerves pass. It should be performed with the neck in flexion. It is suggested that the neck be in 24 degrees of flexion,[5,6] but whether or not this is the best exact angle is not known.

Despite a lack of conclusive evidence of the efficacy of traction it is probably reasonable to give it as a trial in patients with stable spines and no contraindications, such as rheumatoid arthritis involvement of the neck or metastasis to the cervical spine. It is best administered as intermittent manual or mechanical traction.[7] Home traction devices are cumbersome and are not routinely recommended as they may do more harm than good due to improper application. See Chapter 9 for more information on traction.

**Postural Training/Relaxation.**    Much of the dysfunction of neck pain has to do with poor posture, anxiety, and stress. Attacking these elements is ultimately critical to restoring health to the neck. A "head forward" posture stresses the posterior neck muscles which then contract isometrically. Such sustained muscle activity builds up metabolic wastes, causes abnormal neck mechanics, and reduces blood flow to the muscles. Proper posture can help alleviate these problems. Since all three curves of the spine, the lumbar and thoracic as well as the cervical, interact, posture training must address the mid and low back also. Having patients view and correct their postures in front of a mirror is helpful.

Anyone who has ever experienced anxiety or stress knows that it affects the neck muscles. If the emotional state is improved it goes a long way toward relieving neck symptoms.

### Medications and Injections

Medications used for neck pathology are basically the same as for other musculoskeletal disorders. Nonsteroidal antiinflammatory drugs are a mainstay of treatment to reduce pain and inflammation. When necessary, usually after traumatic injury, more powerful analgesics may be necessary for brief periods of time. Some so-called "muscle relaxants" (see Chapter 5) may be useful to reduce pain and anxiety. They also are to be used only for short periods of time. In more chronic states tricyclic antidepressants or anticonvulsants are also helpful (see Chapter 5).

Injections in the neck differ from those in other parts of the body because they are usually into tight muscles, not into painful joints. Myofascial pain is a component of just about any painful neck condition if it lasts long enough. In myofascial pain there are usually tender or trigger points that reproduce some or all of the patient's pain. Injection into these points is often clinically useful, although care must be taken not to cause a pneumothorax. While some say that "dry needling" or saline injection is all that is needed,[8,9] most clinicians inject a local anesthetic or anesthetic-steroid combination. This works well, especially if followed by ultrasound or ice treatment and a therapy session. Another use of injection is fluoroscopy-guided facet joint injection, which may bring about temporary or permanent relief when pain is caused primarily by this joint.

### Examination and Testing Techniques

#### History and Physical Examination

A proper history must, of course, always be taken. It should include information about when and how the neck problem started, what exacerbates or relieves it, how severe it is, as well as any treatments and past medical problems.

Physical examination starts by observing posture, mood, and any abnormal movements. Muscular contour is observed to detect signs of atrophy. The ligaments, joints, and soft tissues of the neck are palpated. The facet joints are felt about 1 inch lateral to the midline. Often palpation of the muscles reveals trigger or tender points.

Range of motion is performed both actively and passively in flexion, extension, lateral bending, and rotation. In addition, passive motion of the individual spinal segments can be assessed by the examiner with the patient lying supine, head and neck relaxed. Both anterior and lateral gliding movements of each vertebra can be performed without exerting much force (Figure 12-6). This examination is pleasant and helps the patient to relax. A good manual examiner can identify specific facet joints that are involved in restricting motion.[10]

Neurologic and muscular strength testing must include sensation, reflexes, and motor strength, not only of the neck but also of the head, upper back, and upper extremities (and possibly lower extremities as well). Obviously, a detailed description of such an examination is beyond the scope of this chapter, but it can be obtained elsewhere.[11,12] What follows are descriptions of a few of the more specialized tests to assess the cervical region.

**Compression Test.**    The compression test (Figure 12-7) is performed by pushing straight down on the sitting patient's head. Pain is a positive though somewhat nonspecific finding. It can be due to a narrowing of the intervertebral foramina but may also be due to increased pressure on the facet joints. When pain is reproduced in a particular radicular distribution, it may help to localize the level of pathology.

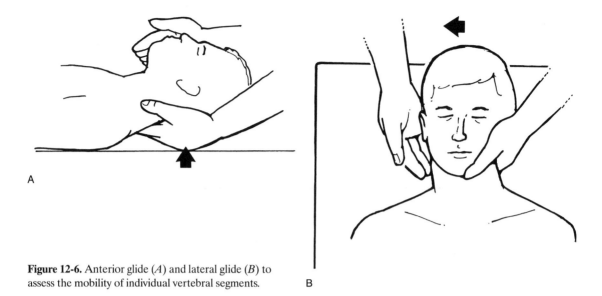

**Figure 12-6.** Anterior glide (*A*) and lateral glide (*B*) to assess the mobility of individual vertebral segments.

A

B

**Distraction Test.** The distraction test (Figure 12-8) is the opposite of the compression test. The examiner pulls up on the head while the patient sits or lies down. Relief of pain can be due to a number of causes such as opening up the intervertebral foramina, unloading the facet joints, or relieving muscle spasm. If pain is reduced, the patient may be a good candidate for traction therapy. Distraction should be sustained for at least 30 seconds to allow the spine time to relax and elongate.

**Spurling Maneuver.** This variation of the compression test is performed by having the patient turn to the side and extend the neck before applying downward pressure. It may help to localize the side of pathology, as the intervertebral foramina and facet joints are more compressed on the side the subject turns to. Again, reproduction of radicular symptoms may help localize the level of dysfunction. If extension causes problems of dizziness, nystagmus, or vertigo it may indicate vertebral artery dysfunction. Caution is in order here, as continuing to stress the neck in extension may result in stroke. A full evaluation, usually by a neurologist, is warranted in such cases.

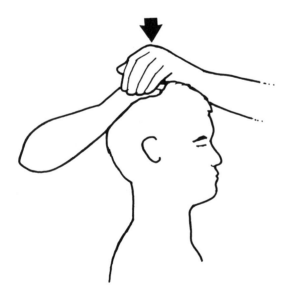

**Figure 12-7.** Compression test.

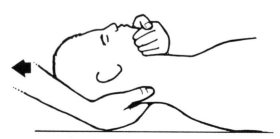

**Figure 12-8.** Distraction test.

**Valsalva Maneuver.**    Increasing venous "back pressure" raises the pressure within the spinal column. This can be done by the Valsalva maneuver, which is basically just holding one's breath and bearing down as if having a bowel movement. The same increase in pressure is elicited by coughing or sneezing. Pain may be due to intraspinal tumor, but it is usually considered a classic sign of a herniated disk.

Valsalva-type maneuvers are not without risk. In patients with cardiac disorders they can cause syncope, so they should be performed with care and not where a fall is likely to result in injury.

**Adson's Test.**    This test is performed by palpating the radial pulse and then extending, abducting, and externally rotating the arm. The patient is asked to turn the head toward the arm being examined, then extend the neck and take a deep breath. Diminution of the pulse is a positive finding and is indicative of intermittent arterial compression. The test is often equivocal or positive in asymptomatic individuals and is insensitive to true compression as well.[13] It is of doubtful value.

**First Rib Mobility.**    Anecdotal evidence suggests that the uppermost rib is sometimes hypomobile. This can be due to muscle tightness or abnormal posture. It is almost never a primary diagnosis but may be associated with other neck problems. Often a therapist can help mobilize this rib with good symptomatic relief (the patient may also be taught home mobilization to be performed by a partner). To assess the mobility of this rib the patient is supine. The examiner places one hand just below the medial clavicle and the other hand on the back medial to the scapula at the level of the first rib. Alternately pushing ventrally and dorsally allows an assessment of the rib mobility.

Recently, Lindgren et al.[14] published evidence of an effective test to detect limitation of first rib mobility. The head is rotated maximally away from the side being tested and is then flexed as far as possible. Limitation of flexion (so as to move the ear to the chest) on one side is considered a positive sign and has been correlated to restricted rib motion under fluoroscopic examination.

**Trigger/Tender Point Palpation.**    Palpating the neck muscles, especially the trapezius, sterno-cleidomastoid and rhomboids, often causes a reproduction of local pain (tender points) or reproduction of pain radiating into the head or limbs (trigger point). Finding such points is indicative of myofascial pain or fibromyalgia (see Chapter 20).

**Shoulder Depression Test.**    If the examiner manually pushes the head to one side while depressing the shoulder, this maneuver can stretch the spinal nerve roots, mainly of levels C5–C7. If radicular pain results it may indicate nerve root or intervertebral foraminal disease.

**Lhermitte's Sign.**    If flexing the neck causes pain to radiate down the spine (Lhermitte's sign)[15] it is indicative of spinal cord or brain pathology. This is sometimes seen after traumatic brain injury and may be due to meningeal adhesions or tumor.

**Blood Pressure.**    While this is not usually considered a specialized test, blood pressure monitoring in both arms can be useful. It may help diagnose subclavian steal syndrome or other conditions of blood flow impairment to one limb.

### Ancillary Diagnostic Testing

In an acute injury where there is a possibility of spinal fracture or subluxation, x-ray studies should be obtained first in neutral, then if cleared to be safe, in flexion and extension. In subacute injury, chronic injury, or when there is no risk of serious bony disruption, the neck should be radiographed in anteroposterior views, open mouth (odontoid) view to visualize the dens, lateral views in neutral, flexion and extension, and oblique views.

The anteroposterior views give a general measure of bony alignment and the structure of the uncovertebral joints. The odontoid view shows whether or not the dens is fractured, which is a potentially life-threatening condition that must be ruled out. Lateral views must include all seven cervical vertebrae. They give information about the intervertebral disks, the facet joints, and signs of soft tissue swelling, as well as subluxation or dislocation. Oblique views are used to visualize the intervertebral foramina.

Other radiologic tests that can be performed are conventional tomography, computerized tomography (CT), myelography, and magnetic resonance imaging (MRI). Conventional tomography is used mainly to demonstrate fractures and subluxations. CT testing gives the best general information to assess bones and detects most fractures, joint disease, and spinal masses. Herniated disks are also well visualized. Myelography gives information about spinal cord or root compression or avulsion. It can be combined with CT to be an even more exact diagnostic tool. MRI is mainly used to visualize soft tissues and is the best test to assess a herniated nucleus pulposus and some spinal cord tumors.

Among other tests that can be helpful are bone scanning to detect stress fractures, bone tumors, and infection; and fluoroscopy to evaluate movement of the cervical spine. Laboratory tests help detect connective tissue disease and infection. Electromyography (EMG) is used to detect neuropathy or myopathy.

## Diagnosis and Treatment of Specific Disorders

The most important initial decision to be made in assessing the neck is whether or not neurologic compromise is present. If it is, it must be addressed. Other important things to keep in mind are whether the pain is a result of intrinsic neck pathology, extrinsic problems referring pain to the neck, or systemic disorders. It is helpful to know whether or not the pain was initiated by trauma and whether it comes from joints or muscles. Referred pain, either to or from the neck, must be differentiated from radicular pain.

This section deals with specific musculoskeletal disorders commonly encountered in a subacute outpatient setting. Medical emergencies such as fractures, dislocations, and spinal cord injury are not covered.

### Acute Cervical Sprain (Whiplash)

The prototypical whiplash injury occurs in the rear-end auto collision and results in hyperextension-hyperflexion injury of the neck. In the past it has gone under a number of names, none of which is universally accepted today. It is safe to say that any condition that has two or more names in common usage is ill-defined, controversial, and may not have a scientifically defensible basis of verifying data. The whiplash syndrome is an example of such a condition. It is also called cervical sprain (better reserved for ligament stretch injury), cervical strain (better reserved for muscle stretch injury), acceleration-deceleration injury, and flexion-extension injury, to name a few.

What is clear about the whiplash syndrome is that it does exist. Any injury that violently hyperflexes or hyperextends the neck will cause some soft tissue damage. When the neck is relaxed, a violent force that pushes the body forward or backward under the head, will cause the neck to suddenly move backward or forward. The muscles involved in such a quick elongation may be partially torn. They may also be injured if contracted forcefully in a stretch reflex. The sternocleidomastoid is often affected. The vertebral bodies and disks may be compressed as the body moves under the head, and the joints and ligaments may be stretched and possibly subluxated at the extremes of motion. Since the cervical vertebrae normally glide on each other during flexion and extension, the intervertebral foramina may be altered sufficiently to compromise the spinal nerves, especially in a spine with preexisting bony spurring or narrowing of the foramina. In addition, the sympathetic nervous system may be damaged, either at the foramina or as the sympathetic fibers pass with the vertebral arteries through the foramina transversaria. The disk is more likely to be damaged if there is a rotatory component to the trauma. It is also sometimes torn from the vertebral body, in which case the anterior longitudinal ligament may be torn as well.[16]

The symptoms of whiplash syndrome vary. Headache, neck pain, neck soreness, muscle tightness, decreased range of motion, dizziness, and difficulty swallowing are common problems. Often they start a day or two after the injury, which can create the impression that they are due to the anticipation of litigation rather than true injury. Radiation of pain is a common complaint and can sometimes be reproduced on the physical examination. Radicular symptoms (not the same thing) imply nerve root or brachial plexus damage. Other neck structures such as the trachea, esophagus, or vocal cords are occasionally damaged.[17]

Hyperextension injury can be more serious in the older individual than in the young. The ligamentum flavum loses elasticity with age, and when a hyperextension injury occurs it may "buckle" the ligament and cause acute spinal cord compression.

Whiplash injuries have a worse prognosis if they are associated with advanced age,[18] neurologic signs, or muscle spasm as manifested by an abnormal spinal curvature, neck stiffness, or preexisting degenerative joint disease even if mild.[19]

*Diagnosis*

Whiplash syndrome is diagnosed mainly by the history. In the acute stage the physical examination is often normal. In the subacute stage there may be signs of muscle splinting, muscle tightness, soreness, and decreased range of motion. Distraction of the neck may relax the neck muscles and relieve pain. In most patients the symptoms resolve in a few weeks. A chronic condition may ensue in more severe injuries or in people who persist in maintaining poor posture and muscle splinting. Rigidly holding the head forward may relieve pain early on, but if maintained, leads to contracture of the posterior spine elements, contracture of the deep anterior neck muscles, chronic isometric muscle contraction, and persistent closing of the intervertebral foramina.

X-ray findings in cervical strain are usually normal or equivocal, but are important in ruling out more structural injury. There are usually no fractures or obvious dislocations present, but there may be a "reduction of the normal cervical lordosis." This is a nonspecific finding that does not really aid much in clinical management, although it may indicate the presence of muscle splinting that can lead to later muscle fatigue and pain. Persons with neck injury often have underlying degenerative change with bony spurring and disk space narrowing. Such x-ray findings are also not of much clinical utility. It is possible that underlying disease predisposed the patient to injury, but often the pain does not correspond to the x-ray findings.

*Treatment*

Acute injury is treated with a few days to a week of rest, possibly aided with a soft collar, analgesia, and treatment with ice. "Muscle relaxants" may also be useful. As symptoms improve, the soft collar is gradually removed as tolerated, antiinflammatory medications are started, and either heat or ice treatment can be used as a modality to reduce symptoms. Range of motion exercises are initiated, avoiding early flexion-extension motion to the extremes of range. Traction may be given a trial. If symptoms do not resolve, the patient may benefit from a physical therapy referral to work on range of motion, posture, relaxation, and neck isometric strengthening. These can be taught as part of a home exercise program with good results.[20] If resolution is slow, further diagnostic studies are considered. Massage, ischemic compression, ice massage, and trigger point injection may also help. If the condition becomes chronic, the patient may benefit from further physical therapy, TENS, heat or cold, aerobic exercise, adjunctive medications, and possibly a referral to a pain clinic.

### Myofascial Pain/Overuse Syndrome/Poor Posture

Almost any situation of overuse, poor posture, or unaccustomed work habits can lead to myofascial pain syndrome, which particularly likes to attack the neck and upper back region. Stress and previous trauma are important contributors to the problem. "Tension headache" often results. Myofascial pain is another one of those disorders with more than half a dozen names. Thus it holds to the rule of being controversial and confusing. It is often confused with fibromyalgia, a distinctly separate disease which is described in detail in Chapter 20. The causes of myofascial pain are unknown but may be due to local muscle tears or ischemia.

*Diagnosis*

The history gives the most information in diagnosing myofascial pain. New activities, stress, complaints of muscle tightness and soreness, and regional pain complaints are the hallmarks of this disorder, and it is common to see at least some element of myofascial pain in any of the problems of the neck. The pain often occurs after prolonged work in an exacerbating posture. Moderate aerobic activity may relieve it.

Trigger points, if present, help make this diagnosis. Palpating such points causes a reproduction of the patient's symptoms and radiation of the pain or paresthesias distally. Trigger points are commonly located in the trapezius, sternocleidomastoid, and rhomboid muscles. Some hold that pain radiation is required to label a point a trigger point, but other experts report that patients often just have local tender spots.

### Treatment

Treatment is aimed first at resolving the symptoms and then removing the underlying cause. These patients usually respond to relative rest, relaxation training, ischemic compression, ice massage, heat, trigger point injection, and a home stretching (with vapocoolant spray) and aerobic exercise program. Sometimes analgesics or nonsteroidal antiinflammatory medications are necessary. In the long run, treatment aims at building muscle strength, improving posture and flexibility, and reducing stress.

### Degenerative Joint Disease/Cervical Spondylosis/Myelopathy/Radiculopathy

Degenerative joint disease (DJD) occurs in the spine just as it does in many other parts of the body. The cause is unknown but may involve aging, overuse, trauma, or genetic predisposition. It is associated with heavy lifting, smoking, diving (from a board), and possibly with operating vibrating equipment or driving.[21] It preferentially affects the C5–C7 vertebrae. In the spine the degeneration affects both the intervertebral disk and the facet joints. Both the nucleus pulposus and the hyaline cartilage of the facet joints contain the same type of collagen fiber, and possibly a degeneration of this collagen is what these structures have in common during degeneration.

As the disk ages and is subject to repetitive trauma and motion, the annulus fibrosus develops small tears, which may gradually coalesce and lead to a weakening. The nucleus, which has a somewhat tenuous nutritional supply mechanism (possibly worsened by constant tension and too-infrequent loading and unloading of the joint) loses water content, develops fissures, and may project into the coalescent radial annular tears. As this degenerative process progresses, the disk loses height and the annulus bulges outward. The vertebral end-plates become sclerotic and grow bony spurs in an attempt to maintain structural strength (Figure 12-9). As the disk loses some of its height, the facet joint surfaces are brought closer together and may shift on each other. This causes synovitis, capsular stretch, and degeneration of these joints as well. They can also degenerate independent of disk disease, primarily by faulty neck motion and repetitive microtrauma, but in most people all these processes proceed together. The overall results are the nonspecific degenerative findings commonly seen on x-ray examination. Sometimes

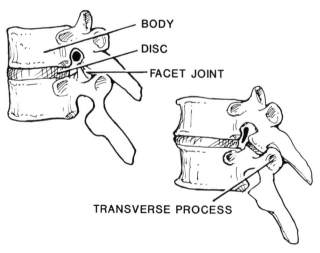

BODY

DISC

FACET JOINT

TRANSVERSE PROCESS

**Figure 12-9.** (*Left*) Normal vertebrae. (*Right*) Bony spurring and reduced disk height in degenerative joint disease can cause a narrowing of the intervertebral canal.

they are a cause of pain and sometimes they are not. The reasons for this are unknown.

When pain occurs, it probably comes to some extent from the disk, the facet joints, the uncovertebral joints, and from the nerves and other spinal column contents that are compressed by the spurs and bulging disk. Symptoms develop insidiously and include morning pain and stiffness. Sometimes DJD of the neck can mimic angina.[22]

If the spurring continues, it eventually compresses the contents of the spinal canal. This process of bony overgrowth is known as cervical spondylosis. If it encroaches upon the spinal cord it is called central (or spinal) stenosis, and if it narrows the intervertebral foramina sufficiently to produce spinal nerve irritation it is called lateral stenosis.

Central stenosis can lead to cervical myelopathy, a condition of ischemic compression of the spinal cord. Lateral stenosis can result in radiculopathy.

*Diagnosis*

The diagnosis of degenerative spine disease is straightforward since almost everyone over 50 years of age has some evidence of it. This can be demonstrated on plain x-rays studies. Determining that the degeneration is the cause of pain is more difficult. The patient may complain of an aching pain in the neck or upper back with intermittent exacerbations. There may be joint crepitus, a lack of signs of radiculopathy, and decreased range of motion (flexion is relatively spared). The facet joints may be tender to palpation. Compression testing worsens symptoms, while distraction may relieve them. X-ray findings reveal diffuse bony spurring and disk space narrowing. In most patients these symptoms and signs stabilize and lessen in time as the spine becomes stiffer (but more stable). In some, however, the bony proliferation produces further problems.

When radiculopathy results, it can occur suddenly or more insidiously. Acute radiculopathy often occurs after prolonged abnormal activity such as painting a ceiling or holding the neck in prolonged extension (in a person with DJD). Such activity may irritate the spinal nerve root to such an extent that it becomes inflamed. Pain, often referred in a dermatomal pattern or to the posterior shoulder, paresthesias, weakness, and reflex changes may occur, although it is important to realize that radiculopathy is not always painful. Compression of the dorsal root ganglion causes a shooting pain down the arm. Usually the symptoms resolve, but occasionally marked segmental muscle weakness and atrophy develop. There may be more than one nerve root involved. Compression testing and the Spurling maneuver reproduce the pain; distraction may lessen it.

Chronic radiculopathy may develop due to progressive narrowing of the intervertebral foramen over time. Posture or trauma may aggravate the symptoms and cause exacerbations. It is rarely incapacitating, and rarely progresses to myelopathy.[23]

Radiculopathy is best diagnosed by electrodiagnostic study. In addition, oblique x-ray films to demonstrate foraminal narrowing and sometimes myelogram or CT are useful to evaluate the extent of bony encroachment. Abduction of the arm may decrease radicular pain in cervical extradural compressive radiculopathy and has been advocated as a diagnostic test for this condition.[24]

Cervical myelopathy can produce far-reaching signs and symptoms. Locally, it may produce pain in the neck from ischemia and spurring. It may cause lower motor neuron damage at the level of pathology which usually results in upper extremity dysesthesias, paresthesias, weakness, and depressed reflexes. These changes have an insidious onset. Upper motor neuron damage at the cervical level causes leg weakness, gait disturbance, and lower extremity spasticity and hyperreflexia. There is also a loss of sensation, and Babinski reflex testing is positive. Reflexes above the level of the spine pathology, such as the jaw reflex, remain normal. The condition is usually mild and most often stabilizes. It rarely progresses rapidly, sometimes in relatively young patients, and sometimes results in bowel and bladder dysfunction. Diagnosis is made by the clinical picture, electromyography, and measurement of the diameter of the spinal canal by radiographs. Affected patients may be developmentally predisposed to the condition by having a narrow spinal canal.

*Treatment*

Conservative treatment is almost always successful in degenerative disease of the cervical spine. In uncomplicated osteoarthritis of the neck, range of motion exercises, nonsteroidal antiinflammatory medications, cervical pillows, soft collars, and modalities such as heat and cold are the mainstays of treatment. Occasionally traction or facet joint injections are required. The patient may expect to have intermittent exacerbations but is unlikely to develop symptoms severe enough to significantly limit function. Exacerbations are minimized by avoiding unaccustomed activity, high impact exercise, or holding the neck in one position (especially extension) for a prolonged period of time.

In radiculopathy, early treatment may combine a few days of rest, traction, and antiinflammatory medication. Physical therapy with range of motion (avoiding excessive extension or extension/ rotation), heat or cold, and minimization of secondary muscle splinting and myofascial pain is added as tolerated. Arm abduction exercise can be incorporated into treatment.[25] Most cases resolve in a few weeks; rarely surgical decompression is indicated.

Patients with predominant complaints of neck pain with no neurologic deficit or radicular symptoms do not get a better long-term outcome from surgery than from conservative care.[26,27] If there is a progressive motor deficit, surgical treatment usually offers good results and is advocated by some,[27] although even patients with motor deficits may still do well with conservative care.[28] It is probably reasonable, when possible, in such cases to work closely in consultation with a spine surgeon who is committed to conservative care.

Cervical myelopathy can be treated similarly to radiculopathy and DJD. Flexion exercises may help to open up the spinal canal. In some cases surgical decompression is necessary, and it may be successful if the narrowing is localized to a small area. In diffuse stenosis surgical results are often poor. Most patients with conservatively treated cervical myelopathy see a stabilization of their symptoms with little long-term disability.

### Herniated Nucleus Pulposus

Herniated nucleus pulposus, also known as a herniated or "slipped" disk, is the result of the type of degenerative disk disease described in the preceding section. It primarily involves cervical levels C5–C7 and affects persons 30 to 55 years of age.

When radial annular tears coalesce, the nucleus pulposus may protrude into the spinal canal to compress the spinal cord or spinal nerves. This can happen suddenly or insidiously. It is much less common in the cervical region than in the lumbar spine. This is due to a number of anatomic reasons: (1) the nucleus is located more anteriorly within the cervical disk; (2) the uncovertebral joints prevent posterolateral herniation; (3) the posterior longitudinal ligament covers the entire posterior disk (unlike the lumbar spine, in which it covers only the central disk); and (4) the posterior annulus is reinforced in the cervical disks.

### Diagnosis

Herniated disks, when they occur, may press either directly on the spinal cord or on the spinal nerves. If they press on the cord they can cause an acute cervical myelopathy, which if severe, can be a medical emergency. Such herniations are rare, however. More likely the herniation occurs laterally and compromises the spinal nerve, causing an acute radiculopathy. Symptoms are the same as for any radiculopathy and include local pain, radicular pain and paresthesia, dysesthesia, weakness, and reflex changes. The symptoms may be worsened or reproduced by a Valsalva maneuver or compression testing. Distraction with manual traction may relieve the symptoms somewhat. MRI, CT, or myelogram confirms the herniation, while the clinical picture and electrodiagnosis will help in diagnosing the radiculopathy.

### Treatment

Herniated nucleus pulposus is treated with rest, analgesia, and traction. Heat or cold, a soft collar, and gradual range of motion exercises are added as needed. Symptoms resolve in time as a rule, but in some cases surgical decompression is necessary. The herniated portion of the disk is phagocytosed and disappears within about 3 to 6 months. This parallels the normal progression of the symptoms, and given such a natural history it is unclear why patients and physicians alike are so eager to surgically remove the disk. With severe symptoms and when myelopathy is present, surgery is considered early, but for most herniated disks, time to heal is all that is needed. Therapeutic interventions mainly serve to maintain neck mobility and strength so that when the disk problem resolves the patient is not left with a contracted, chronically painful neck. Disk surgery is indeed one instance in which the cure can be worse than the disease, as some patients are left with chronic neck pain after the operation. If possible, surgery should be avoided. As described earlier, surgery has not been shown to give a superior outcome compared with conservative care in the treatment of patients with predominant complaints of neck pain,[26,27] and even in patients with strength deficits conservative care may lead to a good outcome. Again, consultation with a surgeon committed to conservative care, when possible, is indicated to plan the best treatment strategy.

### Osteoporosis

Osteoporosis most commonly causes thoracic spinal compression fractures, but it may involve the neck as well. Symptoms develop insidiously with possible exacerbations. Elderly, thin, white women are most at risk. See Chapter 23 for more information on osteoporosis.

*Diagnosis*

Bone scan and x-ray findings make the diagnosis.

*Treatment*

There is no cure for the condition once it has developed. Range of motion should be maintained and a proper diet should be ingested. Estrogen replacement, exercise, and adequate calcium intake can prevent or at least slow the progression.

### Vertebral Artery Insufficiency

The vertebral arteries pass through the transverse processes of the vertebrae on their way to supply the brain with blood. If bony spurs press on the arteries they can restrict blood flow to the brain. This is a potentially life-threatening condition and may cause posterior circulation stroke.

*Diagnosis*

Symptoms of vertebral artery compression include neck pain, headache, lightheadedness, dizziness, vertigo, syncope, ataxia, diplopia, dysphagia, dysarthria, and facial dysesthesia. The symptoms are brought on by positions that compress the arteries, usually turning toward the side of the compression, or extension. This condition should be suspected if the patient experiences the characteristic symptoms during the physical examination, especially on lateral bending, rotation, and the Spurling maneuver. Plain x-ray studies may reveal marked spurring, often at the upper cervical and occipital level. Definitive diagnosis is by arteriography.

*Treatment*

Surgical removal of the offending structures should be considered. Traction and manipulation are absolutely contraindicated. This condition is best managed by a neurosurgeon or other physician well versed in its treatment.

### Thoracic Outlet Syndrome

This condition of neurovascular compromise of the vessels and nerves passing to the arm is rare. It causes symptoms in the shoulder and arm. It is discussed in Chapter 14.

### Occipital Neuralgia

After trauma, the occipital nerve can become irritated at the junction of the skull and neck. This can cause pain radiating from the posterior to the anterior scalp and also pain felt behind the eyes. The headache parallels the sensory distribution of the nerve. The retroorbital pain is due to a looping of some of the nerve fibers around cranial nerve V; thus it is a referred pain.

*Diagnosis*

Diagnosis is made by the clinical symptoms just described and by reproduction of the symptoms with palpation of the nerve. The nerve may be inflamed and swollen.

### Treatment

Treatment is often successful with local anesthetic-steroid injection around the nerve (which also helps to confirm the diagnosis). Care must be taken not to inject the nearby vertebral artery. Other treatment options include ice application, ice and ultrasound, and antiinflammatory medication.

### Temporomandibular Joint Dysfunction

This condition can cause radiation of pain into the neck and can occur after neck extension injury[29] or with no discernible cause.

### Diagnosis

The symptoms of temporomandibular joint dysfunction are pain in the region of the joint, radiation of pain into the neck, a painful "click" on opening the mouth, and painful or restricted range of motion of the jaw. Ultrasound examination of the joint, as well as pressure on the cartilagenous disk of the joint (by manual pressure on the jaw with the joint in neutral), may help make the diagnosis.

### Treatment

This condition can be treated with nonsteroidal antiinflammatory medication, avoidance of hard chewy foods, ice treatment, ultrasound treatment, massage of associated tender points, bite plates, or more definitively, a filing of the teeth to give a better dental occlusion. If symptoms persist despite conservative treatment, a referral should be made to a dentist or other physician specializing in this disorder.

### Connective Tissue Disease

Rheumatoid arthritis, diffuse idiopathic skeletal hyperostosis (DISH), ankylosing spondylitis, and other connective tissue diseases can affect the neck. They are primarily rheumatologic disorders and are not covered in detail in this book; however, a few basic principles are addressed.

Rheumatoid arthritis, as well as the other rheumatologic diseases, is a systemic condition and must be treated as such. Of special interest in the neck is rheumatoid involvement of the atlantoaxial joint at the dens. This joint is, as described earlier, a synovial joint. If it degenerates during the course of connective tissue disease, it can lead to atlantoaxial subluxation. This allows the dens to slip into the spinal cord and brain stem and is potentially fatal. Thus traction, manipulation, and forceful neck mobilization are contraindicated in these individuals.

DISH is a condition characterized by an overproduction of bone, primarily in the spine. It creates a "flowing osteophytosis" seen on radiographs. It presents in middle age with spinal stiffness and tenderness. Occasionally these patients have trouble swallowing due to osteophytes pushing on the esophagus (as well as the immobile cervical spine). Treatment is with general flexibility and conditioning training. Cervical manipulation and traction are again contraindicated.

Ankylosing spondylitis is a disease mainly of young Caucasians, mostly symptomatic in males. It involves calcification and inflammation of spinal tendons and ligaments at their attachments to bone. It typically presents with low back and sacroiliac joint pain and may eventually involve the entire spine. The spine loses mobility and may become fused. Treatment is aimed at maintaining range of motion and avoiding spinal fusion in a stooped posture. Again, traction and manipulation are to be avoided in these patients.

### Other Disorders

A number of other disorders must be kept in mind when diagnosing neck pathology. They include fractures, neoplasm, osteomyelitis, meningitis, referred pain (from myocardial infarction, among many causes), migraine, conversion disorder, Pancoast's tumor, pharyngeal infection, torticollis, malingering, and psychogenic pain. In addition, many shoulder or arm disorders can mimic neck problems. While the list may seem intimidating at first, a systematic approach and an understanding of anatomy and biomechanics usually leads to a correct diagnosis.

## Case Report

A 39-year-old man broke through a wooden staircase, fell onto the back of his head, and was found to have a herniated C5 disk. He underwent surgical disk removal and neck fusion. One and one-half years later he still had significant neck pain and headache, was still on narcotic medication, was sleeping poorly, and was still wearing a soft collar. On examination he allowed almost no movement at the neck. He had a levator scapulae trigger point which caused radiation of his neck pain into the head. He was treated with steroid-anesthetic trigger point injection, amitriptyline, weaning of the narcotic and soft collar, and a home exercise program which he had learned during earlier physical therapy visits. One month after this regimen he had no more headache, only mild neck pain, had discarded the collar, and was moving his neck freely, although not yet with normal range. While his response to treatment could be described as "better than average," it illustrates the power of proper treatment.

## Points of Summary

1. Pain producing structures in the neck are bones, anterior and posterior longitudinal ligaments, facet joints, dura, nerve roots, and probably the outer annulus.
2. The intervertebral foramina narrow with extension and rotation/bending.
3. Myofascial pain accompanies many different neck disorders.
4. Herniated disks are less common in the neck than in the lumbar spine.
5. Injections, ischemic compression, and ice massage are useful in treating myofascial pain.
6. Degeneration of the disk and facet joints may lead to osteoarthritis, radiculopathy, or myelopathy, or may cause none of these disorders.
7. X-ray findings in the spine often do not correlate with symptoms.

8. Proper posture and biomechanics are the keys to preventing chronic neck pain.
9. Most cervical disk herniations do not need surgery; the same is true for spondylosis and stenosis.

## References

1. Bland JH, Boushey DR: Anatomy and physiology of the cervical spine. *Semin Arthritis Rheum* 1990; 20:1–20.
2. Bogduk N: Neck pain: An update. *Aust Fam Physician* 1988;17:75–80.
3. Cailliet, R: *Neck and Arm Pain*, 3rd ed. Philadelphia: FA Davis, 1991.
4. Florian T: Conservative treatment for neck pain, distinguishing useful from useless therapy. *J Back Musculoskel Rehabil* 1991;1(3):55–66.
5. Colachis SC, Strohm BR: A study of tractive forces and angle of pull on vertebral interspaces in the cervical spine. *Arch Phys Med Rehabil* 1965;46:820–830.
6. Geiringer SR, Kincaid CB, Rechtien JJ: Traction, manipulation and massage. In DeLisa JA (ed): *Rehabilitation Medicine: Principles and Practice*. Philadelphia: JB Lippincott, 1988:276–294.
7. Zybergold RS, Piper MC: Cervical spine disorders: A comparison of three types of traction. *Spine* 1985; 10:867–871.
8. Gunn CC, Milbrandt WE, Little AS, et al.: Dry needling of muscle motor points for chronic low back pain: A randomized clinical trial with long-term follow-up. *Spine* 1980;5:279–291.
9. Garvey TA, Marks MR, Wiesel SW: A prospective, randomized, double-blind evaluation of trigger-point injection therapy for low-back pain. *Spine* 1989;14:962–964.
10. Jull G, Bogduk N, Marsland A: The accuracy of manual diagnosis for cervical zygapophyseal joint pain syndromes. *Med J Aust* 1988;148:233–236.
11. McGee DJ: *Orthopedic Physical Assessment*, 2nd ed. Philadelphia: WB Saunders, 1992.
12. Hoppenfeld S: *Physical Examination of the Spine and Extremities*. Norwalk, CT: Appleton-Century-Crofts, 1976.
13. Glassenberg M: The thoracic outlet syndrome: An assessment of 20 cases with regard to new clinical and electromyographic findings. *Angiology* 1981;32:180–186.
14. Lindgren KA, Leino E, Manninen H: Cervical rotation lateral flexion test in brachialgia. *Arch Phys Med Rehabil* 1992;73:735–737.
15. Lhermitte J: Etude de la commation de la moele. *Rev Neurol* 1932;1:210–239.
16. McNab I: Acceleration injuries of the cervical spine. *Spine* 1964;46A:1797–1799.

17. Helliwell M, Robertson JC, Todd GB, et al.: Bilateral vocal cord paralysis due to whiplash injury. *Br Med J* 1984;288:1876–1877.

18. Brooks SH, Nahum AM, Siegel AW: Causes of injury in motor vehicle accidents. *Surg Gynecol Obstet* 1970; 131:185–197.

19. Norris SH, Watt I: The prognosis of neck injuries resulting from rear-end collisions. *J Bone Joint Surg* 1983; 65B:608–611.

20. McKinney LA, Dornan JO, Ryan M: The role of physiotherapy on the management of acute neck sprains following road-traffic accidents. *Arch Emerg Med* 1989; 6:27-33.

21. Kelsey JL, Githens PB, Walter SD, et al.: An epidemiological study of acute prolapsed cervical intervertebral disc. *J Bone Joint Surg* 1984;66A:907–914.

22. Booth RE, Rothman RH: Cervical angina. *Spine* 1976; 1:28–32.

23. Lees F, Turner JWA: Natural history and prognosis of cervical spondylosis. *Br Med J* 1963; 2:988–991.

24. Davidson RI, Dunn EJ, Metzmaker JN: The shoulder abduction test in the diagnosis of radicular pain in cervical extradural compressive mononeuropathies. *Spine* 1981;6:441–446.

25. Fast A, Parikh S, Marin EL: The shoulder abduction relief sign in cervical radiculopathy. *Arch Phys Med Rehabil* 1989;70:402–403.

26. Rothman R, Simeone S: *The Spine*. Philadelphia: WB Saunders, 1982.

27. Dillin W, Booth R, Cuckler J, et al.: Cervical radiculopathy: a review. *Spine* 1986;11:988–991.

28. Honet JC, Puri K: Cervical radiculitis: Treatment and results in 82 patients. *Arch Phys Med Rehabil* 1976; 57:12–16.

29. Roydhouse RH: Torquing of neck and jaw due to belt restraint in whiplash-type accidents. *Lancet* 1985; 1:1341.

## Suggested Reading

Cailliet R: *Neck and Arm Pain*, 3rd ed. Philadelphia: FA Davis, 1991.

Dillin W, Booth R, Cuckler J, et al.: Cervical radiculopathy: A review. *Spine* 1986;11:988–991.

Yunus MB, Kalyan-Raman UP, Kalyan-Raman K: Primary fibromyalgia syndrome and myofascial pain syndrome: Clinical features and muscle pathology. *Arch Phys Med Rehabil* 1988;69:451–454.

Saal JA (ed): Neck and back pain. *Physical Medicine and Rehabilitation: State of the Art Reviews* 1990:4(2).

# Chapter 13
# Back, Spine, and Chest

ANDREA CONTI

Disorders of the back, spine, and thorax are among the most commonly encountered in almost any medical setting. The low back, especially, is becoming the body part complained of most in today's society, and it is said that 80% of the adult population will suffer from low back pain (LBP) at some time.[1,2]

## Anatomy

### The Bony Thorax

The thoracic skeleton is composed of 12 vertebrae, 12 pairs of ribs, and the sternum. The sternum protects the viscera anteriorly and provides stability to the bony cage. It articulates directly with the first seven pairs of ribs at the costosternal joints, which are cartilaginous joints. The eighth through tenth ribs attach to the lower sternum indirectly by means of the costal cartilages of the ribs above them. The lower two (floating) ribs do not articulate with the sternum.

### The Vertebral Column

The bony spine is composed of 7 cervical, 12 thoracic, and 5 lumbar vertebrae sitting on the sacrum. The individual spinal segments move little, but motion of the spine as a whole is remarkable.

During quiet standing the spine is balanced so that virtually no muscular activity is required to maintain its position.

The thoracic and lumbar vertebrae are basically similar, except that the thoracic segments articulate with the ribs. The vertebrae also become larger in the caudal direction. Each vertebra consists of a body to which is attached a ring consisting of two laminae and two pedicles. At the laminopedicular junction bony processes articulate with the corresponding processes above and below them to form the facet joints (zygapophyseal joints). The facet joints are synovial plane joints lined with hyaline cartilage and surrounded by a synovial membrane and capsule. Between these joints and the vertebral bodies (and disks) is a space called the intervertebral foramen through which the spinal nerves exit the spinal canal to reach the periphery (Figure 13-1).

The rings of the vertebrae are stacked on top of one another to form the spinal canal, through which passes the spinal cord and its associated structures. There are lateral and posterior projections of the rings of the vertebrae. They are called the transverse and spinous processes, respectively. They are sites of muscular and ligamentous attachments.

The disks between the vertebral bodies are composed of an inner nucleus pulposus and an outer annulus fibrosus (Figure 13-2). The nucleus is made up of a gelatinous connective tissue with a high water content. It is connected to the

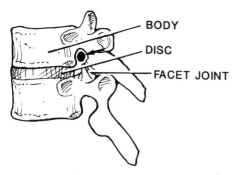

**Figure 13-1.** Functional unit of the spine: two vertebrae and the intervening disk. The intervertebral foramen houses the spinal nerve (*arrow*).

vertebrae on its top and bottom at the vertebral end-plates, which are lined with cartilage. The nucleus has no direct innervation or blood supply. It receives its nutrition through a regular loading and unloading of weight (or force), which pushes water in and pulls it out of the disk by hydraulic pressure. This seems like a somewhat tenuous way to receive nutrition, but it works fairly well most of the time. During a day of standing the disk gradually loses water, which leads to a shortening in body height of about ¾ inch per day. The fluid returns and restores height during sleep.

The annulus fibrosus is composed of collagenous fibers that encircle the nucleus in an angular manner. The structure somewhat resembles a radial tire.

There are several ligaments which help hold the vertebral column together (Figure 13-3). The anterior longitudinal ligament runs along the anterior surfaces of the vertebral bodies and disks. The

posterior longitudinal ligament runs along the posterior vertebral bodies and disks. In the lumbar spine this ligament is narrower and weaker than in the neck, which helps explain why disks herniate more readily in this area. The ligamentum flavum (yellow ligament) runs along the posterior part of the spinal canal.

### Muscles of the Chest and Back

The muscles of the thorax and back are divided into two groups: the extrinsic muscles (Figure 13-4) and the intrinsic muscles (Figure 13-5). For the most part, the extrinsic back muscles are concerned with upper extremity motion and respiration. They are limb muscles that migrate during embryonic development to cover the back. The intrinsic muscles maintain posture and control movement of the vertebral column as a whole.

The intrinsic back muscles are identified by the direction of their fibers. The superficial layer, the splenius muscles of the neck, has fibers that pass superolaterally (from lower spinous process to upper transverse process). The intermediate layer, the erector spinae, run longitudinally in the groove on each side of the vertebral column. The deeper muscles, the multifidus and rotatores, pass superomedially (from lower transverse process to upper spinous process). These deep muscles make up the bulk of the muscles commonly called the paraspinals. They control segmental vertebral motion and spinal stabilization during movement.

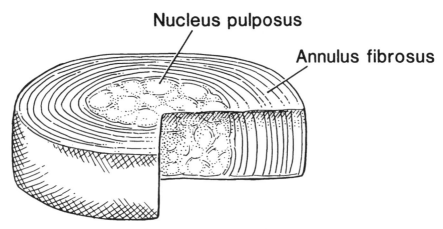

**Figure 13-2.** The intervertebral disk.

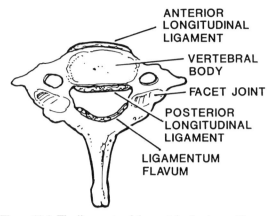

**Figure 13-3.** The ligaments of the vertebral column. The segment shown is from the cervical spine.

*Nerves*

The spinal cord passes through the vertebral canal giving off segmental spinal nerves which exit the spinal canal through the intervertebral foramina. In the thoracic and lumbar spine the nerves are named and numbered after the vertebral body below which they exit the canal. After passing through the foramina, they give off recurrent branches called the sinuvertebral nerves (of von Luschka) which innervate some of the structures within the spinal canal.[3]

The spinal cord ends at vertebral level L1–L2. Below this level the spinal canal contains no cord,

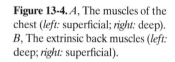

**Figure 13-4.** *A*, The muscles of the chest (*left:* superficial; *right:* deep). *B*, The extrinsic back muscles (*left:* deep; *right:* superficial).

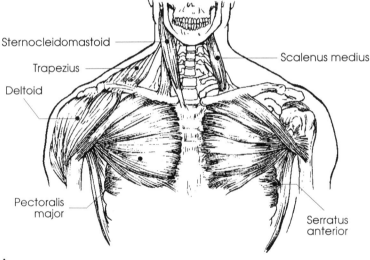

A

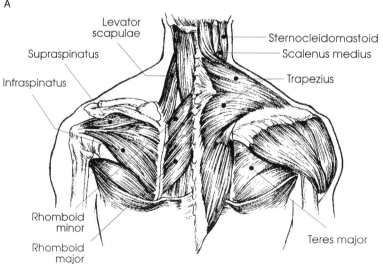

B

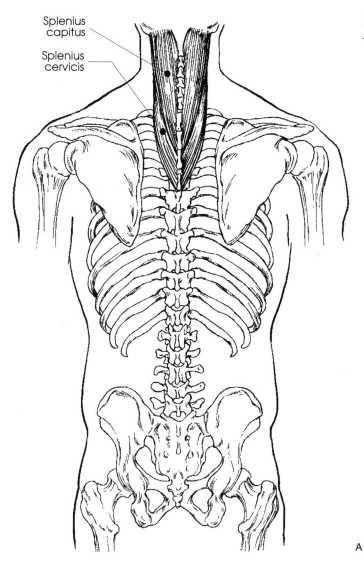

Splenius
capitus

Splenius
cervicis

**Figure 13-5.** The intrinsic back muscles: *A*, superficial.

A

just the nerve roots traveling caudally to the vertebral levels through which they exit. This collection of nerve roots is called the cauda equina (horse's tail).

### Pain-Sensitive Structures

When discussing the spine it is probably easier to focus on the structures that do not cause pain rather than those that do. The adult intervertebral disk is commonly felt not to contain pain-sensitive nerve fibers, although there are pain receptors in the very outer layers of the annulus fibrosus.[3] Also,

with tears of the annulus there may be an ingrowth of nerves into the disk; this may be a cause of pain in disk degeneration.

Another structure which does not have pain sensation is the interior of the vertebral body. The exterior, the periosteum, does contain pain innervation; thus vertebral fractures are painful.

Lastly, the ligamentum flavum is not felt to be pain sensitive. All other structures, including the anterior and posterior longitudinal ligaments, the facet joints, muscles, dura, epidural veins, and spinal nerves can be sources of spinal pain.[3] In addition, pain can be referred to the back from other areas of the body.

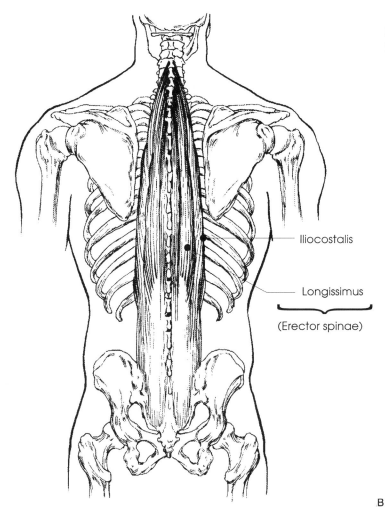

**Figure 13-5.** *(continued) B,* intermediate.

Iliocostalis

Longissimus

(Erector spinae)

B

### Spinal Motion

The thoracic spine has the most limited motion of any area of the vertebral column. The ribs limit motion, as does the nearly frontal orientation of the thoracic facet joints.[4] Side bending is the most free movement allowed. In the lumbar spine all motions are more free than in the thoracic spine, but because of the oblique orientation of the facet joints and the shape of the disks, flexion and extension are the most uninhibited.

When bending forward from a standing position the spine normally flexes to its limit before there is appreciable motion at the hips. As the lumbar spine flexes, the paraspinal muscles contract eccentrically. When full flexion is achieved the back is said to "hang on its ligaments." The paraspinal muscles should relax before the hips

flex. Extension involves a reversal of this sequence. This motion pattern reduces the strain on the low back muscles.

In persons with poor back mechanics the hips tend to flex sooner in forward bending and the paraspinal muscles never fully elongate. This causes the muscles to remain isometrically contracted through the whole motion, which can exacerbate back pain.

When the spine rotates, flexes/extends, or bends to the side, the vertebrae should move on one another in a smooth symmetric manner (Figure 13-6). Local areas of asymmetry, hypermobility, or hypomobility are signs of back dysfunction.

The annular fibers of the disk are designed to resist forces in flexion and extension. Because of their overlapping angled fiber layers, lumbar motion that imposes rotation on a flexed back isolates

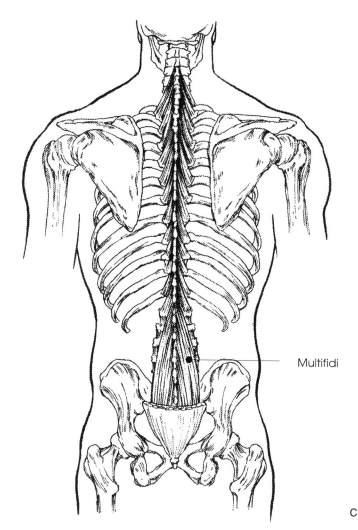

**Figure 13-5.** *(continued) C,* deep muscles.

Multifidi

C

some of the annular layers and may cause them to tear. Thus repetitive rotation of a flexed back is to be avoided. When the back is not flexed, the facet joints prevent the extremes of motion that cause damage.

## Rehabilitative Approach

The basic principles of acute rehabilitation for musculoskeletal injuries of the thorax and back are the same as for other parts of the body: rest, early mobilization, and exercise. In the acute stage ice, rest (the avoidance of exacerbating activities), and antiinflammatory medications are indicated.

## *Early Rest*

The length of time of "rest" for back injuries is continuously debated. Just a few years ago it was not unusual for patients to have prescriptions for 2 to 5 weeks of complete bed rest for any type of back injury. Patients were instructed to arise only for the purpose of toileting and eating. In a randomized clinical trial Deyo et al.[5] studied the effects of work days lost in two groups of patients with nonneurogenic back pain who were assigned to 2 days or 7 days of bed rest. They found that the group with less rest time fared better. Complete bed rest is probably never indicated for back strain. It leads to a loss of muscle mass and strength.[6] It may be prescribed for 5 to 7 days in cases of acutely herniated disks.

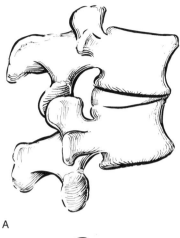

**Figure 13-6.** *A*, Flexion of the spine; *B*, extension; *C*, lateral bending. Flexion opens the intervertebral foramina and compresses the disk. Extension closes the intervertebral foramina. Bending to the side closes the foramina on the side being bent to and opens them on the contralateral side.

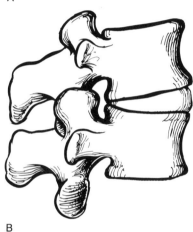

A

B

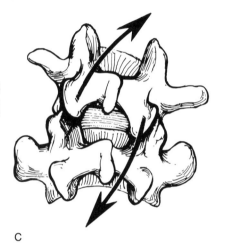

C

### *Surgery Versus Conservative Care*

The recommendations for surgery versus conservative care have also come under scrutiny in the past two decades. After Mixter and Barr[7] first discovered that a herniated disk could cause pain and that removal of the disk could relieve pain, disk surgery became very popular. Even today, patients and physicians alike routinely think of surgery when they are confronted with back pain. Yet only a few of these patients have any need for surgery. (Imagine the parallel: routinely considering surgery when a patient complains of headache.) Furthermore, disk surgery is far from being harmless surgery. It involves cutting important back ligaments and bone, and it is not uncommon for the disk surgery to cause residual back pain that is worse than the pain it was supposed to relieve.

In a prospective study on patients with diagnosed herniated lumbar disks, Weber[8] compared conservative therapy of bed rest, analgesics, and gradual return to activity with surgical excision of the disk. His findings were that after 1 year the surgically treated group fared better, but over the following 9-year period of observation the difference became insignificant. There was a positive correlation between physical activity and favorable results.

Saal and Saal[9] discovered that patients with herniated nucleus pulposus (HNP), leg pain, and radiculopathy, who would ordinarily be considered to have met the criteria for surgery, could be treated just as well with aggressive rehabilitation. They found that a failure of passive nonoperative treatment was not a sufficient reason to operate, and that the presence of weakness did not adversely affect the outcome of conservative treatment. They also noted that conservatively treated patients fared just as well as those treated with surgery, even within the first year. Furthermore, they found that patients treated with delayed surgery (more than 16 weeks) had excellent to good outcomes as well. They considered progressive neurologic deficit to be an indication for surgery and identified a subgroup of patients with HNP plus spinal stenosis who were less likely to respond to conservative care. Patients with simple extruded disks did well without surgery.

In another study Saal et al.[10] found that the natural history of extruded disks was one of eventual resorption with no residual perithecal or perineural fibrosis (often cited as reasons to perform surgery early).

### Disk Pressures

Intradiskal pressure varies with body positioning and with activity. The pressure is least when reclining. This creates about a 50% to 80% drop in pressure compared with standing. Unsupported sitting increases pressure by 40% over standing, while forward leaning and weightlifting increase pressure by more than 100%. Forward flexion and rotation increase the intradiskal pressure by 400%.[11]

While the clinical significance of intradiskal pressure variations is not completely understood, it certainly makes sense that persons with herniated disks would benefit from lower pressures. This may prevent further herniation. Consequently in the early rehabilitation of patients with HNP, lifting while flexing the trunk and practicing flexion exercises are avoided. A trial of back extension exercises may be useful, and isometric abdominal flexion strengthening may be acceptable. Traction, which also reduces disk pressure,[11] may be tried as well.

### Therapeutic Interventions

Important therapeutic interventions in patients with back pain include the various modalities and therapeutic aids described in the following sections. It is important to remember that they must be used in a rational, concerted approach. Using one modality or treatment at a time is rarely successful. Many patients are treated with medications for a few weeks, then exercise for a week, then an injection, then a transcutaneous electrical

nerve stimulation (TENS) unit, etc. Finally they are told that "we've tried everything" and the only other option is surgery. A more appropriate approach is with proper education and whatever medication, modality, injection, etc., is needed to help patients "cure" themselves through a proper exercise program.

### Therapeutic Heat and Cold

Both therapeutic heat and cold (see Chapter 6) have the physiologic effect of ameliorating pain and muscle spasm. Heat also has the benefit of increasing extensibility of collagen when combined with stretching. Cold can decrease swelling and hemorrhage if applied after early trauma.

As a rule, either heat or cold can be used for soft tissue pain depending on patient preference. Cold application may be preferable in the acute stage, but either can be used later on. Myofascial pain often responds to ice massage. This is performed by a helper massaging with an ice block in the direction of the muscle fibers until deep cooling, pain relief, and muscle relaxation are achieved. This can either precede or follow an exercise or stretching session.

One helpful hint for applying ice massage is to put a small paper cup filled with water in the freezer. When the water is frozen, the lip of the cup is torn off and the helper has a nice, comfortable way to hold the ice for the massage.

### Massage and Traction

Massage (see Chapter 9) helps reduce anxiety by relaxing the patient. Often such relaxation helps to break the cycle of muscle tension and pain. Massage can definitely be helpful as part of an overall treatment program.

Traction is also sometimes useful in treating back pain, especially when the pain is due to a herniated disk or radiculopathy. Care must be taken to apply enough force to overcome the friction of the body on the table. Contraindications include osteoporosis, tumor, pregnancy, or spine infection.

### Manipulation and Mobilization

A large segment of the population quickly seeks manipulation when back pain arises. Many report good results, but then again most patients recover regardless of what the treatment is. It is unclear why manipulation works, if in fact it does. It is described in more detail in Chapters 9 and 10.

Mobilization (see Chapter 9) appears to be a more medically accepted form of treatment for the spine. It involves techniques and exercises to restore proper back mechanics and movement and is a more patient-active form of treatment. As distinguished from chiropractic manipulation, mobilization techniques applied by a spine therapist or trained physician generally are viewed as an adjunct to the total program of exercise and patient education.

### Exercise

Exercises prescribed specifically for the back have traditionally been categorized as flexion, extension, and stabilization exercises. Flexion exercises are used to strengthen weak abdominal muscles and to increase the flexibility of the paraspinal muscles. Extension exercise programs, such as McKenzie exercises, are often used to treat patients with herniated disks. They have also been advocated to treat low back strain/sprain.[12]

Stabilization exercises are felt to help the patient attain proper dynamic control of the lumbar spine forces to prevent reinjury.[9] The abdominal muscles are important contributors to protecting the spine, and a basic stabilization program includes exercises to strengthen these muscles. Postural control is developed through a basic and then advanced program of isometric contractions of the intrinsic back muscles to help provide stability to the bony spine. The exercises used rely on a balanced musculature and concentrated effort to relearn proper back motion that will prevent future injury or reinjury (Table 13-1).

Flexibility exercises are an important component of the treatment for back dysfunction. Inflexible paraspinal muscles, hamstrings, piriformis muscles, and others may predispose to back dysfunction and must be addressed.

### Medications and Injections

Medications used for back and thoracic pathology are basically the same as for other musculoskeletal disorders. Nonsteroidal antiinflammatory drugs (NSAIDs) are a mainstay of treatment. When necessary, usually after traumatic injury, more powerful analgesics may be necessary for brief periods of time. Some so-called muscle relaxants (see Chapter 5) may be used to reduce pain and anxiety. They are also to be used only for short periods of time. In more chronic states, tricyclic antidepressants or anticonvulsants may be necessary (see Chapter 5). Tricyclic antidepressants are also used to treat sleep disturbances that often accompany pain.

Steroid medications are also sometimes useful in treating various disorders of the back. In facet arthropathy, steroid-anesthetic joint injection, under fluoroscopic x-ray guidance, can be both a diagnostic and a therapeutic procedure. In acute radiculopathy or nerve root irritation, oral steroids or epidural steroid injection are also helpful in relieving symptoms.[13]

### Back School

Education is the key to understanding and preventing recurrence of low back strain. Back schools were introduced in the 1960s in Sweden to provide education to factory workers on proper body mechanics and prevention of injury. Today, back school curricula range from strictly therapist guided exercises to multifaceted classroom education, exercise prescription, mobilization, and daily posture assessment. They are an important component of the treatment of back pain.

### Pain Clinics/Work Hardening/ Functional Restoration

A complete discussion of treatment of chronic back pain is beyond the scope of this chapter. Suffice it to say that pain clinics, work hardening, or functional restoration programs[14] have been shown to help some persons with chronic pain (usually low back pain). When referring a patient to such a program it is important to steer away from the patient-passive type treatments that emphasize injections and medications. While injections and medications may be useful adjuncts to treatment, chronic pain patients must be taught to take charge of their own bodies with a program that includes exercise, relaxation training, and a change in outlook. Patients must realize that while

**Table 13-1.** Dynamic Lumbar Muscular Stabilization Program

PROGRAM DESCRIPTION

**Treatment Phases**

1. Pain control
   a. Back first aid
   b. Trial extension exercises
   c. Trial of traction
   d. Basic stabilization exercise training
   e. NSAIDs
   f. Non-narcotic analgesics
   g. Corticosteroids
      (1) Oral
      (2) Epidural injection
      (3) Selective nerve root injection
      (4) Facet injection
2. Exercise training
   a. Soft-tissue flexibility
      (1) Hamstring musculotendinous unit
      (2) Quadriceps musculotendinous unit
      (3) Iliopsoas musculotendinous unit
      (4) Gastrocsoleus musculotendinous unit
      (5) External and internal hip rotators
   b. Joint mobility
      (1) Lumbar spine segmental mobility
      (2) Hip range of motion
      (3) Thoracic segmental mobility
   c. Stabilization program
      (1) Finding neutral position (standing, sitting)
      (2) Prone gluteal squeezes
      (3) Supine pelvic bracing
      (4) Bridging progression
         (a) Basic position
         (b) One leg raised
         (c) Stepping
         (d) Balance on gym ball
      (5) Quadruped
         (a) With alternating arm and leg movements (ankle and wrist weights are used during the progression)
      (6) Kneeling stabilization
         (a) Double knee
         (b) Single knee
         (c) Lunges (hand held weights added during the progression)
      (7) Wall slide quadriceps strengthening
      (8) Position transition with postural control
   d. Abdominal program
      (1) Curl-ups
      (2) Dead bugs
      (3) Diagonal curl-ups
      (4) Diagonal curl-ups on incline board
      (5) Straight leg lowering
   e. Gym program
      (1) Latissimus pull-downs
      (2) Angled leg press
      (3) Lunges
      (4) Hyperextension bench
      (5) General upper body weight exercises
      (6) Pulley exercises to stress postural control
   f. Aerobic program
      (1) Progressive walking
      (2) Swimming
      (3) Stationary bicycling
      (4) Cross-country ski machine
      (5) Running
         (a) Initially supervised on a treadmill

(Saal JA: Intervertebral disc herniation: Advances in non-operative treatment. *PM&R: State of the Art Reviews* Philadelphia: Hanley & Belfus, 1990;4:187–188. Reprinted with permission.)

they may never completely be free of pain, they can certainly keep it from dominating and poisoning every aspect of their lives.

## Examination and Testing Techniques

### History and Physical Examination of the Chest Wall

As with any acute or chronic injury, a good history of the chief complaint is essential. Musculoskeletal disorders localized to the chest need to be distinguished from visceral abnormalities causing re-ferred pain or viscerosomatic response. Physical examination should always begin with observation. Inspection of the chest wall should assess the ribs, clavicles, and scapulae at rest and during breathing.

The next step in the examination is palpation. Gentle "springing" pressure is applied at each costosternal junction, noting any pain or audible popping. Segmental examination of the rib cage is performed with the patient supine. The examiner stands at the head of the table and rests his or her hands on the anterior chest wall with the fingertips pointing toward the sternum. It is important to evaluate the ribs during inspiration and expiration to detect any asymmetries.

*History and Physical Examination
of the Back and Spine*

In evaluating disorders of the back and spine it is most important to differentiate neurogenic from nonneurogenic causes. The overwhelming majority of low-back pain patients have nonspecific myofascial or ligamentous injury; however, HNP with radiculopathy, stenosis, or other neurogenic injuries must be ruled out.

The examiner begins with a complete history of the complaint. Specific questions include when and how the problem began. Does the pain radiate from the back into the buttock or legs? What positions make the pain worse (pain which is worse when lying down may be a sign of an intraspinal tumor)? Is the pain aggravated by coughing, sneezing, or straining to have a bowel movement (signs of herniated disk)? Patients with significant psychological components to their disorder report their history either extremely vaguely or in excruciating detail. They may report that "everything hurts," that no position alleviates the pain, or they may report symptoms of a patently nonphysiologic and nonanatomic nature (see Chapters 25 and 28).

Observation proceeds with an examination of the general posture and the curves of the spine. Gait should be observed to assess the fluidity of segmental spinal motion. Range of motion of the back in flexion, extension, rotation, and side bending should be observed and any asymmetries or abnormalities noted (see Hoppenfeld[15] for normal values). If bending forward (in a patient with a complaint of leg pain) causes the patient to bend the knee on the side of the pain, it may be a sign of nerve root compression.[16] A full neurologic examination, including deep tendon (muscle stretch) reflexes, sensory, motor strength, and coordination testing must be performed. Leg length should be measured if there is a suspicion of inequality of length (see Chapter 17 for proper technique).

The back, spine, and buttock must be palpated to detect any abnormalities. The feel of pressing on the individual spinal segments (spinous processes) may reveal areas of abnormal hypermobility, hypomobility, a step-off, spina bifida, or pain.

In addition to this general evaluation, a number of specific testing techniques deserve mention and are presented. Since the sacroiliac joint and pelvis are intimately associated with the low back, the reader is also encouraged to review Chapter 17.

**Straight Leg Raising.**    When the hip is flexed with the knee held in extension, the lumbosacral nerve roots are stretched. Ordinarily there is enough "slack" in the nerves to allow this stretch to be applied without causing any symptoms, but in conditions of nerve root compression, usually due to HNP, the stretching of the nerve roots causes pain to shoot down the leg.[17] This is the straight leg raise (SLR) test.

The patient is asked to lie supine while the examiner passively raises the leg. Pain radiating down the leg is a positive finding, but pain localized to the low back is not. When performing this test, the spinal nerve roots start to be stretched between 20 and 30 degrees of leg flexion. If the patient complains of pain with less than this amount of flexion, it should raise concerns of exaggeration or fabrication. Pain at greater than 60 to 70 degrees of flexion is not as helpful since it may be due to stretching of the hamstrings.

One way to double check the patient's veracity is to perform the straight leg raise while the patient is sitting. This can be incorporated into the muscle strength testing part of the examination without the patient's realizing what is actually being tested. A positive supine test should correlate with a positive sitting test; however, care must be taken to make sure the patient sits straight. Often a person with true nerve root tension slouches to lessen the pain.

Sometimes patients complain of pain shooting down the leg when the contralateral leg is raised. This is called the well-leg SLR (Fajersztajn) test, or cross-leg pain, and if positive, it is also a sign of nerve root tension or compression.

**Passive/Active Back Extension Testing.**    The prone patient is asked to lift the chin and chest off the table. This is an active test of the paraspinal muscles, and pain during this maneuver is a sign of muscle strain. The patient is next asked to prop up on the elbows and allow the back to sag. In conditions of muscle strain this will be painless; however, in facet joint disorders or nerve root compression pain may worsen.

**Cat/Camel Exercises.**    While propped on hands and knees the patient is told to push the back up toward the ceiling and then to let it sag toward the table. This tests whether or not flexion or extension of the back worsens or lessens symptoms and may help in deciding which form of exercise (flexion versus extension) should be prescribed.

**Rectal Examination.**    This test is often performed in patients with back or pelvic pain of insidious onset. It may identify tumors or an enlarged prostate in some cases. It also allows palpation of the undersurface of the piriformis muscle.

**Testing Segmental Mobility.**    When palpating the spinous processes it is useful to apply a firm pressure to evaluate the feel of the individual spinal segments. With practice an examiner can appreciate areas of hypermobility or hypomobility. In hypermobile segments which are painful to palpation the patient is asked to isometrically tighten the paraspinal muscles. If this contraction reduces the pain on palpation it is a sign of an unstable segment.

**Waddell Criteria.**    Assessment of low back pain can be frustrating and confusing when dealing with a patient suspected of having psychological overlay to the physical dysfunction. Waddell et al.[18] have described a simple series of tests to help identify those low back pain patients who have significant nonorganic signs (Table 13-2). Objective recognition of these signs can help to identify patients who may require formal psychosocial evaluation or who are malingerers.

### Ancillary Diagnostic Testing

In an acute injury where there is a possibility of spinal fracture or subluxation, x-ray studies should be obtained. They are also valuable in other conditions to evaluate bony alignment and segmental instability, signs of degeneration, and congenital anomalies. The anteroposterior (AP) view gives a general measure of bony alignment. Lateral views reveal additional information about the state of the disks, the facet joint, and the bony alignment. Oblique views are used to visualize the intervertebral foramina and the pars interarticularis (bone between the superior and inferior zygapophyseal processes). Flexion/extension or side-bending views may help to detect areas of abnormal spinal mobility.

Other radiologic tests that can be performed are computerized tomography (CT) and magnetic resonance imaging (MRI). CT testing gives the best information to assess the bones, and reveals most fractures, joint disease, and spinal masses. Herniated disks are also well visualized. Myelography gives information about spinal cord or root compression or avulsion. It can be combined with CT to be an even more exact diagnostic tool. MRI is mainly used to visualize soft tissues and is the best test to assess HNP and some spinal cord tumors.

Other tests that can be helpful are electromyography (EMG) to detect radiculopathy, and bone scanning to detect stress fractures, bone tumors, and

**Table 13-2.** Waddell's Nonorganic Physical Signs

| |
|---|
| **If three or more of the five categories are positive it is a sign of significant psychological dysfunction or malingering.** |

**Nonorganic tenderness**
   Superficial-skin tenderness to light touch over a wide area of lumbar skin not corresponding to a single dermatome
   *or,*
   Nonanatomic, deep tenderness over a wide area not localized to any particular structure are positive findings.
**Simulation tests**
   If axial loading (on the head) or rotation of the whole body (not the lumbar spine) causes low back pain it is a positive finding.
**Distraction testing**
   If sitting straight leg raise test is negative while supine straight leg raising causes pain, it is a positive finding.
**Regional pain complaints**
   If whole regions of the body, such as the entire leg, are affected in a nonphysiologic manner, it is a positive finding. This includes sensory or motor deficits.
**Overreaction**
   Excessive grimacing, tremor, collapsing, or complaining during the examination is a positive finding.

*Source:* Waddell G., et al.: *Spine* 1980;4:242–250.

infection. Discography involves the injection of saline or radiopaque dye into the disk to see if there is leakage of dye out of a damaged disk or if the injection reproduces pain. It is an invasive test that damages annular fibers in the process and is rarely needed. Laboratory tests help detect connective tissue disease and infection.

## Diagnosis and Treatment of Specific Disorders of the Chest

### Rib Fractures

Fractures of the ribs are usually a result of direct trauma, but in the osteopenic female or in a patient with bone disease they can occasionally occur from sneezing or coughing.

### Diagnosis

Patients complain of localized tenderness or a feeling of being unable to "catch their breath." They have pain on inspiration. Radiographic examination reveals the bony defect.

### Treatment

Healing of the fracture is accomplished by the laying down of new bone and may take 6 to 8 weeks to complete if the fracture is nondisplaced. Analgesics are usually necessary. The use of an abdominal binder for support has questionable benefit as it can limit full inspiration and may cause pulmonary atelectasis. While the rib is healing, it is important to maintain shoulder range of motion to prevent adhesive capsulitis from forming (see Chapter 14).

### Costochondritis

Costochondritis is manifested by painful swelling at one or more of the costosternal articulations. The condition may mimic cardiac pain and some connective tissue disease.

### Diagnosis

The condition is diagnosed by palpation, which reproduces the patient's pain complaints.

### Treatment

Ice massage, NSAIDs, and rest are prescribed in the acute stage. Local steroid injection may help relieve pain and inflammation in chronic cases.

## Diagnosis and Treatment of Specific Disorders of the Back and Spine

### Acute Back Strain/Sprain

This is by far the most common condition of the back. It is usually attributed to a single incident, such as lifting a heavy object while twisting, but the underlying cause is usually a lifetime of improper back motion. The structures that may be injured include the paraspinal muscles, the intervertebral ligaments, the iliolumbar ligaments, the facet joint capsules, or even the annular fibers of the intervertebral disks. Once the injury has occurred the muscles of the low back splint the damaged area in what is commonly called muscle guarding or a back "spasm." This may cause a "listing" of the patient's posture and a functional scoliosis. In time, if the painful muscle splinting and improper posture persist, the patient develops local soft tissue contracture and chronic or recurrent back pain.

It must be remembered that despite the fact that we may not be able to identify its cause in every individual case, low back pain is a symptom and not a diagnosis. In the past it was felt that most cases of low back pain were caused by injury to the intervertebral disk. This led to treating low back pain with prolonged bed rest which was felt to facilitate healing of the disk. We are now hampered by this legacy of treatment. It is now known that prolonged bed rest is contraindicated in the treatment of acute back strain, yet many patients and physicians are still hesitant to proceed with active exercise. There is no reason why we should not aggressively rehabilitate back injury the same way we rehabilitate ankle sprains or other musculoskeletal disorders.

Back strain occurs most in persons 30 to 60 years old, and it appears to have a higher incidence in poorly conditioned persons[19] and in those with poor back extensor muscle endurance.[20] It is also commonly felt to be more prevalent in persons with poor flexibility, coordination, posture, and muscle strength, although a direct cause-and-effect of these factors has not been proved. It has been associated with certain physical activities, mainly lifting, bending, twisting, and truck driving.[21]

### Diagnosis

The patient with back strain or sprain usually relays a history of acute back pain associated with lifting or bending. Often the back is injured when performing unaccustomed activity such as shoveling the first snow or raking leaves. The pain may be minor the day of injury, but the patient may wake up the following day with severe discomfort. Movement is generally restricted in all directions due to pain.

On physical examination the patient may have an antalgic gait, resists quick movements, and resists extremes of range of motion and muscle strength testing due to pain. Neurologic testing is normal. Straight leg raising is negative, and other provocative tests (including those in Chapter 17) are normal except for possibly causing local back pain. Radiographic studies are normal as well.

### Treatment

Acute strains and sprains generally recover within a few days to a week, regardless of treatment. A few days of rest, ice (and later ice or heat), and NSAIDs, followed by a gradual return to activity is most often successful. Sometimes a "muscle relaxant" is also helpful in the early period, especially when prescribed as a single bedtime dose to help the patient get a restful night's sleep. To prevent recurrence of the problem, the patient should be taught proper back motion and lifting technique. Flexibility and strength deficits also need to be addressed, and proper sitting and work-station posture should be taught. As a rule, a vigorous strengthening program should be deferred for about 6 weeks after injury to allow the damaged tissues to heal properly. Less vigorous activity is encouraged prior to this time.

If the back symptoms persist for a longer period of time than expected, it may be necessary to prescribe a more aggressive treatment protocol. Deep heat, soft tissue mobilization, and muscle relaxation techniques are advised. The patient should work with a back therapist to correct posture and back biomechanics and should be started on a progressive stretching and strengthening program. Patients should be reminded that activity is not harmful and that it does not necessarily worsen pain. Exercise can decrease pain, illness behavior, and distress, and will improve function. It may stimulate the release of endogenous opiates to reduce pain perception.[22] Occasionally a lumbosacral corset is helpful, but it should be used only for a brief predetermined period of time to avoid dependency. Shoe inserts may also be used to decrease the force of impact on the spine during walking.[23]

### Acute Disk Herniation

When the annulus fibrosus of the disk develops a defect, the inner nucleus pulposus may protrude outward. This can occur with a traumatic event, such as a fall on the buttocks, but most often the annular tears develop slowly from a lifetime of repetitive trauma. Then one day an acute herniation occurs due to a minor event, or no event at all.

Disk herniation by itself is painful (possibly due to chemical and not mechanical effects),[24] but when the disk protrudes far enough to mechanically compress a nerve root it causes radiculopathy. Chemical release of the inflammatory components of herniation may also cause nerve root irritation and symptoms of radiculopathy.[25] The radiculopathy can cause pain to radiate into the buttock and leg and may cause sensory, motor strength, or reflex changes in the leg as well. The local disk problem causes low back pain.

### Diagnosis

Disk herniation is suspected when the patient complains of both back and leg pain arising over the course of a few hours. Usually there are sensory, reflex, or motor changes in the extremity. The straight leg raising test should be positive. The patient presents with a resistance to movement of the back and associated painful paraspinal muscle splinting. Coughing, sneezing, or straining to have a bowel movement (or any other maneuver that raises intraabdominal and therefore intradiskal pressure) often reproduces the leg pain.

Definitive diagnosis of radiculopathy is made with electromyographic (EMG) testing, while the mechanical disk protrusion can be demonstrated by CT, MRI, or myelography. MRI is the best of these tests if a disk herniation is suspected. When obtaining radiographic confirmation of a herniation, one often receives reports of "bulging" disks. This is not the same thing as a herniation, is not clinically significant, and patients should not be made to worry needlessly about such bulges.

*Treatment*

Almost all herniated disks can be treated conservatively. Treatment is aimed at reducing the intradiskal pressure to prevent a progression of the herniation until the annular tear heals (6 to 8 weeks).

An acute herniation is commonly treated with 5 to 7 days of strict bed rest (except for toilet privileges), analgesia, and local heat to reduce paraspinal muscle pain. Some advocate no bed rest at all, just avoidance of exacerbating activity.[9] "Muscle relaxants" (see Chapter 5) may be prescribed and a lumbosacral corset is sometimes useful. Back flexion is avoided. Any position that raises intradiskal pressure, such as sitting, is avoided. The position of least pressure is supine with the hips and knees flexed. This position also reduces dural tension.

Stool softeners, fluids, and a high fiber diet make it easier to have bowel movements with less straining, which is another cause of increased disk pressure.

A trial of gentle extension exercises may help to reduce symptoms.[9] If it worsens the symptoms, it should be avoided.

Epidural steroid injection or oral steroids should be considered in treatment. They reduce the swelling and inflammation around the nerve root and may hasten recovery.

Traction may be tried in treatment as well. Its benefits are not well documented and it may not be well tolerated, but in some patients it seems to be effective.

After the acute painful period has passed, the patient should start a slowly progressive program of return to activity. Prolonged sitting, excessive back flexion, lifting, bending, and twisting should be avoided for 6 to 8 weeks.

After this initial treatment time, proper back mechanics are taught, strengthening exercises are begun (starting with isometrics and stabilization exercises), and the patient gradually returns to a normal life.

Almost all patients respond to a program as outlined here. One exception is those with herniated nucleus pulposus associated with concomitant lateral stenosis.[9] The presence of such stenosis is not an absolute indication for surgery, but it reduces the success rate for conservative care from around 90% to the 65% to 75% range.[26] Saal feels that if patients have not responded to conservative care by 8 weeks they should be given the option to proceed to surgery.[26] They should be advised that they have not yet "failed" conservative care, just that they are slow responders. It would still be appropriate to continue conservative care, although resolution of symptoms might be faster with surgery. Long-term outcome is probably unchanged, even if surgery is postponed for 3 months.[2]

Other considerations for surgery are persons with central disk herniation with myelopathy (mainly thoracic), persons with intractable pain, and those with progressive neurologic deficits. Patients should always be asked what their worst pain complaint is; back or leg pain. If back pain is the answer then surgery is probably not the cure. Surgery may alleviate leg pain, but it is not as useful for back pain.

*Degenerative Joint Disease (Spondylosis)*

Degenerative joint disease (DJD) (Figure 13-7) occurs in the spine just as it does in many other parts of the body. The cause is unknown but may involve aging, overuse, trauma, or genetic predisposition. As the degeneration takes place the anterior weight-bearing portion of the spine narrows, which causes the facet joints to come closer together and shift on one another. The shear force on these tissues causes capsular thickening and cartilage degeneration. A continuum of the degenerative process leads to spur formation at the posterior vertebral bodies and may lead to narrowing of the intervertebral foramina (lateral stenosis) and radiculopathy or narrowing of the spinal canal (central stenosis).

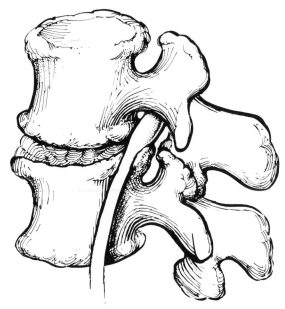

**Figure 13-7.** Degenerative disease of the spine, involving bony spurring, disk space narrowing, and foraminal encroachment.

Kirkaldy-Willis describes a continuum of back degeneration.[27] First is dysfunction, which may be associated with low back strain and sprain. Next comes instability, which often causes back pain or herniated disk. Lastly comes the stabilization phase in which disk space narrowing and bony spurring lead to a stable but relatively immobile spine. It is this last phase that is associated with lateral and central stenosis.

### Diagnosis

The symptoms of DJD include nonspecific complaints of back pain, often exacerbated by extension and relieved by moderate activity. The condition usually has an insidious onset with increased prevalence associated with advancing age. Patients complain of morning stiffness, have decreased back range of motion, and have pain on the extremes of their range. These patients may have unstable spinal segments that are tender to palpation. Isometric muscle splinting relieves the tenderness as it prevents the abnormal motion. In advanced cases x-ray studies show signs of disk space narrowing, facet degeneration, and bony spurring. If radiculopathy is present, it can be studied with EMG.

### Treatment

Since DJD is not generally reversible, patients often have a series of recurring flare-ups of their back pain. These exacerbations become less frequent and less severe with aging as the spine stabilizes. Treatment is aimed at alleviating pain and maintaining mobility.

Acute exacerbations are treated with rest, heat, and NSAIDs. This is followed by a maintenance program of gentle strengthening, flexibility, and aerobic exercises, and back school.

### Spinal Stenosis

When DJD causes sufficient narrowing of the spinal canal, especially in a congenitally narrow canal, it can compress the nerve roots and other contents of the canal. The compression of the spinal contents can cause symptoms of leg pain, numbness, and weakness which are brought on or worsened by spine extension. These patients often complain of pain when walking or standing. This condition is often confused with intermittent claudication, a condition of poor arterial blood supply to the legs which causes ischemic leg pain with exercise. The symptoms of stenosis, sometimes called pseudoclaudication, are due to position,[28] not exercise. Thus, rest does not relieve symptoms (as it does in vascular claudication) unless the patient also sits or squats or somehow flexes the back. Such patients often tolerate bicycling better than walking, because bicycling is done with a flexed back.

Because of the spinal bony narrowing, a multilevel radiculopathy is not uncommon in stenosis. Lateral stenosis may accompany HNP.

### Diagnosis

The characteristic history of symptoms as described helps in making the diagnosis. These patients often have signs of radiculopathy with mild reflex, sensory, or motor changes as well. X-ray findings, CT, or myelography reveals the spinal narrowing, while EMG can help detect the nerve damage.

## Treatment

Strengthening flexion exercises can often keep symptoms of pseudoclaudication tolerable. Patients also benefit from using NSAIDs, a cane or walker, and soft shoe inserts. In some cases, if symptoms are limiting enough, a surgical decompression of the spinal canal is necessary.[29]

## Spondylolisthesis

Spondylolysis is a defect of the pars interarticularis of the arch of the vertebrae. As such, it involves a break in the bony circle around the spinal canal and may allow the upper vertebra to slip forward on the lower one, a condition known as spondylolisthesis.

Spondylolysis is not present at birth. At age 6 it has a prevalence of 4.4% and in adults is seen in 6% of the population. It occurs twice as often in males as in females.[30] The spondylolysis in children is not usually associated with pain or spondylolisthesis. It occurs more frequently in children with spina bifida occulta and appears to be passed on genetically.[30]

Spondylolisthesis may be due to a number of causes, including congenital deformity, degeneration, trauma, pathologic bone disease, or pars interarticularis defect as just described (called isthmic spondylolisthesis).[31] It most commonly occurs at the L5–S1 junction and less frequently at L4–L5.

Isthmic spondylolytic spondylolisthesis is due to a bony stress fracture. It is usually asymptomatic, except in some athletes who repetitively engage in lumbar hyperextension (gymnasts and football linemen). The severity of the condition is classified according to the degree of displacement of the superior vertebral body on the inferior one. Grade I is a displacement of less than 25% of the diameter of the vertebral body. Grade II is a 26% to 50% displacement. Grade III is a 51% to 75% displacement, and Grade IV is a displacement of greater than 75%. Patients with symptomatic spondylolisthesis complain of low back pain and possible sciatica. This may not be associated with trauma although exacerbation is possible following a traumatic incident involving the lumbar spine and pelvis. The forward slippage is caused by the anterior shear forces present at the L5–S1 interface.

A defect in the posterior element of the spine allows forward motion of the body of the superior vertebra, a narrowing of the intervertebral foramina, and a traction on the spinal nerve roots.

## Diagnosis

This condition is diagnosed by x-ray study or CT, which shows a displacement of the vertebra and a disruption of the bony vertebral arch. Sometimes a step-off can be palpated from one vertebral spinous process to the next, and this may raise the suspicion that a spondylolisthesis is present.

In young athletes with stress fractures of the pars interarticularis, a bone scan is the earliest way to detect the defect.

In patients with degenerative spondylolisthesis, symptoms of back pain are more likely due to their underlying DJD rather than to the vertebral arch disruption.

## Treatment

Grade I or II slippages often cause no symptoms, and since persons with such displacement may have back and pelvic pain due to other causes, it is important to exclude other sources of pain. Spondylolisthesis also predisposes to developing disk disease above the level of the defect, and this may be the actual source of the symptoms. Asymptomatic individuals need no treatment; however, they might well be advised not to engage in activities that require forceful back extension or excessively jarring motion (especially in adolescents who are not yet skeletally mature).

Symptomatic Grade I or II slippages may be treated with weight loss, flexion exercise,[32] rest, proper posture, possibly a lumbar orthosis, and avoidance of jarring motions and excessive back extension. The conservative approach involves remaining physically fit with specific exercises to stabilize the lumbar spine. High-risk activity is again avoided.

Surgery is indicated for symptomatic individuals with grade III or higher slippage and in those with progressive neurologic deficit, a worsening deficit, or severe pain.

Athletes with symptomatic spondylolisthesis may not be able to return to their sports.

Children with spondylolysis or spondylolisthesis should probably be evaluated with periodic radiographs to make sure that their vertebral displacement is not progressing. If progression is seen, surgery is an option.

### Facet Syndrome

There appears to be a subset of low back pain patients who have primary facet joint pathology. These patients often complain of a sudden "catch" in their back associated with certain movements or positions. They may respond to rest, NSAIDs, facet joint injection, or manipulation.[33] The attacks are often recurrent.

The patient should be taught a maintenance program of flexion exercises and should be instructed in proper body mechanics.[34]

### Scoliosis

This condition is described in Chapter 21 on Pediatric issues.

### Other Causes of Back Pain

Numerous other conditions may cause or be associated with back and spinal pain. They include Scheuermann's disease (thoracic vertebral wedge fractures in teenage boys), osteoporotic vertebral compression fractures, and spina bifida. In addition, myofascial pain, fibromyalgia, tumors, disk infections, and referred pain syndromes, among others, may cause back pain. Cutaneous nerves from the upper lumbar levels pass over the iliac crest and may be sites of nerve entrapment and pain as well.[35,36]

### Chronic Back Pain/Failed Back Syndrome

It is no surprise that chronic back pain and failed back syndrome are often considered to be synonymous, as a "failed back" is generally considered to be one that has not responded to surgery. Indeed it is hard to find a patient with chronic back pain who has not had back surgery; many have had several operations. This is not to say that surgery necessarily causes all chronic back pain; just that it is not a particularly good treatment for it.

Chronic back pain is the end result of back dysfunction in some individuals who never recover normal function, flexibility, and strength after acute back strain, disk herniation, or surgery. They generally wind up with inflexible spines, excessive muscle splinting, and poor back biomechanics. These patients often become obsessed with their pain, allowing it to dominate their private and working lives.

Once a person has developed chronic back pain it is difficult to treat. Therefore it is important to make sure that acute back patients are not allowed to slip into a passive role where they "protect" their backs from any activity or exercise, where they rely on narcotic analgesia, injections, or indefinite physical therapy, and where the back pain becomes the focus of their existence.

When chronic pain has developed, it must be treated with a multidisciplinary approach to restore mobility and strength, teach relaxation, regain a sense of proportion, and help the patient to regain control over his or her life. Chapters 25 and 28 describe some of the treatment strategies in more detail.

Pain clinics, work hardening, and functional restoration programs may be useful in these patients. They should be referred to a specialist in physical medicine and rehabilitation or other physician dedicated to the restoration of function through exercise.

### Case Report

A 35-year-old man presented with a several-year history of intermittent low back pain. The episodes were usually triggered by performing an unaccustomed activity. His latest episode had started 8 weeks before his visit to the office, and it was by far his worst to date. He complained of inability to sleep, to perform his usual exercise, or to play with his children. He was able to continue his work as an accountant. On physical examination he was completely normal except for asymmetry of the lower lumbar segments on side bending, improper lumbosacral bending rhythm, and inflexibility of the paraspinal muscles. In the office he was taught a few simple back flexibility exercises and was referred to physical therapy for instruction in a more complete flexibility and conditioning program as well as back school. On 1 month followup he reported that after 2 days of stretching, even before physical therapy, his symptoms were nearly completely resolved. He had continued with therapy to learn the rest of his maintenance program. On examination he still had a bit of asymmetry on side bending, but otherwise was moving well. He was advised that he must learn to correct his asymmetry to prevent a future recurrence of pain. While his progress was a bit more dramatic than could routinely be hoped for, he does illustrate what a few simple exercises can do to overcome faulty back motion.

## Points of Summary

1. Acute low back sprain or strain should not be treated with prolonged bed rest.
2. Back schools are an important part of the education process for patients with back pain.
3. Almost all herniated disks, even when they are associated with weakness and neurologic deficits, can be treated without surgery.
4. Surgery involves the cutting of important connective tissues of the back.
5. The subset of patients with herniated disks and lateral stenosis may respond more slowly to conservative care, but do not necessarily require surgical treatment.
6. Positions of back flexion, which increase intradiskal pressure, are avoided in early herniated disk rehabilitation.
7. Degenerative joint disease of the spine causes the insidious onset of low back pain, decreased and painful range of motion, and morning stiffness.
8. Spondylolysis is a defect in the pars interarticularis.
9. Spondylolisthesis is a forward slippage of one vertebra on the one below it.

## References

1. Waddell G: A new clinical model for the treatment of low-back pain. *Spine* 1987;12:632–644.
2. Shvartzman L, Weingarten E, Sherry H, et al.: Cost-effectiveness analysis of extended conservative therapy versus surgical intervention in the management of herniated lumbar intervertebral disc. *Spine* 1992;17:176–182.
3. Bogduk N: The innervation of the lumbar spine. *Spine* 1983;8:286–293.
4. Jenkins DB: *Hollinshead's Functional Anatomy of the Limbs and Back*, 6th ed. Philadelphia: WB Saunders, 1991.
5. Deyo RA, Diehl AK, Rosenthal M: How many days bed rest for acute low back pain? A randomized clinical trial. *N Engl J Med* 1986;315:1064–1070.
6. Kottke FJ, Lehmann JF (eds): *Krusen's Handbook of Physical Medicine and Rehabilitation*, 4th ed. Philadelphia: WB Saunders, 1990.
7. Mixter W, Barr J: Rupture of the intervertebral disk with involvement of the spinal canal. *N Engl J Med* 1934;2:210.
8. Weber H: Lumbar disc herniation: A controlled, prospective study with ten years of observation. *Spine* 1983;8:131–140.
9. Saal JA, Saal JS: The nonoperative treatment of herniated nucleus pulposus with radiculopathy: An outcome study. *Spine* 1989;14:431–437.
10. Saal JA, Saal JS, Herzog RJ: The natural history of lumbar intervertebral disc extrusions treated nonoperatively. *Spine* 1990;15:683–686.
11. Nachemson AL: Disc pressure measurements. *Spine* 1981;6:93–99.
12. Stankovic R, Johnell O: Conservative treatment of acute low-back pain. *Spine* 1990;15:120–123.
13. Benzon HT: Epidural steroid injection for low back pain and lumbosacral radiculopathy. *Pain* 1986;24:277–295.
14. Mayer TG, Gatchel RJ, Mayer H, et al.: A prospective two-year study of functional restoration on industrial low back injury. *JAMA* 1987;13:1763–1767.
15. Hoppenfeld S: *Physical Examination of the Spine and Extremities*. Norwalk, CT: Appleton-Century-Crofts, 1976.
16. Rask M: Knee flexion test and sciatica. *Clin Orthop* 1978;134:221.
17. Breig A, Troup JDG: Biomechanical considerations in the straight-leg-raising test: Cadaveric and clinical studies of the effects of medial hip rotation. *Spine* 1979;4:242–250.
18. Waddell G, McCulloch JA, Kummel E, et al.: Nonorganic physical signs in low-back pain. *Spine* 1980;5:117–124.
19. Cady LD, Bischoff DP, O'Connell ER, et al.: Strength and fitness and subsequent back injuries in firefighters. *J Occup Med* 1979;21:269–272.
20. Biering-Sorenson F: Physical measurements as risk factors for low back trouble over a one year period. *Spine* 1984;9:106–119.
21. Cassidy JD, Wedge JH: The epidemiology and natural history of low back pain and spinal degeneration. In

Kirkaldy-Willis WH (ed): *Managing Low Back Pain*, 2nd ed. New York: Churchill Livingstone, 1988:3–14.

22. Carr DB, Bullen BA, Skrinar GS: Physical conditioning facilitates the exercise-induced secretion of beta-endorphin and beta-lipotrophin in women. *N Engl J Med* 1981;305:560–563.

23. Wosk J, Voloshin AS: Low back pain: Conservative treatment with artificial shock absorbers. *Arch Phys Med Rehabil* 1985;66:145–148.

24. Rosomoff HL: Do herniated disks produce pain? *Clin J Pain* 1985;1:91–93.

25. Saal JS, Franson RC, Dobrow R, et al.: High levels of inflammatory phospholipase $A_2$, activity in lumbar disc herniations. *Spine* 1990;15:674–678.

26. Saal JA: Intervertebral disc herniation: Advances in nonoperative treatment. *Physical Medicine and Rehabilitation: State of the Art Reviews* 1990;175–190.

27. Kirkaldy-Willis WH (ed): *Managing Low Back Pain*, 2nd ed. New York: Churchill Livingstone, 1988.

28. Dyck P: The stoop-test in lumbar entrapment radiculopathy. *Spine* 1979;4:89–92.

29. Turner JA, Ersek M, Herron L et al.: Surgery for lumbar spinal stenosis: Attempted meta-analysis of the literature. *Spine* 1992;17:1–8.

30. Fredrickson BE, Baker D, McHolick WJ, et al.: The natural history of spondylolysis and spondylolisthesis. *J Bone Joint Surg* 1984;66A:699–707.

31. Wiltse LL, Newman PH, MacNab I: Classification of spondylolisis and spondylolisthesis. *Clin Orthop* 1976;117:23–29.

32. Gramse RR, Sinaki M, Ilstrup DM: Lumbar spondylolisthesis: A rational approach to conservative treatment. *Mayo Clin Proc* 1980;55:681–686.

33. Kirkaldy-Willis WH, Hill RJ: A more precise diagnosis for low back pain. *Spine* 1979;4:102–109.

34. Hanson TJ, Merritt JL: Rehabilitation of the patient with lower back pain. In DeLisa JA (ed): *Rehabilitation Medicine: Principles and Practice*. Philadelphia: JB Lippincott, 1988:726–748.

35. Maigne R: Low back pain of thoracolumbar origin. *Arch Phys Med Rehabil* 1980;61:389–395.

36. Maigne JY, Maigne R: Trigger point of the posterior iliac crest: Painful iliolumbar ligament insertion or cutaneous dorsal ramus pain? An anatomic study. *Arch Phys Med Rehabil* 1991;72:734–737.

## Suggested Readings

Cailliet R: *Soft Tissue Pain and Disability*, 2nd ed. Philadelphia: FA Davis, 1988.

Herring SA (ed): Low back pain. *Phys Med Rehabil Clin North Am* 1991;2(1).

Kirkaldy-Willis (ed): *Managing Low Back Pain*, 2nd ed. New York: Churchill Livingstone, 1988.

Saal JA (ed); Neck and back pain. *Physical Medicine and Rehabilitation: State of the Art Reviews* 1990;4(2).

Waddell G: A new clinical model for the treatment of low-back pain. *Spine* 1987;12:632–643.

# Chapter 14
# Shoulder Girdle and Arm

RALPH BUSCHBACHER

The shoulder is the most mobile connecting structure in the body. It moves in several planes with motion occurring at many joints and involving several bones. In a larger sense, it can be thought of as the "shoulder girdle," of which the shoulder proper is just a small part.

## Shoulder and Arm Anatomy

### Bones of the Shoulder (Figure 14-1)

**Scapula.** This triangular bone is split into two sections by the "spine of the scapula." The upper section is the supraspinatus fossa; the lower is the infraspinatus fossa. The inner surface of the scapula is known as the subscapular fossa. All three fossae are sites of muscle attachment. The lateral projection of the spine ends as the acromion or "tip of the shoulder." The lateral angle of the scapula widens into an articulating surface, the glenoid fossa, and projecting anteriorly from the scapula is the coracoid process.

**Clavicle.** This S-shaped bone is convex anteriorly in its medial section and is concave laterally. It provides the only bony attachment of the shoulder and arm to the axial skeleton.

**Humerus.** The humerus is a long bone and has an articulating head superiorly. Anteriorly, the humerus has a prominence known as the lesser tubercle, which is separated from the lateral greater tubercle by the intertubercular groove.

### Joints of the Shoulder

**Glenohumeral Joint.** This is the articulation between the humerus and the scapula. The glenoid fossa has an upward tilt which helps hold the humerus in place without active muscle contraction. The fossa is surrounded by a rim called the glenoid labrum which was once described as a discrete piece of fibrocartilage, but which is now felt to be a fold of the joint capsule.[1] The labrum increases the depth of the joint and increases the surface of articulation, both of which improve the stability of the joint.

To maintain mobility, the glenohumeral joint capsule is relatively loose in all directions. It does, however, have some areas that are reinforced for stability. Superiorly, it is reinforced by the coracohumeral ligament, and anteriorly, it has three thickened areas known as the superior, middle, and inferior glenohumeral ligaments.

**Acromioclavicular Joint.** This is a plane joint which is strengthened by the superior and inferior acromioclavicular ligaments. More importantly, the clavicle is kept in place in relation to the acromion by the coracoclavicular ligament (Figure 14-2).

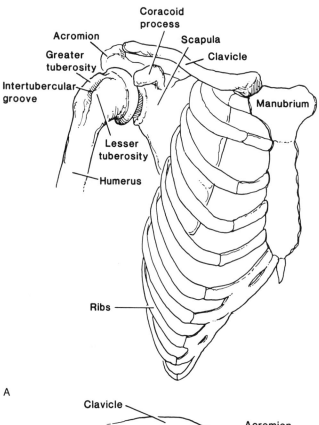

Coracoid
process

Acromion

Scapula

Greater
tuberosity

Clavicle

Intertubercular
groove

Manubrium

Lesser
tuberosity

Humerus

Ribs

A

**Figure 14-1.** Anterior bones (*A*) and posterior bones (*B*) of the shoulder girdle.

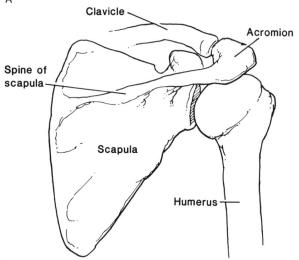

Clavicle

Acromion

Spine of
scapula

Scapula

Humerus

B

**Scapulothoracic Joint.** This is a gliding joint between the scapula and the thoracic wall. It is lubricated by a bursa at its inferomedial pole.

**Other Joints.** Other joints involved to a lesser extent in shoulder motion are the sternoclavicular, costovertebral, sternocostal, and vertebral joints.

*Muscles of the Shoulder (Figure 14-3)*

The muscles of the shoulder can be divided into intrinsic and extrinsic muscles (Table 14-1). The intrinsic muscles arise on and insert on the shoulder girdle. Four of the intrinsic muscles, the supraspinatus, infraspinatus, subscapularis, and teres minor are collectively known as the rotator

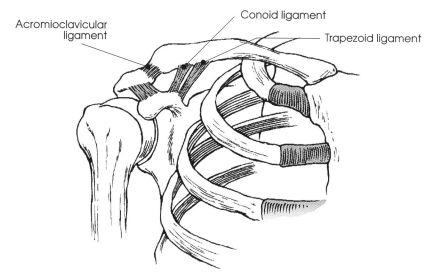

**Figure 14-2.** The supporting ligaments of the acromioclavicular joint.

cuff. They surround the glenohumeral joint. In addition to performing specific actions, the rotator cuff, as a group, serves two main purposes:

Depression of the humeral head to prevent upward migration of the humerus.
Centering of the humeral head in the glenoid fossa during motion.

In addition, the supraspinatus is important in the initiation of abduction.

The rotator cuff tendons contain areas of relative avascularity. This predisposes them, especially the supraspinatus, to injury. When in the recumbent position this area becomes hyperemic, which explains the common finding of night pain when this area is injured.

### Other Important Structures of the Shoulder

**Coracoacromial Arch.**    (Figure 14-4). This arch is formed by the acromion, the coracoid process, the coracoacromial ligament, and the scapula below. It contains the supraspinatus, subacromial (subdeltoid) bursa, the tendon of the long head of the biceps, and the coracohumeral ligament. It protects the enclosed structures as well as the humeral head below, but since it has a fixed volume, it is subject to problems that increase the pressure within the arch. Any condition that causes inflammation, edema, or bleeding can result in such a pressure increase.

**Brachial Plexus.**    The brachial plexus (see Chapter 2) is a group of interconnecting nerves that emerges from the neck. It passes between the clavicle and first rib to reach the axilla where it forms the great nerves of the arm.

**Bursae.**    The subacromial (subdeltoid) bursa (Figure 14-5) lies between the rotator cuff and the coracoacromial arch and deltoid muscle. It does

**Table 14-1.** Muscles of the Shoulder

| **Intrinsic Shoulder Muscles** | |
| --- | --- |
| Supraspinatus | |
| Infraspinatus | |
| Teres minor | Rotator cuff |
| Subscapularis | |
| Teres major | |
| Deltoid | |
| Coracobrachialis | |

| **Extrinsic Shoulder Muscles** |
| --- |
| Pectoralis major |
| Pectoralis minor |
| Sternocleidomastoid |
| Trapezius |
| Levator scapulae |
| Latissimus dorsi |
| Rhomboid major |
| Rhomboid minor |
| Serratus anterior |
| Biceps |
| Triceps |

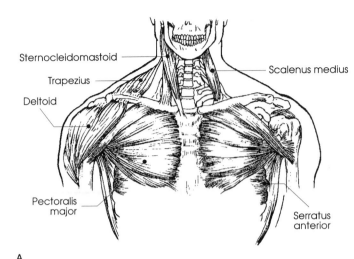

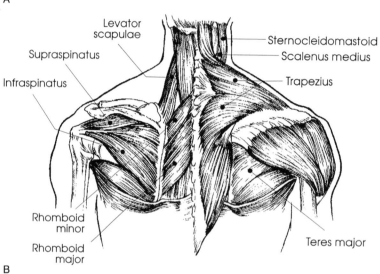

**Figure 14-3.** The shoulder girdle muscles: *A,* Anterior view (*left:* superficial; *right:* deep). *B,* Posterior view (*right:* superficial, *left:* deep).

not normally communicate with the glenohumeral joint cavity. The scapulothoracic bursa lies between the inferomedial angle of the scapula and the chest wall.

### Glenohumeral and Scapulothoracic Motion

Ordinarily scapulothoracic motion complements glenohumeral motion in what Codman described as the "scapulohumeral rhythm."[2] During abduction the scapula rotates 1 degree for every 2 degrees of glenohumeral motion. When assessing shoulder motion, the exact ratio of motion is unimportant. What is important is that the motion is smooth and symmetric on both

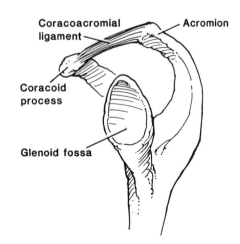

**Figure 14-4.** The coracoacromial arch, a lateral view.

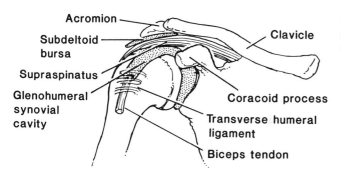

**Figure 14-5.** The glenohumeral synovial cavity and subdeltoid (subacromial) bursa in an anterior shoulder view.

sides. Scapular movement keeps the deltoid operating near its maximal power length and therefore it is sorely missed when defective. The humerus can be fully abducted only when it is rotated externally.

At rest the humeral head is kept from drifting downward by the upward angle of the glenoid fossa and by the coracohumeral ligament, which is taut in this position. In conditions of motor weakness in which the scapula is allowed to rotate downward, the shoulder may subluxate.

**Rehabilitative Approach**

As described in Chapter 4, the rehabilitation of disorders of the shoulder, as well as of other parts of the body, can be divided into four overlapping phases.

Phase I involves the control of pain and inflammation. In the acute stage of Phase I this is done with ice, rest, and in overuse syndromes with nonsteroidal antiinflammatory agents (NSAIDs). Ice can be applied for 20 minutes three times a day for 1 to 2 days.

In the subacute stage, superficial heat, ice, or alternating heat and ice may be used. Again 20 to 30 minutes three times a day for the next few days to a week is most often sufficient. Occasionally ultrasound treatment is helpful.

Immobilization is usually avoided except in conditions of acute injury, usually joint dislocation. The shoulder is particularly susceptible to complications of immobility; thus relative rest from exacerbating activities is preferred if feasible. For most conditions, overhead activities are curtailed.

During early treatment of a shoulder disorder the rest of the body should not be allowed to deteriorate. General aerobic conditioning is easily maintained with an exercise bicycle. Flexibility of the healthy body parts should be maintained, and atrophy of the muscles distal to the injured shoulder is prevented with isometrics. The hand can be exercised with putty or a tennis ball for grip. Wrist and elbow isometrics contracting against the good arm are started as soon as pain allows. Five to ten contractions are performed at two-thirds maximal effort. They are held for 6 seconds, with 2 to 3 seconds of relaxation between contractions. This sequence is repeated twice a day.

Phase I usually lasts 1 to 3 weeks, possibly up to 6 weeks in some cases. It is similar after surgery but is usually a bit longer, averaging around 6 weeks.

Phase II is started after pain and inflammation have subsided. The goal of this phase is to provide full painless range of motion to the shoulder. When beginning this phase, first it is important not to lose the gains made in phase I. Pain and inflammation are controlled and general conditioning is maintained. Added to this is a flexibility program. Flexibility is best improved or maintained with several short stretching sessions a day rather than one long one. Heat or ice application may be used prior to stretching depending on the patient's preference. NSAIDs before stretching may prevent recurrence of inflammation as well as reduce pain and secondary muscle splinting. Good stretching should cause some discomfort, but it should not be pushed to test the patient's pain tolerance. Toward the end of a stretching session heat may again be applied to the shoulder. Then the stretch is held while the shoulder cools down. This type of stretching has been shown to increase flexibility with minimal weakening of the soft tissues for the best long-lasting results.[3] Deep heat such as ultrasound is preferred.

If the shoulder was immobilized during phase I with a sling, then early in phase II the sling should be removed only for the exercise sessions. One to two weeks later it can be discarded altogether.

The flexibility program is begun with warm-up Codman (pendulum) exercises (Figure 14-6). These are performed forward and back, side to side, and clockwise and counterclockwise, using the body motion to swing the arm passively. The patient must be counseled to do these exercises without active shoulder movement.

When tolerated, active assistive ROM exercises are begun using either a therapist or the good arm for assistance. Movement is started in the directions of flexion, extension, adduction, abduction, internal rotation, external rotation, and total elevation (in the scapular plane). As the patient progresses, diagonal and more functional movements are performed, and the patient progresses to more vigorous stretching. When either the glenohumeral or the scapulothoracic joints are relatively inflexible, it is often useful for a therapist to help with the early stretching program. Patients, if left to themselves, will often end up stretching the parts or joint that is already flexible, while the tight areas get even tighter.

The goal of stretching is to achieve equality of range of motion (ROM) with the good side. In some cases, such as in anterior instability, 10 to 15 degrees' less excursion (in external rotation in this instance) is acceptable to help prevent reinjury.

The methods of stretching the various shoulder structures are nearly infinite. It is best to stick with

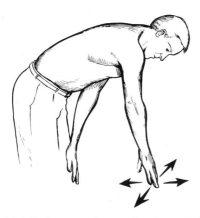

**Figure 14-6.** Codman exercises are done by passively swinging the arm using body motion. Forward and back, side to side, and circular motions are performed. (Lillegard WA, Rucker KS: *Handbook of Sports Medicine.* Stoneham, MA: Andover Medical Publishers, 1993. Reprinted by permission.)

a few simple easy stretches using the simplest devices to ensure patient compliance. Door frames are a ubiquitous simple stretching machine. So are corners, walls, and doorknobs. The shoulder protractors are stretched by leaning into a corner (Figure 14-7A). The internal rotators are stretched using a door frame or doorknob. Walls can be used for finger climbing exercises (Figure 14-7B) (there are also special wall mounted gadgets for this). Shoulder shrugs and slow punching movements from the supine position are good scapular mobilization exercises. In addition, a short wand (Figure 14-7C) can be used to push the arm into external rotation with the good hand. Wand exercises are also used for total elevation stretching. Reciprocating pulley exercises are also useful, but must be done slowly and gently and should be discontinued if they worsen symptoms.

The stretching program is probably the most critical phase of shoulder rehabilitation. More than any other joint, the shoulder is prone to losing mobility quickly. Any such loss takes an inordinate amount of time and effort to recoup.

Isometric exercises of the shoulder are started, as tolerated, late in phase II. All directions are strengthened, including the scapular stabilizers and elevators. Resistance is provided by a therapist, the good arm, or a wall.

Phase III may overlap somewhat with phase II. It is the strengthening phase. Isotonic exercises are added to the isometrics already described. They are started below-shoulder level with light free weights, pulleys, or against resistance from surgical tubing. Initially low-resistance, high-repetition exercises are done. This is gradually switched to high resistance, low repetition.

As the patient progresses, above-the-shoulder exercises are instituted, first in flexion/extension and abduction/adduction, then in functional diagonal planes. Isokinetics are also begun, starting with high speed arcs (180 to 300 degrees/second). When possible, therapist-assisted proprioceptive neuromuscular facilitation (PNF) techniques are helpful in improving functional strength. A few specific exercises in a strengthening program are described in Table 14-2.

When the patient has progressed to regaining enough strength to prevent recurrence of the

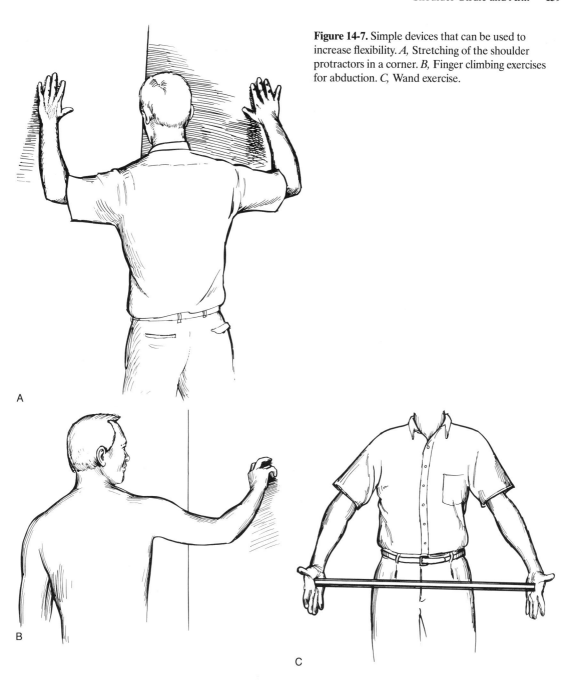

**Figure 14-7.** Simple devices that can be used to increase flexibility. *A,* Stretching of the shoulder protractors in a corner. *B,* Finger climbing exercises for abduction. *C,* Wand exercise.

A

B

C

shoulder injury, phase IV may be started. This is a functional progression of activities to demonstrate that he or she is ready to return to normal activity. Any trunk motion abnormalities or poor techniques are corrected to prevent reinjury. The patient is advised to continue a maintenance strength and flexibility program year-round.

## Examination and Testing Techniques

### *History*

Before proceeding with a physical examination and diagnostic tests, a good history of the nature of the shoulder complaint is indicated. Included in the history should be a description of when and

**Table 14-2.** Sample Muscle Strengthening Exercises

| Exercise | Muscle Strengthened |
|---|---|
| Shoulder shrugs | Upper trapezius |
| Pushups | Serratus anterior |
| Chin up/pull-down | Latissimus dorsi, pectoralis major |
| Internal rotation | Subscapularis, latissimus dorsi, teres major, pectoralis major |
| External rotation | Infraspinatus, teres minor |
| Flexion | Anterior deltoid, coracobrachialis, biceps |
| Extension | Posterior deltoid, pectoralis major, latissimus dorsi, teres major |
| Horizontal adduction with a pulley | Pectoralis major, anterior deltoid |
| Abduction performed with the arm at 90° abduction, 30° flexion and internal rotation (see Figure 14-11) | Supraspinatus |
| Abduction | Deltoid, supraspinatus |

where the dysfunction or pain began, what activity caused it and exacerbates it, and any past history of injury or surgery to the area. This often leads the examiner to the most productive line of inquiry and testing. Discussing functional limitations such as dressing, eating, and hair combing may be useful. Discussing a general review of systems is also helpful, since abdominal or other diseases may cause pain to be referred to the shoulder.

### Physical Examination

As always, the physical examination must include the following: inspection, palpation, passive range of motion, active range of motion, and stability testing.

**Cervical Spine.**    A complete shoulder examination must include testing of the cervical spine, as disorders here can cause pain radiation to the shoulder and arm. Flexion, extension, rotation, and lateral bending are all assessed. Extension and lateral bending close the intervertebral foramina and may reproduce pain arising from the vertebral structures. When combined with axial compression, i.e., Spurling's maneuver (see Chapter 12), this test helps to diagnose neck pathology.

**Glenohumeral and Scapulothoracic Joints.**    Inspection may reveal signs of muscular atrophy such as a prominent scapular spine. Atrophy may result from cervical nerve root compression, from bra-

chial plexus or peripheral nerve damage, or from muscular tears or inactivity. If the biceps tendon is ruptured, the muscle retracts and creates a distal lateral enlargement of the biceps.

Anterior dislocation is accompanied by prominence of the humeral head anteriorly with a depression in back. Posterior dislocation has a posterior bulge and the coracoid becomes prominent anteriorly. Inferior subluxation, seen after cerebrovascular accident, brachial plexus, or axillary nerve injury causes a step-off between the acromion and the humeral head.

Palpation of the shoulder structures may reveal tenderness at the site of injury, either at a cuff tear, in calcific tendonitis, or with other damage. Tenderness at the intertubercular groove is common in noninjured people, and bicipital tendonitis should not be overdiagnosed by this isolated finding.

Active range of motion should be assessed in the seated, not standing, position to avoid trunk and leg contribution to range of motion. Passive range of motion is tested in the supine position. Tables of normal range of motion are found in other sources.[4]

An easy functional way to assess range of motion is the Apley scratch test (Figure 14-8). The patient is asked to touch to the opposite scapula across the opposite shoulder, behind the neck, and from behind the lower back. Active ROM testing reveals areas of inflexibility, specific muscle weakness, and painful arcs. Active abduction and external rotation are decreased in rotator cuff disease. In cuff problems the patient tends to shrug the shoulder when asked to abduct the arm.

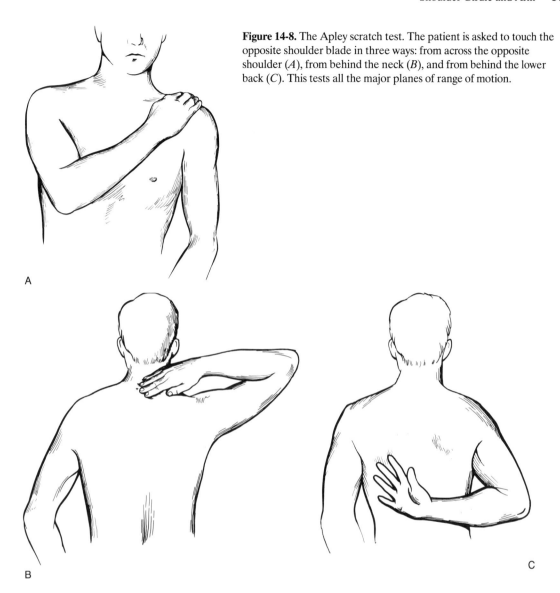

**Figure 14-8.** The Apley scratch test. The patient is asked to touch the opposite shoulder blade in three ways: from across the opposite shoulder (*A*), from behind the neck (*B*), and from behind the lower back (*C*). This tests all the major planes of range of motion.

A

B

C

Discrepancies between active and passive range of motion are noted. If both active and passive range of motion are limited, there is likely to be a joint contracture, adhesive capsulitis, fixed dislocation, or a bony abnormality. When passive motion is greater than active, a rotator cuff tear is suspected.

Range of motion of the scapulothoracic joint is observed along with that of the glenohumeral joint. The scapulohumeral rhythm is evaluated using the nonaffected side as a control. Excessive scapulothoracic motion is a sign of glenohumeral stiffness and is commonly seen in rotator cuff tears, adhesive capsulitis, and in degenerative joint disease.

To test stability of the shoulder, the patient is asked to lie supine at the edge of the table. The arm is held over the edge of the table in a position of abduction and external rotation. The examiner tries to move the humeral head anteriorly by exerting pressure on the proximal humerus (Figure 14-9A). Pain on attempting this maneuver is a sign of anterior subluxation; apprehension is indicative of a prior dislocation and is called a *positive apprehension test*. Pushing the humeral head back into place relieves the pain and apprehension.

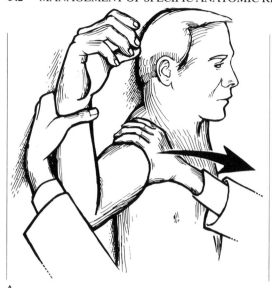

A

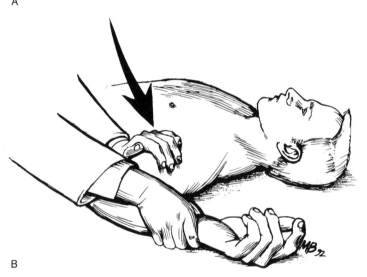

B

**Figure 14-9.** Test for shoulder stability. *A,* Anterior stability. *B,* Posterior stability. (Lillegard WA, Rucker KS: *Handbook of Sports Medicine.* Stoneham, MA: Andover Medical Publishers, 1993. Reprinted by permission.)

Pushing the proximal humerus posteriorly tests for posterior subluxation (Figure 14-9B). This is less likely to cause pain or apprehension, and the degree of posterior movement may be subtle. Relocating a subluxated humerus may cause a snap. Posterior stability can also be evaluated by directing a posterior force on the flexed and internally rotated humerus. This may produce a posterior subluxation which is accompanied by a snap when the arm is relocated by extending the arm. In either test, a posterior translation of the humeral head of up to 50% of its diameter has been described as being normal.[5]

Inferior stability is assessed by applying inferior traction to the relaxed arm. If this causes a "step-off" to appear between the humeral head and the acromion, it is called a *positive sulcus sign* and indicates inferior instability. Strength testing at the shoulder must systematically isolate the various muscle groups. The deltoid is tested in its anterior, middle, and posterior portions. The biceps is tested by Yergason's test of resisted forearm supination (Figure 14-10).[6] The internal rotators are tested with the arm held across the chest resisting the examiner's pull away from this position. External rotation is tested with the arms by the side with elbows flexed. While carrying out these motions it is helpful to palpate the origins of the muscles being tested to detect any musculotendinous ruptures.

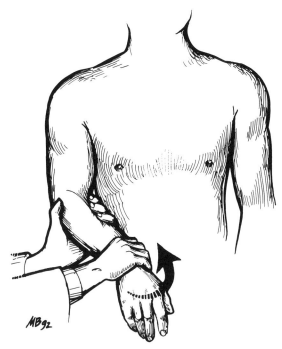

**Figure 14-10.** Yergason's test for bicipital tendonitis. The arm is held at the side with the elbow flexed to 90 degrees and the forearm pronated. The examiner resists, while the patient attempts to supinate the forearm. Pain at the intertubercular groove at the shoulder is a positive finding.

The supraspinatus can be isolated and tested by holding the arm abducted to 90 degrees, flexed to 30 degrees, and internally rotated so the thumbs point down (Figure 14-11). Pain or weakness to downward pressure in this position is indicative of supraspinatus pathology.

Serratus anterior weakness is accompanied by winging of the medial scapula when pushing against a wall (Figure 14-12). Trapezius weakness may cause a similar winging with the same maneuver and leads to a weak shoulder shrug. The scapular retractors are tested by pushing posteriorly with the arms across and behind the lower back (palm facing to the rear).

After assessing the basics as just described, a number of more specialized tests and observations may be indicated.

**Impingement Testing** (for supraspinatus pathology). In the Neer test the arm is internally rotated and then flexed to its limit (Figure 14-13). Pain is a positive finding. The Hawkins test is per-

formed by flexing the arm to 90 degrees and then internally rotating it to its limit (Figure 14-14). Impingement is again painful. In both of these maneuvers pain is relieved after injection of 10 ml of lidocaine (xylocaine) into the subacromial space.[7] This *impingement injection test* rules out other causes of shoulder pain, such as acromioclavicular pain and adhesive capsulitis, which are not relieved by the injection. Also, pain relief allows more accurate muscle and ROM testing.

**Adson's Test.** This is a test of thoracic outlet obstruction. The examiner palpates the radial pulse and abducts, extends, and externally rotates the patient's arm. Then the patient takes a deep breath while turning the head toward the arm being tested. A positive sign is indicated by a diminution of the pulse. This test is insensitive to true thoracic outlet syndrome and often gives false-positive results.[8] It is of doubtful value.

**Drop Arm Test.** The "drop arm test" is used to evaluate a possible rotator cuff tear, specifically in the supraspinatus muscle. The patient sits or

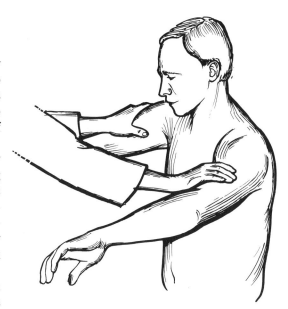

**Figure 14-11.** Supraspinatus testing: the arm is abducted 90 degrees, flexed forward 30 degrees and the thumbs point down. This lines the humerous up in the plane of the scapula and isolates the supraspinatus for testing. (Lillegard WA, Rucker KS: *Handbook of Sports Medicine.* Stoneham, MA: Andover Medical Publishers, 1993. Reprinted by permission.)

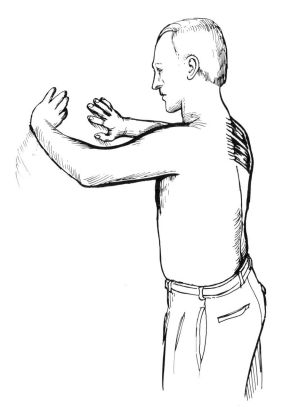

**Figure 14-12.** Serratus anterior weakness causes a "winging" of the scapula when pushing against a wall. The elbows point laterally.

stands while the examiner abducts the arm. The patient is asked to hold the arm in place and to lower it slowly. Severe pain or inability to lower the arm slowly is a positive finding. In impingement or partial rotator cuff tear the muscle forms a mass that passes under the coracoacromial arch in the arc of 70 to 120 degrees of abduction. Therefore, pain in this range is suggestive of an inflamed or swollen supraspinatus.

*Ancillary Diagnostic Testing*

There are numerous ancillary diagnostic procedures that may be performed to test the shoulder musculature. They include x-ray studies, magnetic resonance imaging (MRI), diagnostic ultrasound, computerized tomography, electromyography, arthroscopy, and arthrography. Arthrography is especially good at detecting full-thickness rotator cuff tears (see Chapter 8).

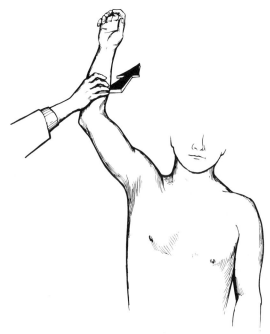

**Figure 14-13.** The Neer test for impingement. (Lillegard WA, Rucker KS: *Handbook of Sports Medicine.* Stoneham, MA: Andover Medical Publishers, 1993. Reprinted by permission.)

It is difficult to know when an x-ray study is needed. There are no hard and fast rules, but Table 14-3 gives some general guidelines of when an x-ray evaluation might be appropriate. Three basic x-ray views should be obtained. They are the anteroposterior view in both internal and external rotation and the axillary view.

**Table 14-3.** Guidelines on When to Order X-Ray Studies

| |
|---|
| When there is severe, unremitting, or prolonged pain. |
| When there is joint swelling. |
| When range of motion is decreased (active or passive). |
| After any dislocation to rule out associated fracture. |
| When the shoulder is unstable. |
| If there is evidence of a mechanical block or articular "grinding." |
| When the joint is incongruent to examination. |
| After a clavicular or acromial "contusion" to rule out fracture or acromioclavicular separation. |
| In adolescents or preadolescents with a diagnosis of "ligamentous" sprain to rule out growth plate injury (ligaments may be stronger than growth plate). |

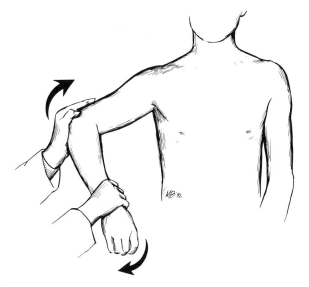

**Figure 14-14.** The Hawkins test for impingement. (Lillegard WA, Rucker KS: *Handbook of Sports Medicine.* Stoneham, MA: Andover Medical Publishers, 1993. Reprinted by permission.)

## Diagnosis and Treatment of Specific Disorders

### Impingement Syndrome

Impingement syndrome is a condition of pain, inflammation, and edema of the structures within the coracoacromial arch. It occurs mostly at the supraspinatus muscle. It is due to repetitive microtrauma, usually from overhand arm motions and is exacerbated by motions that increase the encroachment of the humeral head into the coracoacromial arch, most notably internal rotation. Impingement may progress to rotator cuff tear. True impingement of the supraspinatus is almost always intertwined with rotator cuff tendonitis, subdeltoid (subacromial) bursitis, or bicipital tendonitis, although isolated overuse of the biceps may occur in some repetitive underhand motions.

As described previously, the supraspinatus tendon is chronically ischemic.[9] Repetitive use of the hands at or above shoulder height increases the load on the shoulders and worsens the ischemia. Degeneration occurs slowly with age and repetitive movement, making the cuff muscles weaker. As they weaken, the deltoid overpowers the cuff and pulls the humerus into the coracoacromial arch, thereby compressing the supraspinatus and damaging it even more.

Sometimes calcific deposits form within the rotator cuff tendons. This is also a part of the continuum of overuse injury and is most common in middle age. Presentation is identical to impingement. While calcific deposits are found in some patients with shoulder pain, they are not always the cause of the pain. It is important to remember that such deposits are formed as the body reacts to impingement and damage; they are not the primary cause of the damage. There are three stags of impingement (Table 14-4).[7]

### Diagnosis

Pain in impingement is localized to the superior lateral shoulder, anterior and lateral to the acromion. Impingement signs may be positive and abduction in the arc between 70 to 120 degrees may be painful. There may be signs of rotator cuff muscular atrophy.

In the early stage of impingement, pain occurs only after strenuous activity. Later it may occur

**Table 14-4.** Stages of Impingement[7]

| | |
|---|---|
| *Stage 1:* | Edema, swelling, pain, hemorrhage |
| *Stage 2:* | Fibrosis, tendonitis, incomplete cuff tears |
| *Stage 3:* | Small complete cuff tears, bony changes such as acromial and greater tuberosity sclerosis, cyst and spur formation. If left untreated, these progress to "cuff tear arthropathy" with a large cuff tear leading to upward migration and erosion of the humeral head into the acromion. |

with almost any movement, and if not treated it can progress to nearly constant pain, especially night pain. When the biceps tendon is involved, it is tender to palpation and Yergason's test is positive. Isolated tenderness over the biceps tendon is common in normal individuals and care must be taken not to overdiagnose this condition.

X-ray findings of impingement are usually minimal. In advanced cases bony spurring may be detected, but in general this is purely a soft tissue disorder. Underpenetrating x-rays are best at detecting calcific deposits.

*Treatment*

In the early stages of impingement, before rotator cuff tear has occurred, the main goals of treatment in phase I are to reduce pain and inflammation. Rest, with no overhead activity, is indicated. NSAIDs and ice are used in this stage. If symptoms are severe, 3 to 4 days of immobilization with a sling may ease the pain and inflammation. Steroid injections are considered. They are not a definitive treatment by themselves but may allow the patient to participate more fully in therapy. Shoulder isometrics can be started early, in 3 to 5 days.

Phase II of rehabilitation is started in about a week if the patient tolerates it. It lasts approximately 2 weeks and starts with Codman exercises, gentle stretching, and moist heat. Movement in forward flexion and external rotation is emphasized in a tight shoulder, and abduction is avoided in the early stages as this may worsen impingement. Phase III strengthening exercises are initially limited to below shoulder level but rapidly progress to include all shoulder motions.

The goal of the strengthening exercises is to improve the function of the humeral head depressors. Thus the rotator cuff muscles and the latissimus dorsi are targeted. Strengthening and flexibility in the direction of external rotation is stressed, since a position of internal rotation tends to worsen the impingement. Corner pushups, wand, and pulley exercises are valuable. If the flexibility program does not bring a return of full range of motion, mobilization by a therapist may be indicated.

The rotator cuff muscles can be strengthened with a few specific exercises. Internal and external rotation are practiced with the arm by the side to strengthen the subscapularis and the infraspinatus/teres minor, respectively. This can be done with weights while lying on the side or with elastic bands tied to a doorknob or other support. The supraspinatus is strengthened by holding the arm abducted 90 degrees and flexed forward 30 degrees, with the thumb pointing down. The arm is slowly lowered and then brought back up. The patient should be instructed not to raise it above horizontal level. At first no weights are used, later 1- to 5-lb weights can be added (preferably strapped to the wrists rather than held), but heavy weights are avoided since they aggravate the inflammation. Ten to twenty repetitions done one to two times a day are adequate.

If conservative treatment fails to improve symptoms rapidly, or if symptoms worsen with this program, it is best to avoid waiting too long before considering surgery. Too long a wait can allow a rotator cuff tear to develop. More advanced stages of impingement (stages II and III) are also initially treated conservatively, as described previously. Partial or small rotator cuff tears may respond to this treatment as well, but when conservative treatment fails for a period of 3 months or so, an arthrogram should probably be performed to rule out a larger rotator cuff tear. Up to 18 months of conservative treatment in the absence of a rotator cuff tear has been advocated.[7]

Large rotator cuff tears usually require surgical repair, and the end stage, cuff tear arthropathy may well require surgery, including possibly a joint replacement.

In addition to the guidelines presented, bicipital tendonitis or chronic bursitis may respond to ultrasound deep-heat treatment. Calcific tendinitis may respond to puncture of the tendon with a needle to allow the contents to spill into the bursa and from there be resorbed.[10] This relieves the intratendinous pressure and reduces its swelling.

Steroid injections into either the biceps tendon sheath or the subacromial bursa may be necessary, but they are limited to a maximum of three injections spaced 1 to 2 months apart. Tendon strength is decreased for up to 6 weeks after an injection, and even though pain may be improved, activity should be light during this period to avoid tendon rupture.

## Rotator Cuff Tears

A tear of the rotator cuff may, of course, be caused in a healthy shoulder by a macrotraumatic injury such as a glenohumeral dislocation. More commonly, however, this injury is superimposed on chronic pathology. Overuse, age, tendonitis, and inflammation all take their toll on the rotator cuff. The weakened cuff tendon is more easily torn when a traumatic event comes along, and since it is weak, it is less able to avoid such a traumatic event.

Rotator cuff tears may occur in young athletes who are active in sports that stress repetitive motion or in middle-age athletes who have been sedentary for a long time. Typically, they decide to "get in shape," overdo it, and end up tearing their rotator cuff in their enthusiasm. Training principles such as "no pain, no gain" and "work through the pain" only worsen the condition of the shoulder. Older patients are more likely to have degenerative change in the shoulder. This predisposes them to injury from a macrotraumatic event that would not harm a younger, healthier shoulder.

Rotator cuff tears occur in the tendons of the cuff muscles, most often in the supraspinatus. The tear can be partial or full thickness. A full-thickness tear is classified by size: small ones are less than 1 cm in length, and large ones are greater than 1 cm.

### Diagnosis

Acute rotator cuff tears are associated with acute onset of pain and tenderness of the greater tuberosity. There may be weakness in the initiation of abduction, and there may be a positive drop arm test. Supraspinatus strength testing elicits pain and weakness, and impingement testing may be positive. On x-ray study there may be superior migration of the humeral head.

Chronic tears are the most common rotator cuff tears, especially in older individuals. They can be due to an old macrotraumatic injury, but more likely are due to chronic degenerative disease of the tendons. There is often a gradual onset of symptoms including night pain and weakness. Overhead arm activities cause discomfort and fatigue. The drop arm test is often positive, and there is usually weakness in external rotation. Atrophy of the shoulder muscles, especially the su-

praspinatus and deltoid, is common. Supraspinatus testing is painful, and there is a positive impingement sign. X-ray findings are nonspecific but may show degenerative bony changes and upward migration of the humeral head.[11] The diagnosis should be confirmed with MRI or arthrography[12] which is almost always positive in complete tears. In partial tears, MRI or diagnostic ultrasound testing may detect a defect missed by arthrography.

### Treatment

Conservative care of rotator cuff tears is similar to that for impingement. After controlling pain and inflammation, flexibility is restored. Then isometrics are started with progression to isotonic exercises as tolerated. Again, rotator cuff muscles and external rotators are strengthened to reduce impingement. Judicious use of intrabursal steroid injection is considered. In acute rotator cuff tears the patient may be followed conservatively with rest for the first 1 to 2 weeks. If strength returns and pain resolves, a program of rehabilitation may be commenced. If there is no improvement, an arthrogram or MRI should be obtained. If this reveals a rotator cuff tear then surgery should probably be performed. Surgical outcome is best if the repair is done within the first 3 weeks after injury.[12,13]

In chronic rotator cuff tears, planning the best treatment can be difficult. Massive tears are usually surgically repaired. Partial tears may initially be treated with rest, ice, and NSAIDs. Subsequently, when the pain and inflammation have subsided, a rehabilitation course is instituted. If the symptoms recur, the patient may need surgery. The treatment of smaller complete tears depends on the activity level of the patient. An active, motivated individual will probably benefit from surgery, although a 3-month trial of conservative treatment as discussed earlier for impingement syndrome may be tried first. Some patients, those who are unlikely to use the shoulder vigorously in the future, those who pose a greater surgical risk, or those who are likely to develop postoperative complications of immobility may be treated conservatively. After surgery for a massive tear the patient may be immobilized for 6 weeks in an abduction brace to facilitate healing. After this, phase II of rehabilitation is started and progresses to phase III as tolerated. The total rehabilitation after repair of a rotator cuff tear takes 9 to 12 months.[14]

### Instability

Glenohumeral instability is the most prevalent shoulder problem in young athletes. While anterior instability is most common, instability can also be present in other directions: posterior, inferior, anterosuperior, and multidirectional.

Instability can be limited to subluxation, in which the humeral head slips over the glenoid rim but spontaneously relocates. It can also result in frank dislocation, in which the humeral head lodges outside the glenoid rim. Instability can result from macrotrauma, repetitive microtrauma, or from congenital or neuromuscular abnormalities of the joint.

Anterior dislocation or subluxation occurs when the arm is forcibly abducted, externally rotated, and elevated (Figure 14-15A). The anterior labrum is often torn in the process and the rotator cuff and axillary nerve may be damaged. Posterior dislocations or subluxations may occur from a fall on the outstretched arm or in car accidents (Figure 14-15B). They may also occur during seizures when the stronger internal rotators overpower the external rotators. Once a shoulder has dislocated or subluxated it is likely to do so again in the future, especially in younger patients.

### Diagnosis

Stability testing reveals abnormal laxity in the affected directions, and apprehension testing is positive. In acute dislocations, the patient may be unable to move the arm out of the locked position.

X-ray study, including the axillary view, confirms the diagnosis. Radiographic films should always be obtained, even after a dislocation has been reduced, to rule out any associated fractures.

### Treatment

Dislocations must of course be reduced, and for a discussion of such reduction the reader is referred elsewhere.[14] Postreduction treatment is controversial. Some clinicians believe that the arm should not be immobilized in a sling to prevent resulting joint stiffness. Most, however, would probably agree that the shoulder should be immobilized from 1 to 6 weeks (probably 3 to 6 weeks is reasonable) in a position of having the arm slightly anterior and internally rotated.[15] A shorter period (7 to 10 days), or no immobilization at all, may be indicated in older patients who are less likely to have a recurrence and who are more susceptible to problems of

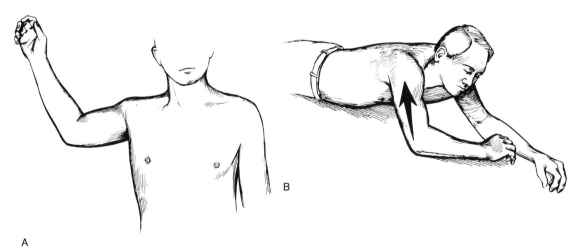

**Figure 14-15.** *A,* Anterior dislocation is caused by forcible abduction and external rotation. *B,* Posterior dislocation may be caused by a fall on the internally rotated adducted arm.

immobility.[16] Recurrent dislocation or subluxation can also be immobilized for a shorter period of time.

The shoulder is treated in phase I with ice and distal arm isometrics. In phase II the ice is continued, while heat and gentle range of motion, with the arm below shoulder level, are started. External rotation is limited to 10 degrees less than the good arm, and since this is a condition of joint laxity, the stretching program is relatively nonaggressive. Posterior shoulder structures, if they are tight, are stretched more vigorously. In phase III, strengthening is begun. This is done first with the arm below shoulder level, stressing the internal rotators, then adding other motions, isotonics, isokinetics, and diagonal strength exercises. In all the strengthening exercises the extremes of range of motion are avoided.[17]

If the patient does not improve with conservative treatment within 3 months, surgery can be considered. The surgery usually involves a capsular shift procedure to tighten the anterior shoulder, with a labral repair if indicated. Postoperatively the shoulder is usually immobilized for 6 weeks and then the whole rehabilitative process is started over again. Stretching of the anterior shoulder is restricted.[15]

Recurrence of shoulder dislocations is high, up to 94% in athletes under age 20.[18] A rehabilitation program may decrease this rate of recurrence to as low as 25%.[19]

Anterior subluxation does not require prolonged sling immobilization. It is treated similar to a dislocation. Posterior dislocation or subluxation is also treated similarly, although in this condition the anterior shoulder muscles are stretched more, while the posterior muscles are strengthened relatively more.

### Adhesive Capsulitis

This is a painful condition of decreased range of motion of the glenohumeral joint. The cause is unknown, but it often follows an injury or a period of immobilization of the shoulder or arm. There appears to be fibrosis of the lower glenohumeral joint capsule, the inferior axillary fold, which restricts range of motion. This condition is usually described as being self-limited, with restoration of normal to near-normal function within 1 to 2 years. However, during this time span there is much morbidity and loss of function. Muscles atrophy and the patient's lifestyle changes. Occasionally this condition may progress to even more severe reflex sympathetic dystrophy. Clearly, early aggressive treatment is indicated.

### Diagnosis

Almost any other injury can lead to the development of adhesive capsulitis; thus this condition should always be looked for even when the shoulder has other obvious disorders. The hallmark of adhesive capsulitis is that both passive and active range of motion are restricted, especially in abduction and external rotation. Pain is evident, often at rest, but especially when attempting range of motion. The patient moves the shoulder mainly at the scapulothoracic joint, a sign that the glenohumeral joint is stiff. Local anesthetic injection into the glenohumeral joint relieves the pain but does not change joint mobility.

### Treatment

At the first signs of adhesive capsulitis aggressive pain control and mobilization are indicated. NSAIDs or intraarticular steroids may be prescribed. Frequent ROM exercises just short of producing pain are indicated. Treatment may start with a home program of wand exercises, door frame stretches, and "wall walking," but if improvement does not begin within the first week or so, therapist assisted exercises are warranted. Moist heat, slow gentle stretching, ultrasound treatment, as well as joint glide mobilizations, are all helpful and should be performed once or twice daily. Pulley exercises may be used, but only with caution. The long lever arm of the pulley may actually injure the shoulder and cause impingement. In cases refractory to even aggressive physical management, manipulation under anesthesia is an option.

Adhesive capsulitis may occur after any surgery or period of joint immobilization; thus it is clear that the shoulder should always be mobilized as soon as is feasible. Prevention is important, especially in the elderly or debilitated, and is done with twice-daily shoulder range of motion exercises.

### Reflex Sympathetic Dystrophy

Also known as shoulder-hand syndrome (see also Chapter 16), reflex sympathetic dystrophy (RSD) involves an abnormal sympathetic nervous system response to often trivial injury. Problems ranging from nerve trauma to wrist sprain to stroke may cause this abnormal response. The underlying etiology and pathogenesis are not fully understood at this time.

#### Diagnosis

RSD should be suspected whenever the patient's complaints of pain are out of proportion to the stimuli being applied. Light touch to the skin, or seemingly minor joint movement, may cause such pain. The joints of the hand and wrist are often tender and swollen. Shoulder range of motion is limited by pain. There may be skin and temperature changes in the limb. It is often warm and swollen early on, then becomes cool and clammy, and later tight and atrophic. A bone scan may be positive.

#### Treatment

Early aggressive treatment is indicated. Medications that may be used are NSAIDs, a short burst of rapidly tapering high-dose oral steroids, or alpha-adrenergic blockers, among others. All may work in the early stages of the disorder; few work well later on. In addition, sympathetic nerve outflow to the limb may be interrupted with an anesthetic stellate ganglion block. This is both a therapeutic and a diagnostic procedure.

Physical modalities are a crucial adjunct to the medications and are described in Chapter 16. When signs of RSD become evident the patient needs to be evaluated by a physician well versed in this disorder. Delays may worsen long-term outcome.

### Neurovascular Compromise/Thoracic Outlet Syndrome

A number of causes of neurovascular compression can cause shoulder and neck pain. Compression of the brachial plexus between the anterior and middle scalene muscles (scalenus anticus syndrome), compression between the clavicle and the first rib (costoclavicular syndrome), an abnormal shape of the first rib, and a cervical rib, among others, have been described. They tend to affect the ulnar distribution predominantly, although the median nerve may also be affected. They occur only rarely and are probably overdiagnosed.

#### Diagnosis

These problems cause a burning pain and numbness in the shoulder or the arm. Blood flow studies with a Doppler device or an arteriogram, as well as nerve conduction studies may be helpful in making the diagnosis.

#### Treatment

The shoulder elevators and retractors are strengthened, and the anterior chest and neck structures are stretched. Surgery may occasionally be necessary, although it is probably performed more often than it should be. When the compression involves only the vasculature to the arm (by far the more common situation), surgery often provides no relief. If there is evidence of nerve damage by electromyography, then surgical outcome is more promising.

### Degenerative Joint Disease

Arthritis of the glenohumeral and acromioclavicular joints may occur, especially in patients with prior injury to these joints. It also occurs in aging, overuse, and in rheumatic conditions.

#### Diagnosis

Joint crepitus, decreased range of motion, and diffuse pain are seen in these disorders. Often mild activity lessens the symptoms. X-ray findings confirm the diagnosis with signs of bony degeneration, spurring (which may be felt also), and sclerosis.

#### Treatment

Proper joint mechanics and energy conservation techniques are helpful. NSAIDs and occasional steroid injections are also often used. Rarely, surgical excision of the acromioclavicular joint or joint replacement of the glenohumeral joint are indicated.

## Case Report

A 42-year-old right-handed man had been suffering from right-sided shoulder pain since his teens due to a baseball overuse injury. He was able to do most activities but was limited in athletic participation and overhead activities by a dull aching pain deep in the shoulder. On examination he had moderate tenderness over the supraspinatus tendon; this muscle was moderately atrophic. His supraspinatus was weak compared with his asymptomatic side and he had positive signs of impingement. He had nearly full active range of motion but scapulothoracic contribution to abduction was excessive, and external rotation was decreased. Stability testing revealed no defect. He was diagnosed as having a chronic impingement syndrome, very likely with a partial or small rotator cuff tear. Since his shoulder was not acutely inflamed he was started immediately on a flexibility program emphasizing external rotation and a strengthening program for the rotator cuff. He was started on NSAIDs to minimize the possibility of an exacerbation and was instructed to apply ice to the rotator cuff tendons before and after his strengthening exercises. He responded well. He now has full range of motion and normal strength throughout. He still has occasional pain with overhead activity but has returned to recreational golf. He may develop later arthritic problems and if his symptoms worsen in the future, arthrography or arthroscopy should be performed.

## Points of Summary

1. The rotator cuff muscles depress the head of the humerus and help prevent impingement.
2. The supraspinatus muscle is predisposed to overuse syndromes.
3. Impingement of the supraspinatus is usually combined with subdeltoid bursitis and bicipital tendonitis.
4. Scapulohumeral rhythm describes motion of the scapula of 1 degree for every 2 degrees of glenohumeral abduction.
5. The shoulder is uniquely susceptible to problems of immobility.
6. In anterior instability, the internal rotators are strengthened.
7. In posterior instability, the external rotators are strengthened.
8. Thoracic outlet syndrome is overdiagnosed.
9. Arthrography detects complete rotator cuff tears.
10. Adhesive capsulitis should be treated with early aggressive therapy.

## References

1. Mosley HF, Övergaard B: The anterior capsular mechanism in recurrent anterior dislocation of the shoulder: Morphological and clinical studies with special reference to the glenoid labrum and the glenohumeral ligaments. *J Bone Joint Surg* 1962;44B:913–927.
2. Codman EA: *The Shoulder*, Boston: Thomas Todd, 1934.
3. Lehmann JF, deLateur BJ: Theraputic heat. In Lehmann JF (ed): *Theraputic Heat and Cold*, 4th ed. Baltimore: Williams & Wilkins, 1990.
4. Hoppenfeld S: *Physical Examination of the Spine and Extremities*. East Norwalk, CT: Appleton-Century-Crofts, 1976.
5. Jobe FW, Bradley JP: The diagnosis and nonoperative treatment of shoulder injuries in athletes. *Clin Sports Med* 1989;8:419–437.
6. Yergason RM: Supination sign. *J Bone Joint Surg* 1937;13B:160.
7. Neer CS: Impingement lesions. *Clin Orthop* 1983;173:70–77.
8. Glassenberg M: The thoracic outlet syndrome: An assessment of 20 cases with regard to new clinical and electromyographical findings. *Angiology* 1981;32:180–186.
9. Caillet R: *Shoulder Pain*, 2nd ed. Philadelphia, FA Davis, 1989.
10. Neviaser RJ: Painful conditions affecting the shoulder. *Clin Orthop* 1983;173:63–69.
11. Hamada K, Fukuda H, Mikasa M, et al.: Roentgenographic findings in massive rotator cuff tears: A long-term observation. *Clin Orthop* 1990;254:92–96.
12. Neviaser RJ: Ruptures of the rotator cuff. *Orthop Clin North Am* 1987;18:387–394.
13. Bassett RW, Cofield RH: Acute tears of the rotator cuff: The timing of surgical repair. *Clin Orthop* 1983;1975:18–24.
14. Skyhar MJ, Warren RF, Altdek DW: Instability of the shoulder. In Nicholas JA, Hershman EB (eds); *The Upper Extremity and Spine in Sports Medicine*. St. Louis: CV Mosby, 1990:181–212.

15. Mendoza FX, Nicholas JA, Sands A: Principles of shoulder rehabilitation in the athlete. In Nicholas JA, Hershman EB (eds): *The Upper Extremity and Spine in Sports Medicine*. St. Louis: CV Mosby, 1990:251–264.

16. O'Brien SJ, Warren RF, Schwartz E: Anterior shoulder instability. *Orthop Clin North Am* 1987;18:395–408.

17. Jobe FW, Moynes DR, Brewster CE: Rehabilitation of shoulder joint instabilities. *Orthop Clin North Am* 1987;18:473–482.

18. Rowe CR, Sakellarides HT: Factors related to recurrences of anterior dislocations of the shoulder. *Clin Orthop* 1961;20:40–47.

19. Aronen JG, Regan K: Decreasing the incidence of recurrence of first time anterior shoulder dislocations with rehabilitation. *Am J Sports Med* 1984;12:283–291.

## Suggested Readings

Brems J: Rotator cuff tear: Evaluation and treatment. *Orthopedics* 1988;11:69–81.

Neviaser RJ: Adhesive capsulitis. *Orthop Clin North Am* 1987;18:439–443.

Neviaser RJ: Painful conditions affecting the shoulder. *Clin Orthop* 1983;173:63–69.

Jobe FW, Bradley JP: The diagnosis and nonoperative treatment of shoulder injuries in athletes. *Clin Sports Med* 1989;8:419–437.

# Chapter 15
# Elbow and Forearm

ROBERT P. WILDER,
ROBERT P. NIRSCHL,
AND JANET SOBEL

Disorders of the elbow and forearm are commonly encountered in clinical practice. Evaluation of these injuries is dependent upon an understanding of anatomy, the mechanism of injury, history, and presentation. Establishment of a correct pathoanatomic diagnosis is the basis for implementing rehabilitative, and if needed, surgical management.

## Anatomy of the Elbow and Forearm

The elbow complex consists of three articulations: the humeroulnar, humeroradial, and proximal radioulnar joints. The humeroulnar and humeroradial joints are hinge joints which act together in flexion and extension. The proximal radioulnar joint is a pivot joint which allows pronation and supination. Stability is provided by ligamentous and muscular support.

### Osseous Structures (Figure 15-1)

**Humerus.**   The long bone of the arm, the humerus, flares medially and laterally at its distal end, terminating in rounded medial and lateral epicondyles. The epicondyles serve as origins for the flexor and extensor forearm musculature. The distal end of the humerus bears two articulating surfaces: the capitellum which articulates laterally

with the head of the radius, and the trochlea which articulates medially with the ulna.

**Ulna.**   The ulna is the medial bone of the forearm. At its proximal and posterior aspect is the olecranon, a large process which articulates posteriorly with the olecranon fossa of the humerus. When the elbow is flexed, the coronoid process of the ulna fits in the coronoid fossa of the humerus. This fossa is located anteriorly and proximal to the trochlea.

**Radius.**   The radius is the lateral bone of the forearm. At its proximal aspect the radial head is expanded and flattened to articulate with the capitellum.

### Ligamentous Structures (Figure 15-2)

**Lateral Collateral Ligament.**   The lateral (radial) collateral ligament extends from the lateral epicondyle to the annular ligament. It provides lateral support to the elbow complex.

**Medial Collateral Ligament.**   The medial (ulnar) collateral ligament extends from the medial epicondyle to the ulna. It provides medial support to the elbow complex. It is divided into three bundles: anterior, posterior, and transverse, with the

153

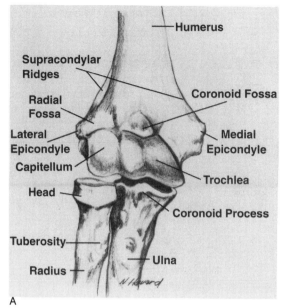

A

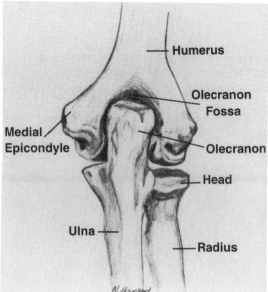

B

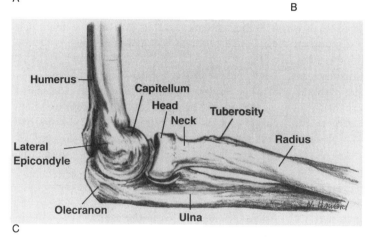

C

**Figure 15-1.** Osseous structures of the elbow. *A,* Anterior view. *B,* Posterior view. *C,* Lateral view.

anterior bundle providing the greatest degree of stability.

**Annular Ligament.** The annular ligament cups the radial head and neck, holding them in place at the radioulnar articulation.

*Muscles of the Elbow and Forearm (Figure 15-3)*

The muscles of the elbow and forearm can be divided into four groups based on their anatomic location.

**Lateral.** The muscles of the posterolateral or extensor surface of the elbow can be divided into two groups. The superficial group includes the brachioradialis, extensor carpi radialis longus, extensor carpi radialis brevis, extensor digitorum, extensor digiti minimi, and extensor carpi ulnaris. The deep group includes the supinator, abductor pollicis longus, extensor pollicis brevis, extensor pollicis longus, and extensor indicis. The extensor carpi radialis brevis, extensor digitorum, extensor digiti minimi, and extensor carpi ulnaris arise from a common aponeurosis near the lateral epicondyle. This is of clinical importance in

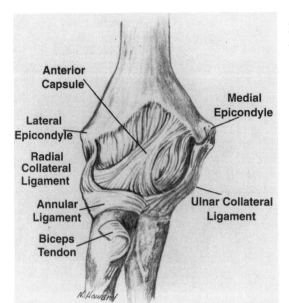

Figure 15-2. Ligamentous structures of the elbow. *A*, Anterior view. *B,* Lateral view. *C,* Medial view.

Anterior Capsule

Medial Epicondyle

Lateral Epicondyle

Radial Collateral Ligament

Annular Ligament

Biceps Tendon

Ulnar Collateral Ligament

*N. Howard*

A

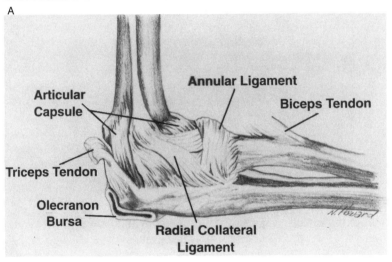

Articular Capsule

Annular Ligament

Biceps Tendon

Triceps Tendon

Olecranon Bursa

Radial Collateral Ligament

*N. Howard*

B

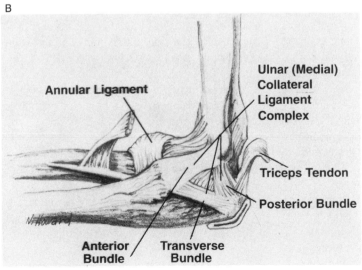

Annular Ligament

Ulnar (Medial) Collateral Ligament Complex

Triceps Tendon

Posterior Bundle

Anterior Bundle

Transverse Bundle

*N. Howard*

C

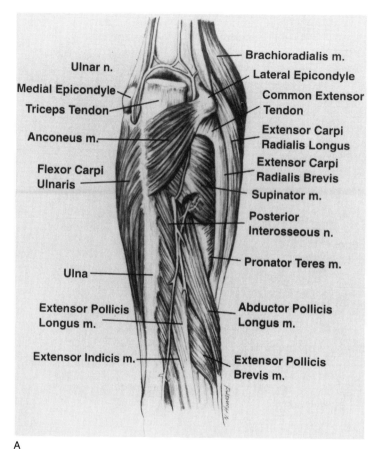

**Figure 15-3.** Muscles of the elbow and forearm: *A,* Posterior group.

Ulnar n.

Medial Epicondyle

Triceps Tendon

Anconeus m.

Flexor Carpi Ulnaris

Ulna

Extensor Pollicis Longus m.

Extensor Indicis m.

Brachioradialis m.

Lateral Epicondyle

Common Extensor Tendon

Extensor Carpi Radialis Longus

Extensor Carpi Radialis Brevis

Supinator m.

Posterior Interosseous n.

Pronator Teres m.

Abductor Pollicis Longus m.

Extensor Pollicis Brevis m.

A

lateral tennis elbow, as the tendons of these muscles may be involved in overuse injury.

**Medial.**    The flexor muscles of the forearm can be divided into three groups. The superficial group includes the pronator teres, palmaris longus, flexor carpi radialis, and flexor carpi ulnaris. These four muscles arise from a common aponeurosis near the medial epicondyle. Chronic overuse of this group can result in medial tennis elbow. The intermediate mass is made up of one muscle, the flexor digitorum superficialis. The deep group includes the flexor digitorum profundus, the flexor pollicis longus, and the pronator quadratus.

**Anterior.**    The anterior elbow muscles, the biceps brachii and brachialis, arise from the shoulder and upper arm. The biceps is a flexor and supinator of the forearm. Its two heads unite in the biceps tendon, which inserts on the radial tuberosity, the proximal radius, and the forearm fascia. The brachialis

arises from the anterior humerus and inserts on the ulnar tuberosity just distal to the coronoid process. The brachialis functions as a flexor of the forearm.

**Posterior.**    Posteriorly, the three heads of the triceps provide extension to the elbow and insert on the proximal olecranon. The anconeous is attached to the lateral epicondyle, the lateral side of the olecranon, and the adjacent part of the ulna. It provides extension to the elbow and stabilizes against flexion and pronation-supination.

*Neurovascular Structures*

**Brachial Artery.**    The brachial artery can be palpated just medial to the biceps tendon at the level of and just proximal to the antecubital fossa.

**Median Nerve.**    At the elbow, the median nerve lies medial to the brachial artery. It passes between

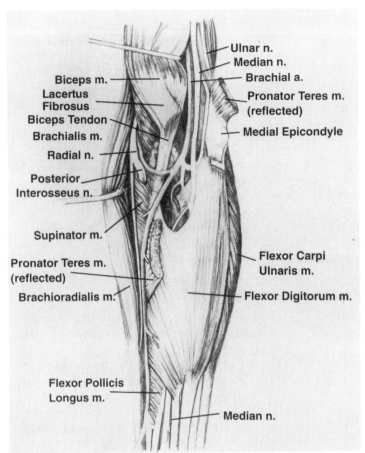

Biceps m.
Lacertus Fibrosus
Biceps Tendon
Brachialis m.
Radial n.
Posterior Interosseus n.
Supinator m.
Pronator Teres m. (reflected)
Brachioradialis m.
Flexor Pollicis Longus m.

Ulnar n.
Median n.
Brachial a.
Pronator Teres m. (reflected)
Medial Epicondyle
Flexor Carpi Ulnaris m.
Flexor Digitorum m.
Median n.

B

**Figure 15-3.** *(continued) B,* Anterior group.

the two heads of the pronator teres to enter the volar forearm.

**Ulnar Nerve.** The ulnar nerve runs in a sulcus between the medial epicondyle and the olecranon process. It passes between the heads of the flexor carpi ulnaris to enter the medial forearm.

## Rehabilitative Approach

A comprehensive rehabilitation program following elbow injuries emphasizes the stages outlined by the management system pyramid of the Virginia Sportsmedicine Institute (Figure 15-4).[1-8]

### Pathoanatomic Diagnosis

Establishing a correct diagnosis forms the basis for all rehabilitation programs. The history is the most important aspect of establishing the diagnosis and is designed to ascertain the specifics of injury. Pain phase scales may be useful in establishing prognosis and gauging rehabilitation progress (Table 15-1). For example, in the authors' experience, patients with lateral or medial tennis elbow who present with pain rated as phase 5 or less on the Nirschl Pain Phase Scale are more likely to respond favorably to a rehabilitative program. Physical examination identifies muscle imbalances and structural malalignment, and assists in reaching a

**Table 15-1.** Nirschl Pain Phase Scale

| | |
|---|---|
| Phase 1 | Stiffness or mild soreness after activity. Pain is usually gone within 24 hours. |
| Phase 2 | Stiffness or mild soreness before activity which is relieved by warm-up. The symptoms are not present during activity, but return after activity (lasting for 48 hours or less). |
| Phase 3 | Stiffness or mild soreness before specific sports or occupational activity. Pain is partially relieved by warm-up. It is minimally present during activity, and does not cause an alteration of the activity. |
| Phase 4 | Pain is similar, but somewhat more intense than phase 3 pain. Phase 4 pain causes a change in the performance of the attempted specific activity. Mild pain may also be noticed with activities of daily living (ADLs). |
| Phase 5 | Significant (moderate or greater) pain before, during, and after a specific activity which alters the activity. Pain occurs with ADLs, but does not cause a major change in ADLs. |
| Phase 6 | Phase 5 pain which persists even with complete rest. Phase 6 pain disrupts simple ADLs, and household chores are usually eliminated. |
| Phase 7 | Phase 6 pain which also causes a disruption of sleep on a consistent basis. Pain is aching in nature and intensifies with activity. |

Courtesy Nirschl Orthopedic & Sportsmedicine Clinic, Arlington, VA; used with permission.

proper diagnosis and preparing a well-constructed rehabilitation program.

### *Control of Inflammation*

Relief of pain and inflammation is achieved through the principles of PRICEMM, which stands for *p*rotection, *r*est, *i*ce, *c*ompression, *e*levation, *m*edication, and *m*odalities. It is important to note that rest does not mean immobilization, but rather elimination of the specific activities that cause pain (abuse). So, for example, if lateral ten-

nis elbow symptoms occur only with the tennis backhand stroke, the player is not instructed to stop playing tennis, but rather to avoid the backhand (Figure 15-5). Nonsteroidal antiinflammatory drugs (NSAIDs) are helpful, as can be oral steroids (if symptoms are acute or particularly intense). Cortisone injections are used sparingly, as intratendinous injections can result in tendon atrophy or dissolution. Injections are generally reserved for those cases in which pain interferes with rehabilitative progress. Modalities which are helpful include high voltage electrical stimulation, ultrasound, ice, and heat. For tendonosis/tendonitis, electrical stimulation is effective in reducing

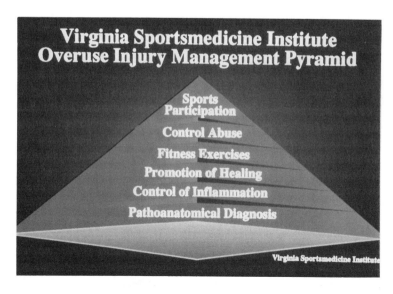

**Figure 15-4.** The Overuse Injury Management Pyramid developed by the Virginia Sportsmedicine Institute.

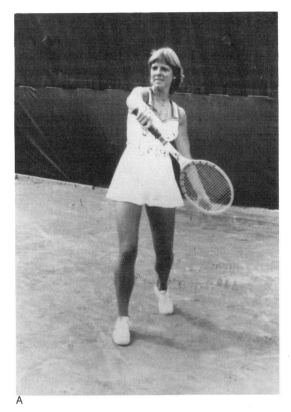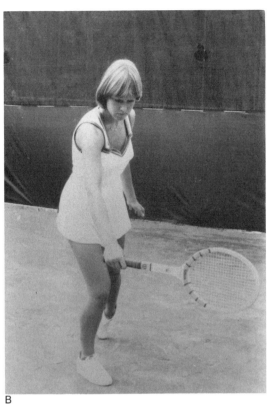

A                                                          B

**Figure 15-5.** *A,* Faulty backhand stroke. Poor lower body mechanics increase forceful stresses on small forearm wrist extensors. *B,* Correct backhand stroke. Proper lower body mechanics with forward weight transfer and shoulder circumduction enhance the quality of tennis play and decrease the potential for forearm muscle-tendon overload. (Courtesy Medical Sports, Inc., Arlington, VA.)

pain, inflammation, and spasm as well as enhancing circulation. A continuous sensory stimulation at a submotor intensity with a high pulse rate (greater than 100 pulses per second) for 20 to 40 minutes is recommended. Four to six sessions over 2 to 3 weeks is usually sufficient. Electrical stimulation is theorized to enhance healing because of its piezoelectric effect, which may facilitate proper alignment of the new tissues based on electrical charge orientation. Ultrasound is effective in facilitating flexibility exercises and for applying deep heat in chronic muscle injury.

*Promotion of Healing*

Promotion of healing is advanced by rehabilitative exercises, aerobic exercise, and general conditioning. The goal of rehabilitative exercise is to replace degenerative tissue with a more normal tissue state

(i.e., biologically healthy healing scar). As lateral and medial tennis elbow are the most common elbow overuse injuries encountered in clinical practice, the following rehabilitation program pertains most specifically to these injuries. The principles can be applied, however, to other elbow injuries as well. Further details are provided in the sections describing specific injuries.

Rehabilitative exercises begin with isometric strengthening of the elbow flexors, wrist extensors, and the pronators and supinators for lateral elbow injury, as well as wrist flexors for medial injury. Exercises are performed throughout the day following a rule of 5's: five repetitions, five seconds/repetition, five times/day, avoiding any position which is particularly painful. Daily isotonic exercises without weights are also started within pain-free arcs of motion. Full-range exercises and weights are gradually added to tolerance. Exercises are performed first with the elbow bent, and when tolerated, with the elbow extended. Exercises with Isoflex resistance tubing are initiated when the patient is able to perform isotonic exercises with 3 lb. Isoflex exercises are performed for wrist extension (and wrist flexion in medial injury), pronation, supination, and radial and ulnar deviation. They are started at five repetitions and progress to ten. Throughout this phase, patients are instructed to squeeze a tennis ball and open their fingers against the resistance of a rubber band throughout the day, first with the elbow bent and when tolerated, with the elbow extended. In competitive racquet sport athletes, isokinetics are started concurrently with Isoflex exercise. They are performed throughout a velocity spectrum from 60 degrees/second up to 210 degrees/second, then back down to 60 degrees/second. Early 5-second bouts progress to 30-second bouts. Arm cycling (i.e., with use of the Cybex UBE) encourages vascular flow and is incorporated throughout the program. Flexibility exercises are essential; however, they should not be initiated until 80% of normal strength is achieved, as experience has demonstrated poor patient tolerance to aggressive stretching programs in the early stages of rehabilitation. Pain-free activities of daily living serve as one endpoint of the rehabilitative program. Strength testing assists in monitoring progress. On grip testing with a spring loaded dynamometer, the dominant arm should be 20% stronger than the nondominant arm. With isokinetic testing, the dominant arm should be approximately 5% stronger in noncompetitive players and 10% stronger in competitive athletes. Patients are generally able to tolerate competitive activity well when they can complete isotonic exercises using at least 5 lb for fifteen repetitions of each exercise without pain. Some athletes choose to return to their sport sooner; however, the rehabilitation program should continue until they can tolerate this level of rehabilitative exercise. At this point, the rehabilitation process is decreased to a maintenance program emphasizing isotonic and Isoflex exercises three times a week.

### Fitness Exercises

Aerobic exercise and general body conditioning maintain body fitness in addition to promoting tissue healing. They offer advantages in enhancing rehabilitation as follows:

1. Central and peripheral aerobics increase regional tissue perfusion.
2. Neurophysiologic synergy and overflow provide neurologic stimulus to injured tissue.
3. Exercise minimizes the development of weakness of adjacent uninjured tissue.
4. Exercise minimizes the development of negative psychological effects of injury.

Fitness exercise is designed to take repaired normal tissue to a supranormal level and is best accomplished by sport-specific rehabilitative exercise and further development of general body conditioning. Sport-specific rehabilitation can begin once pain-free range of motion is attained and strength/endurance testing indicates a nearly complete return to preinjury levels. Sport-specific exercise consists of actual sport activity performed in a progressive, controlled fashion. Proper biomechanical technique is mandatory. In throwing sports, long tossing precedes short tossing. Velocity is gradually increased. Full windup is attempted later, and fastball and curveball throwing are added last.[9] Return to tennis is initiated with nonabusive strokes.[8] Patients with lateral tennis elbow start with the forehand only, and increase their time of play before adding the backhand stroke. Patients with medial tennis elbow start with the backhand and lobs, adding the forehand stroke later. Service and competitive play are added last. Plyometric exercise (i.e., medicine ball exercises) and transitional exercises (i.e., pulley exercises) may be added in this phase as needed.

### Control Abuse

Control of force loads is achieved by strict adherence to the use of proper sport technique, control of intensity and duration of activity, and counterforce bracing. Such bracing constrains the muscle groups while maintaining muscle balance (Figure 15-6). Elbow counterforce bracing has been shown by Groppel to decrease electromyographic (EMG) muscle activity and elbow angular acceleration and may therefore be of value in treating tennis

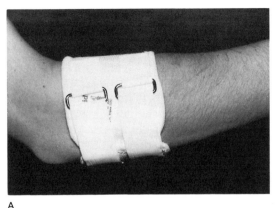
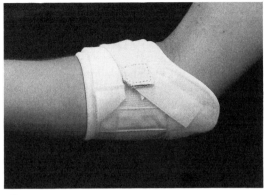

A                                                                          B

**Figure 15-6.** Elbow counterforce braces. Counterforce bracing constrains key muscle groups while maintaining muscle balance, thus controlling intrinsic overload of the elbow tendons. *A,* Lateral tennis elbow counterforce brace. *B,* Medial tennis elbow counterforce brace. The medial brace extends over the medial epicondyle, thus providing additional support to the pronator teres and flexor carpi radialis.

elbow.[10] Assessment of sport technique should include attention to biomechanics, equipment, and sport-specific activities, which when faulty may cause concentrated force loads that lead to overuse injuries. Lateral tennis elbow seems to be closely related to a faulty backhand or delayed forehand with a late wrist snap. Medial tennis elbow appears to be related to overhead serves as well as a late forehand. Control of intensity and duration of activity is of utmost importance. Intensity and duration represent the two principal training errors that lead to overuse injury, and athletes therefore must follow the training principle of gradual progression. Proper equipment is important to avoid overuse injury. Appropriate racquet grip size should be measured as described by Nirschl (Figure 15-7).

### Sports Participation

Return to sport activity may commence when the patient has attained full range of motion and 80% to 90% of strength compared with the uninjured side. Sport activity should initially be limited to every other day, then increased as tolerated. Rehabilitative exercises should continue upon return to the sport activity for up to 6 weeks. It may then be decreased as tolerated. Some degree of maintenance rehabilitative exercise assists in decreasing the likelihood of reinjury.

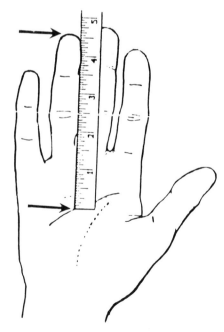

**Figure 15-7.** Grip size measurement (Nirschl technique). Place tapemeasure on radial border of ring finger and measure from proximal palmar crease to tip of ring finger. Measurement reflects functional working length of ring finger and is an excellent guide for proper handle size of sports or occupational implements. (Nirschl RP: Soft-tissue injuries about the elbow. *Clin Sports Med* 1986;5:637–652. Reproduced with permission.)

## Examination and Testing Techniques

### History

As with all musculoskeletal injury, evaluation of the elbow begins with a thorough history. The precise location, quality, frequency, duration, and incitement of pain must be established. Determining activities that exacerbate or relieve the pain aids in diagnosis. Past history of injury must be reviewed. For the athlete, training schedules, technique, and equipment should also be reviewed. Prior interventions, including self-treatments, should be investigated.

### Physical Examination

Physical examination must include inspection, range of motion testing, palpation, provocative testing, and neuromuscular testing. Any asymmetry in size or positioning between the extremities should be noted. The arms should be examined in the anatomic position, noting the carrying angle, the angle formed between the arm and forearm (Figure 15-8). Normal carrying angles measure up to five degrees of valgus in males and ten to fifteen degrees in females. An excessive carrying angle, known as cubitus valgus, may be congenital or due

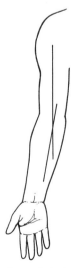

**Figure 5-8.** The carrying angle is the angle formed between the arm and forearm. Normal carrying angles measure up to 5 degrees of valgus in males and 10 to 15 degrees in females.

to traumatic causes such as fracture or epiphyseal damage. Cubitus varus may result from a supracondylar fracture of the humerus. Posterior elbow swelling should be noted. It may be a sign of olecranon bursitis or fracture.

Range of motion should include both active and passive testing.[11] Passive limitation warrants further investigation to determine the source of mechanical blockade. Normal values for forearm range of motion are as follows: extension (0 degrees), flexion (150 degrees), pronation (70 degrees), and supination (90 degrees).[12] Coronal plane stability should be assessed with both valgus and varus testing in 10 to 15 degrees of flexion as well as in full extension. Anterior-posterior stress should be applied to test for sagittal plane instability. Palpation with the elbow held at 90 degrees identifies areas of tenderness. When examining the elbow, it is helpful to concentrate on specific areas such as the lateral, medial, anterior, and posterior regions. What follows is a brief description of some of the techniques of examining these regions.

**Lateral.** The lateral epicondyle, supracondylar line of the humerus, tendon origins, and radial head should be palpated. Rotation of the radial head is noted with pronation and supination. The extensor forearm muscle group is often subject to overuse injury, and palpable tenderness over the extensor carpi radialis brevis is common in this condition. Pain is intensified with resisted wrist and finger extension with the elbow extended, and in advanced cases with the elbow flexed as well. The lateral collateral ligament and annular ligament (located deep to the extensor aponeurosis) are not directly palpable, although the area should be examined for tenderness. Varus stress testing (force applied medially to stress the lateral structures) exacerbates instability and pain secondary to lateral collateral ligament sprain. Provocative testing with resisted wrist and finger extension distinguishes pain due to extensor tendonosis from that originating from other structures.

**Medial.** The medial epicondyle, medial supracondylar line of the humerus, and the ulnar border should be palpated. Overuse of the flexor mass results in pain and palpable tenderness at the medial epicondyle (and for approximately 1 to 3 centimeters distal to the epicondyle). Pain is intensified with provocative testing such as resisted wrist flexion with the elbow extended (and in advanced cases with the elbow bent as well). The ulnar nerve is located in the sulcus between the medial epicondyle and the olecranon. Tinel's sign (tapping the area of the nerve in the ulnar groove, which results in a tingling sensation down the arm in the ulnar nerve distribution) may be present in patients with nerve entrapment. Laxity or pain at the underside of the medial epicondyle which is exacerbated by valgus stress testing (force applied laterally to stress the medial structures) suggests a sprain or tear of the medial collateral ligament.

**Anterior.**    Located medially to laterally in the cubital fossa are the median nerve, brachial artery, biceps tendon, and brachialis insertion. A ruptured biceps tendon can result in exquisite tenderness and a painful retracted mass in the mid to distal arm.

**Posterior.**    The tip of the olecranon and the olecranon fossa should be palpated, as should the triceps insertion. The olecranon bursa is not palpable unless inflamed or thickened. The examiner should asses for crepitus in the olecranon fossa as well as for subtle extension blockade, which is suggestive of synovitis or the presence of intraarticular loose bodies. Valgus stress testing may demonstrate crepitus (associated with chondromalacia) in the olecranon fossa.

### Ancillary Diagnostic Testing

X-ray studies should include anteroposterior and lateral views. Special views such as an oblique view to examine the radial head or an axial projection to examine the olecranon fossa are obtained as deemed necessary. Arthrography and magnetic resonance imaging (MRI) can identify loose bodies. Arthroscopy is a final diagnostic approach for intraarticular inspection, join débridement, and removal of loose bodies as indicated. Electromyography (EMG) can help detect areas of nerve compression.

## Diagnosis and Treatment of Specific Disorders

Injuries to the elbow can be divided into those resulting from overuse and those resulting from single-event trauma. Overuse injuries are caused by repetitive loads which result in chronic pathologic changes in the tissues involved.[1,13] Several factors have been identified which contribute to such injury (Table 15-2). Intrinsic factors are unique to the individual and include forearm muscle insufficiencies such as weakness, imbalance, or inflexibility, as well as instability of the elbow complex and prior injury. Extrinsic factors are related to training error and include improper conditioning, techniques, and equipment. Rehabilitative management includes correction of such inadequacies in addition to promoting healing of the injured tissues. As overuse injuries comprise the majority of elbow disorders seen in a rehabilitative practice, this discussion focuses on such injuries. In addition to overuse and traumatic injuries, compartment syndrome can result in elbow and forearm pain and is also discussed. Overuse injuries are conveniently classified according to their anatomic location (i.e., lateral, medial, anterior, or posterior).

### Lateral Overuse Injuries

#### Lateral Tennis Elbow (Lateral Epicondylitis)

Lateral tennis elbow results from chronic overuse activity which causes pathologic changes in the forearm extensor tendons. The actual tissue changes have been termed *angiofibroblastic tendonosis*. Histologically, the changes appear as invasion of young vascular and fibroblastic tissue in a characteristic pattern with collagen formation in

**Table 15-2.** Overuse Injury Risk Factors

| Intrinsic Factors | Extrinsic Factors |
| --- | --- |
| Malalignment | Training errors |
| Muscular imbalance | Equipment |
| Inflexibility | Environment |
| Muscular weakness | Technique |
| Instability | Sports-imposed deficiencies |

an unorganized fashion. The extensor carpi radialis brevis tendon is the structure most commonly involved. The extensor communis, and rarely the extensor carpi radialis longus and extensor carpi ulnaris, may be involved as well. It should be noted that this condition represents a primarily degenerative rather than inflammatory process (inflammatory cells are rarely present in histologic specimens). Furthermore, changes occur within the tendon tissue itself, not specifically at the epicondyle. Therefore, the term *epicondylitis* is really a misnomer. Most commonly seen in racquet sports and in occupations requiring repetitive extensor forearm use, lateral tennis elbow has been related to poor sport and occupational mechanics, conditioning, and equipment use.

**Diagnosis.** Patients with lateral tennis elbow present with localized tenderness medial and distal to the lateral epicondyle. Pain and tenderness extend distally along the muscle mass of the extensor brevis. Symptoms are exacerbated with provocative stress testing such as resisted wrist and finger extension with the elbow extended (and in advanced cases with the elbow flexed).

**Treatment.** The rehabilitative effort has been described earlier in detail. Surgical management, which includes resection of the pathologic tissue while leaving all normal tendon origins in place, is considered only if the patient fails to respond to an adequate rehabilitation program (generally lasting a minimum of 3 to 4 months).[14] When treating a patient for lateral tennis elbow, it is important to address weakness and biomechanical abnormalities in other parts of the upper extremity which may be related to this condition. For instance, weak rotator cuff muscles may cause the patient to overstress the wrist extensors during tennis in order to compensate for the deficiency.

### Posterior Interosseous Nerve Entrapment

The posterior interosseous syndrome is an entrapment neuropathy. It involves damage to the posterior interosseous branch of the radial nerve at the fibrous arch of the supinator muscle or more distally within the muscle itself.

**Diagnosis.** In posterior interosseous nerve compression, lateral elbow pain radiates into the distal forearm and is aggravated by pronation and supination. Tenderness is noted 3 to 4 cm distal to the lateral epicondyle where the radial nerve crosses the radial head and penetrates the supinator muscle. Tinel's sign may be present and there may be weakness of the wrist and finger extensors. Numbness is not normally present as this is a motor nerve at this level. Confirmation of this condition can be obtained electromyographically (see Chapter 8).

**Treatment.** Treatment of posterior interosseous nerve entrapment emphasizes rest, NSAIDs, and flexibility and endurance training. Surgical decompression may become necessary in refractory cases.

### Radiocapitellar Chondromalacia

Repetitive valgus forces, such as those encountered in throwing sports, cause lateral elbow joint compression and may lead to damage to the radial head and humeral capitellum.

**Diagnosis.** Pain in radiocapitellar chondromalacia is localized to the radiocapitellar joint and is exacerbated by activity. Crepitus or "catching" may be present. X-ray studies demonstrate a loss of radiocapitellar joint space, osteophytes, or sometimes loose bodies.

**Treatment.** Mild cases of this condition respond to NSAIDs and rehabilitation. Exercises are similar to those described for lateral tennis elbow; however, special caution to perform exercises only within pain-free arcs ensures joint safety. Surgical debridement is often necessary, especially in more severe cases.

### Posterolateral Synovitis

A potential and not uncommon companion to lateral tennis elbow is synovitis and (probable) chondromalacia of the posterolateral joint in and around the lateral olecranon gutter. This most likely represents an impingement phenomenon of the inflamed synovium.

**Diagnosis.** In posterolateral synovitis, pain and tenderness are localized to the lateral olecranon gutter to the level of the radial head. Joint crepitus may be present, but motion is rarely restricted. Posterolateral synovitis is most often associated with lateral tennis elbow, but may present independently or in association with other elbow maladies.

**Treatment.** Conservative treatment for this condition emphasizes antiinflammatory measures (NSAIDs, ice, relative rest). Rehabilitative exercises are similar to those described for lateral tennis elbow; however, exercises are initiated with the elbow straight. Exercises performed with the elbow bent are generally poorly tolerated by patients with posterolateral synovitis. Recalcitrant cases require surgical débridement.

### Osteochondritis Dissecans Capitellum

Lateral compressive forces on the elbow joint can lead to focal avascular necrosis of the capitellum. This is known as osteochondritis dissecans.

**Diagnosis.** In osteochondritis dissecans, pain at the radiocapitellar joint is increased with pronation and supination. Patients often lack full active and passive elbow extension. X-ray films may reveal a flattening or focal distortion of the capitellum and perhaps even loose bodies. Tomograms or MRI can confirm the diagnosis.

**Treatment.** Osteochondritis dissecans of the capitellum often responds to rest (3 to 4 months of nonabusive activity) and rehabilitative effort. Exercises are directed toward minimizing strength loss during the rest period. The specific exercises are similar to those described for lateral tennis elbow with added emphasis on biceps and triceps strength. Surgery is required if loose bodies are present. Preliminary evidence suggests that electrical bone stimulation may stimulate vascular supply and healing and is recommended by the authors.

### Medial Overuse Injuries

### Medial Tennis Elbow (Medial Epicondylitis)

Medial tennis elbow, or golfer's elbow, results from chronic overuse of the flexor forearm muscu-

lature. Primary injury occurs in the pronator teres and flexor carpi radialis and to a lesser degree in the palmaris longus, flexor carpi ulnaris, and rarely the flexor digitorum sublimis.

**Diagnosis.** In medial tennis elbow localized tenderness at the tip of the epicondyle extends distally for approximately 1 to 3 cm along the pronator teres and flexor carpi radialis. Pain is exacerbated by resisted wrist flexion and/or pronation with the elbow in extension (and in advanced cases with the elbow flexed).

**Treatment.** Rehabilitative management for medial tennis elbow has been described previously. Surgical management is considered only after failure of adequate rehabilitative effort.

### Ulnar Nerve Compression/Subluxation

Nirschl has divided the medial epicondylar groove into three zones:[5]

Zone I: Proximal to the medial epicondyle
Zone II: The level of the medial epicondyle (retrocondylar groove)
Zone III: Distal to the medial epicondyle (cubital tunnel)

Repetitive overuse can result in compression of the ulnar nerve in zone III by a tight flexor carpi ulnaris muscle. Entrapment can also be precipitated in zones II and III by a subluxating ulnar nerve (a nerve that slips around the epicondyle during elbow flexion), in zone II by elbow synovitis, in zone I or II by cubitus valgus deformity, or in zone I by the medial intermuscular septum.

**Diagnosis.** In ulnar neuropathy at the elbow, numbness and weakness may be present in the zone of entrapment. Intrinsic hand muscle wasting may be noted in long-standing cases. Confirmation of the disorder is made electromyographically.

**Treatment.** Conservative management of an ulnar entrapment neuropathy includes the use of NSAIDs, protection with an elbow pad, avoidance of extreme repetitive flexion (in cases of a subluxating nerve), and exercise emphasizing elbow flexibility and forearm flexor strength and endurance. Failure to respond to conservative management after 3 to 4 months, chronic subluxation, or progressive motor or sensory deficit calls for surgical decompression of the nerve. In some cases an anterior transposition of the ulnar nerve is indicated. Surgical transposition may be suboptimal, however, if blood supply to the nerve is compromised.

*Medial Collateral Ligament Sprain*

Medial collateral ligament (MCL) sprain can result from repetitive valgus stress and is common in racquet and throwing sports, especially in baseball pitchers.

**Diagnosis.** In MCL sprain, elbow pain of insidious onset is increased by valgus stress testing at 30 degrees of elbow flexion. MCL sprain must be differentiated from complete ligamentous rupture which is more often associated with acute trauma. Instability on examination and abnormal calcifications on plain X-rays suggest the presence of ligament rupture. This diagnosis can be confirmed by MRI.

**Treatment.** Most cases of MCL sprain respond to rehabilitative management. Emphasis is placed on isometric exercises of the forearm flexors and pronators in order to enhance their role as secondary stabilizers of the medial joint. Chronic cases, especially if accompanied by heterotopic ossification (abnormal bone deposition), bone spurring, or loose bodies may require surgery. Ligamentous rupture necessitates surgical repair (usually with an autogenous tendon graft).

*Medial Epicondyle Apophysitis*
*(Little League Elbow)*

Repetitive valgus stress in an adolescent whose growth plates have not yet fused can result in an avulsion injury of the medial epicondyle. This is called an apophysitis. A single traumatic event can also result in a complete avulsion of the epicondyle. This is associated with rupture of the medial capsule.

**Diagnosis.** In apophysitis, pain and tenderness is located to the medial epicondyle. The symptoms are intensified by throwing. A widening of the ap-

ophyseal line or even complete apophyseal separation will be seen on X-ray.

**Treatment.** Lesions involving less than 0.5 to 1 cm of apophyseal separation are initially treated with rest for 2 to 3 weeks. This is followed by rehabilitative effort which is similar to that described for medial tennis elbow; however, resistance exercises are avoided until isotonic exercises without weight can be performed without pain (generally 2 to 3 weeks). Throwing is avoided for 6 to 12 weeks. Separation greater than 0.5 to 1 cm, failure to respond to conservative measures, or sudden traumatic avulsions are indications for surgery.

*Anterior Overuse Injuries*

*Biceps Tendonitis*

Biceps tendonitis is an overuse injury resulting from repetitive elbow flexion and forearm supination.

**Diagnosis.** In this tendonitis, localized pain of the biceps tendon in the anterior elbow is exacerbated by resisted flexion and supination.

*Treatment*

Rehabilitative effort for biceps tendonitis emphasizes rest, NSAIDs, and later, restoration of strength and flexibility of the flexor mechanism. The biceps rarely ruptures at the elbow, and such injury is generally attributable to a traumatic event. If it occurs, immediate surgical repair is indicated.

*Pronator Syndrome*

The pronator syndrome is an entrapment neuropathy of the median nerve distal to the antecubital fossa. In most cases, the median nerve pierces the two heads of the pronator teres prior to passing under the muscle. Muscle hypertrophy, trauma, or entrapment by an anomalous fibrous band may injure the nerve at this point.

**Diagnosis.** In this condition, pain at the pronator teres is exacerbated by resisted pronation. Weakness of the wrist and finger flexors, numbness, and

Tinel's sign may be present. Diagnosis is confirmed electromyographically.

**Treatment.**    Rehabilitation emphasizes removal of the causative activity, rest, NSAIDs, ice, and restoration of proper flexibility and strength of the wrist flexors and forearm pronators. Rehabilitation most benefits those cases in which compression is related to medial elbow tendonosis. Gentle massage along the fibers may aid in breaking up adhesions. Surgical release may be needed in recalcitrant cases (i.e., those cases related to muscle hypertrophy or entrapment by a fibrous band).

### Anterior Capsule Strain

Repetitive hyperextension activity results in small tears of the anterior capsule. Associated brachialis muscle tears with myositis may also occur. Anterior elbow pain may also occur after a single traumatic hyperextension event.

**Diagnosis.**    Anterior elbow pain is worsened with passive extension or with hyperextension stress testing of the elbow. Radiographs are advisable to rule out myositis ossificans of the brachialis muscle.

**Treatment.**    Rehabilitative management of anterior capsule strain emphasizes active range of motion exercise to avoid the formation of a flexion contracture. A gradual strengthening program for the biceps and brachialis accompanies the flexibility program.

### Posterior Overuse Injuries

### Triceps Tendonitis

Triceps tendon overload injury results from repetitive extension of the elbow.

**Diagnosis.**    In triceps tendonitis, posterior elbow pain is caused or worsened by resisted extension. X-ray evaluation is indicated to rule out olecranon apophysitis in adolescents and an avulsion fracture in adults.

**Treatment.**    Initial management includes rest, NSAIDs, and ice. Rehabilitative exercises emphasize flexibility and strength of the extensor mechanism.

A violent triceps contraction may result in tendon rupture or olecranon avulsion fracture. These conditions are associated with severe pain and often a palpable defect at the triceps insertion. Surgical reattachment is followed by a short period of immobilization, then gradual range of motion and strengthening exercise.

### Olecranon Bursitis

Inflammation of the olecranon bursa may be caused by repetitive or single-event trauma.

**Diagnosis.**    Repetitive irritation, contusion, or direct trauma to the olecranon bursa results in swelling of the posterior elbow. Pain or associated redness may be signs of an associated intrabursal infection. X-ray studies are indicated to rule out loose fragments, prominent exostosis, or chip fractures.

**Treatment.**    Treatment of bursitis involves ice, NSAIDs, and the use of elbow pads. In refractory cases the bursal fluid should be aspirated. This should also be done in cases in which infection is suspected. Recurrent swelling may necessitate surgical referral for bursectomy.

### Olecranon Impingement Syndrome

Repetitive impingement of the olecranon in the olecranon fossa may occur with valgus stress in throwing sports. Stress to both articular surfaces of the joint may result in the formation of loose bodies, osteophytes, chondromalacia, and synovitis.

**Diagnosis.**    In olecranon impingement, posterior elbow pain may be associated with catching, clicking, and crepitus which are worsened by elbow extension. Full extension may be limited by mechanical blockade. X-ray findings confirm loose bodies, olecranon osteophytes, and commonly associated anterior elbow changes.

**Treatment.**    Mild cases of olecranon impingement respond to rehabilitative management to reestablish normal motion, strength, and endurance; however, continued pain, loose bodies, and mechanical blockade are indications for surgery.

*Olecranon Stress Fracture/Apophysitis*

Repetitive overload may result in olecranon stress fracture or separation of the olecranon apophysis.

**Diagnosis.** In these conditions, pain over the olecranon is exacerbated by resisted elbow extension. Swelling may be present, and the bone may be tender to percussion. X-ray studies may confirm the diagnosis; however, a bone scan may be necessary to detect early stress fractures.

**Treatment.** Treatment involves relaxed immobilization for 4 to 6 weeks with a 90-degree elbow immobilizer. Daily range of motion exercises are performed. Rehabilitative effort commences after 4 to 6 weeks if x-ray evaluation and clinical examination show evidence of healing. Separation of the olecranon apophysis is an indication for surgical referral for possible open reduction and internal fixation.

*Traumatic Skeletal Injuries*

Sudden acute trauma must alert the health practitioner to the likelihood of fractures or dislocations of the elbow. Such injuries are best treated by immediate splinting and prompt referral to an orthopedic surgeon. Neurovascular status must be evaluated, as nerve or artery damage may be associated with fractures. In particular, brachial artery damage may be caused by a supracondylar humerus fracture. Radiographic evaluation includes anteroposterior, lateral, oblique, and opposite-side comparison views. A posterior fat pad sign may assist in the diagnosis of subtle fractures.

Some of the more common traumatic injuries of the elbow include fractures of the supracondylar humerus, medial epicondyle, lateral condyle, radial head, olecranon, and radial and ulnar shafts as well as posterior elbow dislocation. Rehabilitative management to ensure adequate flexibility, strength, and endurance as well as optimum sport technique is important following any necessary surgical management or period of immobilization.

*Compartment Syndrome*

Increased pressure within the volar and dorsal compartments of the forearm may compromise circulation to the tissues in these spaces. This may result from trauma, bleeding, or muscle hypertrophy. Chronic exertion compartment syndrome is a condition in which excessive intermittent pressure during activity decreases blood flow to the compartment. Intense pain, weakness, and sensory symptoms can result. Compartment pressure may be measured with a catheter. Pressures exceeding 35 to 40 mmHg mandate surgical decompression.

**Case Report**

A 41-year-old right-handed man presented with dull pain in his right lateral elbow. Pain had been present for 6 months, but just recently started to interfere with his tennis, which he played three to four times per week. He also noticed pain during yard work and typing. Pain was rated as a 4 on the Nirschl Pain Phase Scale. Physical examination was significant for tenderness to palpation just distal to the lateral epicondyle, extending 2 cm along the extensor muscle mass. Pain was increased with resisted wrist extension with the elbow extended. Tenderness was also noted over the anterior shoulder. Weakness was present in the elbow extensors and shoulder abductors and external rotators. Elbow and shoulder range of motion was normal. Plain films of the elbow were unremarkable. Dynamometer grip testing measured 71 lb on the right and 85 lb on the left. A diagnosis of lateral tennis elbow and associated rotator cuff tendonosis was made. The patient was given a 10-day course of NSAIDs and was instructed to apply ice to the elbow three times per day, particularly after challenging activity. A lateral counterforce brace was worn during sport and other activities which exacerbated the pain. He was advised that he could continue tennis with light ground strokes if the pain was not worsened. A daily rehabilitative program was initially supervised by a physical therapist twice a week for 2 weeks, then performed at home. Throughout this phase, a general conditioning program (jogging and stretching) was continued. After 6 weeks, exercise frequency decreased to three times per week. By this time he had resumed all tennis strokes. By 10 weeks he was able to resume competitive play.

## Points of Summary

1. Injury to the elbow and forearm can most easily be classified as overuse or traumatic.
2. Overuse injuries are the result of repetitive microtrauma, which over time can result in inflammation and cellular degeneration.
3. In lateral tennis elbow, the tendon most commonly involved is the extensor carpi radialis brevis. This is followed in frequency by the extensor communis and extensor carpi radialis, and to a lesser degree the extensor carpi ulnaris.
4. In medial tennis elbow, the most commonly involved tendons are those of the pronator teres and flexor carpi radialis. The palmaris longus, flexor carpi ulnaris, and flexor sublimis may also be affected.
5. Provocative testing for lateral tennis elbow consists of resisted wrist and finger extension with the elbow in extension. Testing for medial tennis elbow consists of resisted wrist flexion and/or pronation with the elbow in extension. Advanced cases elicit pain when tested with the elbow in flexion.
6. The management of overuse injury follows a stepwise rehabilitative approach as outlined by the Virginia Sportsmedicine Institute's management pyramid.
7. Cortisone injection plays a limited role in elbow rehabilitation due to the danger of tendon injury and lack of curative capacity.
8. The goal of rehabilitative exercise is to restore injured tissue to a normal or near-normal state; fitness exercise is directed toward training normal tissue to a supranormal state.
9. All rehabilitative programs should include assessment of intrinsic and extrinsic risk factors in addition to injury-specific management.
10. Surgical management of tennis elbow, conducted after failure of an adequate trial of rehabilitation, is directed toward removal of degenerated tissue, thus providing an optimum environment for more normal healing.

## References

1. O'Connor FG, Nirschl RP, Sobel JR: Five-step treatment for overuse injuries. *Physical Sportsmed* 1992;20:128–142.
2. Nirschl R, Sobel J: Conservative treatment of tennis elbow. *Physical Sportsmed* 1981;9:42–54.
3. Nirschl R: Tennis elbow. *Orthop Clin North Am* 1973;4:787–800.
4. Nirschl R: Tennis elbow: Surgery and rehabilitation of the professional athlete. In Pettrone F (ed): *AAOS Symposium on Upper Extremity Injuries in Athletics*. St. Louis: CV Mosby, 1986:244–265.
5. Nirschl R: Soft-tissue injuries about the elbow. *Clin Sports Med* 1986;5:637–652.
6. Nirschl R: Prevention and treatment of elbow and shoulder injuries in the tennis player. *Clin Sports Med* 1988;7:289–308.
7. Nirschl R: Tennis injuries. In Nicholas J, Hershman E (eds): *The Upper Extremity in Sports Medicine*. St. Louis: CV Mosby, 1990.
8. Sobel J, Pettrone F, Nirschl R: Prevention and rehabilitation of racquet sport injuries. In Nicholas J, Hershman E (eds): *The Upper Extremity in Sports Medicine*. St. Louis: CV Mosby, 1990.
9. Saal JA: Rehabilitation of throwing and tennis related shoulder injuries. *Physical Medicine and Rehabilitation: State of the Art Reviews* 1987;1:610.
10. Groppel J, Nirschl R: A mechanical and electromyographical analysis of the effects of various joint counterforce braces on the tennis player. *Am J Sports Med* 1986;14:195–200.
11. Hoppenfeld S: *Physical Examination of the Spine and Extremities*. Norwalk, CT: Appleton-Century-Crofts, 1976:35–57.
12. Mehloff T, Bennett J: Elbow injuries. In Mellion M, Walsh W, Shelton G (eds): *The Team Physician's Handbook*. Philadelphia, Hanley & Belfus, 1990.
13. Herring SA, Nilson KL: Introduction to overuse injuries. *Clin Sports Med* 1987;6:225–239.
14. Nirschl R, Pettrone F: Tennis elbow: The surgical treatment of lateral epicondylitis. *J Bone Joint Surg* 1979;61A:832–839.

## Suggested Readings

Hoppenfeld S: *Physical Examination of the Spine and Extremities*. Norwalk, CT: Appleton-Century-Crofts, 1976.

Mehlhoff T, Bennett J: Elbow Injuries. In Mellion M, Walsh W, Shelton G (eds). *The Team Physician's Handbook*. Philadelphia: Hanley & Belfus, 1990.

Morrey BF (ed): *The Elbow and Its Disorders*. Philadelphia, WB Saunders, 1985.

Nirschl RP: Soft-tissue injuries about the elbow. *Clin Sports Med* 1986;5:637–652.

Nirschl R: Tennis injuries. In Nicholas J, Hershman E (eds): *The Upper Extremity in Sports Medicine*. St. Louis, CV Mosby, 1990.

Sobel J, Pettrone F, Nirschl R: Prevention and rehabilitation of racquet sport injuries. In Nicholas J, Hershman E (eds): *The Upper Extremity in Sports Medicine*. St. Louis: CV Mosby, 1990.

# Chapter 16
# Wrist and Hand

BARBARA E. MCNEIL,
RALPH BUSCHBACHER

The hand and wrist complex is a complicated structure capable of performing movements requiring a combination of flexibility, power, dexterity, and fine sensibility. Dependent on the upper extremity for positioning, the hand can function as a tool, or it can use objects to manipulate the environment. Impairment of the wrist and hand result in significant changes in daily living, vocational, and recreational function.

Few physicians see enough hand and wrist disorders to become experts at treating this region. This chapter serves as an introduction to the field. The interested reader is referred to the suggested readings at the end of the chapter for more information.

## Wrist and Hand Anatomy

### Bones, Joints, and Ligaments

The bones of the hand and wrist are divided into the carpals, metacarpals, and phalanges (Figure 16-1). There are numerous joints between the bones. Three are of special interest: the radiocarpal, first carpometacarpal, and the metacarpophalangeal joints, and deserve further mention (Figure 16-2).

The radiocarpal joint is an ellipsoid joint, a modified spheroid joint (see Chapter 2) which extends into the area between the ulna and the carpal bones. The ulna does not articulate directly with the carpal bones, nor does it contribute to the radiocarpal joint. Instead, it is separated from the radiocarpal joint by a structure called the triangular fibrocartilaginous complex.

The first carpometacarpal joint (of the thumb) is a sellar joint (see Chapter 2) which provides most of the mobility of the thumb. It is subject to degenerative change. The metacarpophalangeal joints (MCP) of digits 2 through 5 are condylar joints (see Chapter 1). They are reinforced medially and laterally by collateral ligaments. These ligaments are in a relaxed position when the digits are extended but become taut when the MCP joints are flexed (Figure 16-3). Thus it is easy to abduct and adduct the fingers when they are extended, but this motion is not normally allowed when the MCP joints are flexed. This is important when positioning the hand during immobilization, as debilitating contractures may occur if the joints are splinted in extension.

### Muscles

The muscles of the hand and wrist can be divided into intrinsic and extrinsic muscles depending on where they originate. The extrinsic muscles arise from the elbow or forearm, and their tendons insert onto the hand and wrist to control movement. The tendons of the flexors and extensors of the digits are interestingly arranged. The tendon of

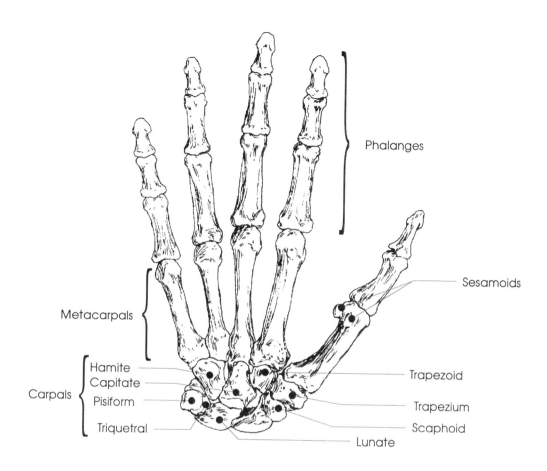

the flexor digitorum superficialis (FDS) splits at the proximal interphalangeal (PIP) joint to allow the tendon of the flexor digitorum profundus (FDP) to pass distally to the distal phalanx (Figure 16-4). The FDS flexes the PIP joint, while the FDP flexes the distal interphalangeal (DIP) joint. The extensor tendons also split (Figure 16-5), with insertions on the middle and distal phalanges. Because there is only one extensor tendon for each finger, the tendons extend both the PIP and DIP joints (as well as the MCP joints).

Some of the intrinsic muscles of the hand, the lumbricals and the interossei, insert onto the extensor tendons. They flex the MCP joints, extend the PIP and DIP joints, and provide abduction/adduction force. The other intrinsic hand muscles make up the prominent masses of the hand, namely the thenar eminence around the base of the thumb and the hypothenar eminence at the fifth metacarpal (Figure 16-6).

### Nerves

The radial, ulnar, and median nerves all pass into the hand (Figure 16-7). The radial nerve is purely a sensory branch in the hand. It supplies sensation to the dorsum of the hand. The median and ulnar nerves also provide sensation to the hand. In addition, the median nerve controls most of the thenar muscles, while the ulnar nerve innervates the rest of the muscles of the hand.

### Carpal Tunnel

The carpal tunnel is the space enclosed by the carpal bones and the transverse carpal ligament. This ligament is a fascial sheath which lies beneath the flexor retinaculum (Figure 16-8). The carpal tunnel contains nine ligaments, an artery (median

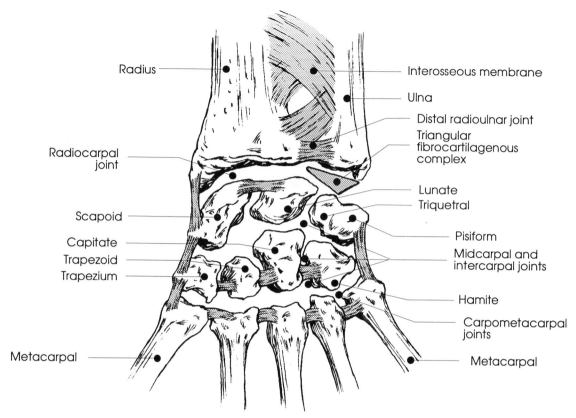

**Figure 16-2.** The joints of the hand and wrist.

artery), and the median nerve. Because it is constrained by relatively unyielding structures, any condition that increases pressure within the carpal tunnel can injure the median nerve.

### Rehabilitative Approach

The basic goals of rehabilitation of hand and wrist impairments should focus on the following:

Reduction of inflammation and edema
Reduction of pain
Restoration of strength and range of motion
Restoration of function
Protection against further injury

A few specific techniques to help accomplish these goals are described below. Since the hand and wrist are so important and complex, it is often worthwhile to enlist the aid of a dedicated hand therapist in treating this area.

### Heat and Cold

As in other parts of the body, local heat or cold application is sometimes useful in treating the wrist and hand. However, because of the limited

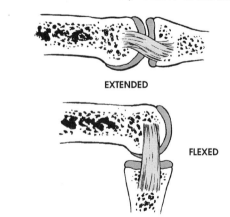

**Figure 16-3.** The metacarpophalangeal collateral ligaments. When the finger is extended these ligaments are lax and allow motion in abduction and adduction. When the finger is flexed the ligaments are taut.

program might include immersing the hand in buckets of beans or rice or rubbing progressively coarser materials over the skin. Care must be taken not to overstimulate the limb, especially in patients with reflex sympathetic dystrophy, so symptoms are not exacerbated. Contrast baths, as just described, are also used.

### Edema Management

The hand is susceptible to edema. Education of patients with edema should encourage positioning of the hand above the heart to facilitate the fluid's return to the circulation. Immobilization of the hand in a sling usually worsens edema because it places the arm in a flexed, adducted, static, and dependent posture. If a sling is necessary, it should support the hand at or slightly above the level of

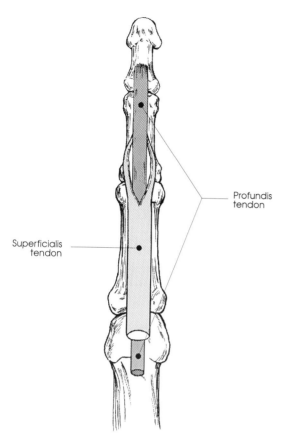

Profundis tendon

Superficialis tendon

**Figure 16-4.** Flexor tendons of the fingers. The flexor digitorum superficialis splits to allow the flexor digitorum profundus to pass underneath to the distal phalanx.

thickness of this part of the body, superficial heating modalities may actually penetrate to the deep tissues. While any of the modalities described in Chapter 6 may be used, paraffin baths are especially useful in treating rheumatoid arthritis hand involvement. Ultrasound treatment, with the hand held under water and the applicator several centimeters away, is also useful, especially in treating multiple joints and hand structures.

Contrast baths, the alternate application of heat and cold, is also often used in the hand. This technique can be used to control edema or to desensitize the area in conditions of skin hypersensitivity.

### Desensitization

In conditions of hyperalgesia, a progressive desensitization program can help relieve pain. Such a

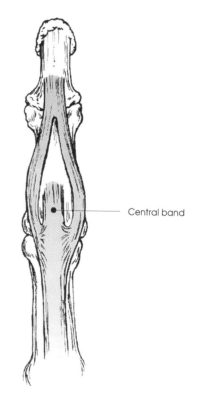

Central band

**Figure 16-5.** The extensor tendons of the fingers. The tendon splits into a central band that inserts on the middle phalanx and lateral bands that pass to the distal phalanx.

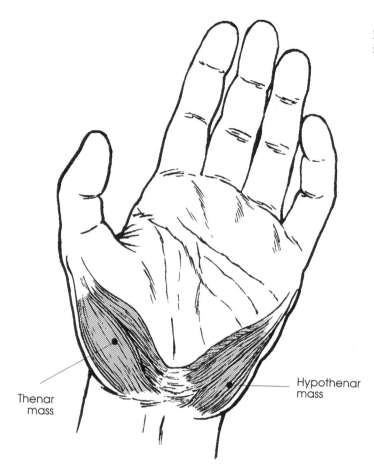

**Figure 16-6.** The thenar and hypothenar muscle masses.

Hypothenar mass

Thenar mass

the heart. Swelling unresponsive to elevation may need aggressive therapeutic intervention. Massage may help to push the excess fluid out of the hand.[1] Compressive garments, such as Isotoner gloves or Jobst custom fitted wraps, provide constant pressure and prevent fluctuating edema. Coban (3M, Minneapolis, MN) is an elastic tape that is wrapped distally to proximally to combine a "milking" of the tissue with constant pressure. Patients can be taught to wrap the hand with Coban at home. It can be used in conjunction with ice water immersion. In addition, active exercises, such as "making a fist" help to reduce edema and should be performed with the hand elevated.

*Positioning*

Proper positioning of the hand and wrist is important after injury, surgery, or in patients with muscle imbalances. An improperly positioned hand will become contracted in a functionally useless posture. Proper positioning may facilitate healing, and even in patients who have no improvement of strength or sensation, it may allow the hand and wrist to maintain a position of function, so that they can be useful to the patient.

A complete description of proper positioning and orthotic use is beyond the scope of this chapter but can be obtained elsewhere (see Chapter 24).[2-4] Orthoses (splints) are either static or dynamic.

A static splint prevents motion across a joint. Indications for such a splint may be to immobilize the hand to ensure healing, to decrease inflammation, to protect the hand, or to provide a functional position. Other uses are to maintain or increase range of motion and to decrease muscle tone. As a rule, static splints should maintain the following joint positions:

Wrist—extended 30 degrees
MCP joints 2 through 5—flexed 70 to 90 degrees

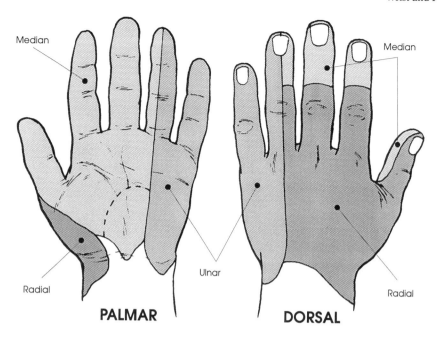

**Figure 16-7.** Sensory innervation patterns of the hand.

PIP joints—flexed 10 to 20 degrees
Thumb—fully abducted

The splint should be constructed to maintain the first (thumb) web space. Such positioning prevents ligamentous contracture. It may, however, lead to contracture of the intrinsic hand muscles. Therefore, these muscles must be stretched at least twice a day. This is done by combined MCP extension and interphalangeal (IP) joint flexion, a position which maximally elongates these muscles. Care must be taken to construct splints to support the arch of the palm; volar splints do this best.

Dynamic orthoses use an external source of traction such as hinges, rubber bands, springs, or pneumatic devices to provide passive range of motion. They can be used to maintain mobility, increase function, and apply longitudinal stretch.

When using orthoses, only those joints which are injured or being treated should be splinted. When possible, unaffected joints should be allowed to move freely.

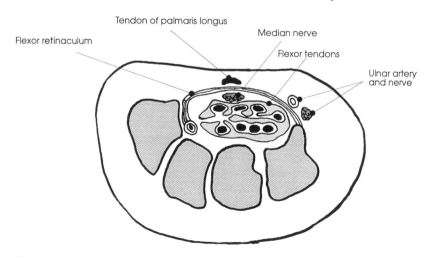

**Figure 16-8.** The contents of the carpal tunnel: median nerve and the flexor tendons of the digits.

### Workplace Modification

Adequate rehabilitation involves removing the cause of the injury to prevent its recurrence. Workplace assessment and, if needed, job modification or improved ergodynamics are recommended.

## Examination and Testing Techniques

### History and Physical Examination

A good evaluation should start with a complete history. Hand dominance can be useful in evaluating disability or an overuse injury. A brief review of symptoms may lead the examiner to establish a working diagnosis of a general connective tissue disease such as rheumatoid arthritis, which often presents with hand complaints. If an injury is being evaluated, the mechanism of injury should be established.

The physical examination should include observations for atrophy and skin and vascular changes as well as general hand posture. The hand and wrist are palpated to detect nodules, joint swelling, and tenderness. Strength testing is performed with care to avoid further injury in the case of structural damage. Grip strength may be quantified with the use of a hand held dynamometer. Sensory testing is also important. Range of motion is assessed passively and actively. Decreased passive and active range is indicative of joint pathology or contracture. Isolated loss of active range of motion may be a sign of ligamentous tear. Range of motion of the forearm, especially in supination/pronation, should be assessed, as the distal radioulnar joint may be limited in range. In addition, a complete upper extremity and neck examination is important to rule out more proximal problems that may be causing hand or wrist symptoms. A number of specific tests may also be performed.

**Weber's Two-Point Discrimination Test.** It is important to document and follow loss of sensation during the clinical course, especially in compressive neuropathies. The hand should be firmly immobilized on a flat surface. Equal pressure is exerted using a two-pronged object with a known distance separating the two points. There are many commercially available devices to do this, but an unfolded paper clip may also be used. Normal digital two-point discrimination should be 6 mm or less when measured longitudinally on either side of the distal digits.[5] The pressure applied should not be enough to blanch the skin.

**Froment's Sign.** The patient is asked to hold a piece of paper between the thumb and hand in the first web space. An inability to do so without flexing the IP joint is considered a positive sign. It is indicative of weakness of the thumb adductor, a muscle innervated by the ulnar nerve.

**Tendon Isolation Testing.** When flexion of the fingers is impaired it may be difficult to determine which tendon, the flexor digitorum profundus, the flexor digitorum superficialis, or both, is damaged. The tendons can be tested in isolation according to their function. The flexor digitorum profundus, which inserts on the distal phalanx, is tested by stabilizing the PIP joint and asking the patient to flex the finger. If the flexor digitorum profundus tendon is intact, the distal phalanx should flex.

The flexor digitorum superficialis is isolated by the examiner by stabilizing the adjacent fingers. The purpose of this stabilization is to remove the contribution of the flexor digitorum profundus to PIP flexion. Since the flexor digitorum profundus tendons arise from a common muscle, it is impossible to flex one DIP joint without also flexing the neighboring ones. Therefore, the examiner stabilizes the adjacent finger PIP and DIP joints and asks the patient to flex the finger being tested. Normally the PIP (but not the DIP) bends. If it does not, it indicates possible FDS rupture (*note: some persons without obvious injury have difficulty passing this test, especially in the fifth digit; therefore it must be interpreted in conjunction with the rest of the examination*).

**Intrinsic Muscle Flexibility Testing.** As described earlier, the intrinsic hand muscles that insert on the extensor tendons of the digits flex the MCP and extend the PIP and DIP joints. To test for tightness, the patient is asked to hyperextend the MCP and maximally flex the IP joints (this puts muscles at maximal stretch). Then the MCP joints are flexed (relaxes the muscles). If this flexion allows the IP joints to flex further, it is a sign of intrinsic muscle inflexibility.

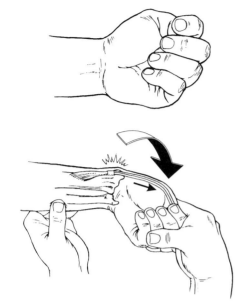

**Figure 16-9.** Finkelstein's test for DeQuervain's tenosynovitis of the extensor pollicis brevis and abductor pollicis longus.

**Finkelstein's Test** (Figure 16-9).    This is a test to detect tendon sheath inflammation of some of the thumb muscles. Specifically, the tendons of the extensor pollicis brevis and the abductor pollicis longus are tested. Together they form the anterior border of the anatomic snuffbox (Figure 16-10). The patient holds the thumb clasped in a fist and ulnarly deviates the wrist. Pain over the tendons at the wrist and distal forearm is a positive finding.

**Phalen's Test.**    This is a test for carpal tunnel syndrome (CTS). The patient is instructed to hold the hands together, back to back, for 1 minute (Fig-

ure 16-11). Pain or numbness in the distribution of the median nerve is a positive finding.[6,7] The sooner these symptoms are produced, the worse the condition is felt to be.

**Tinel's Test.**    Tapping over the median nerve at the wrist with either a finger or a reflex hammer sometimes causes pain and numbness to be felt in the hand in the median nerve distribution. This test is adjunctive in making the diagnosis of carpal tunnel syndrome, but it is insensitive and not of much clinical value.[8]

**Edema Measurement.**    To quantify the extent of hand swelling, the fingers and wrists can be measured circumferentially. Another, more accurate, technique is to measure hand volume by water displacement. This allows serial measurement of the progression of edema.

**Allen's Test.**    This is a test to evaluate the patency of the radial and ulnar arteries to the hand. The patient is asked to clench the hand in a fist while the examiner occludes one artery with firm pressure. The patient opens the fist. The hand should quickly turn pink. If it remains pale, it is a sign that the opposite artery is occluded.

### Ancillary Diagnostic Testing

Most ancillary radiographic studies involve plain x-ray films to look for fractures or abnormal bone alignment and to detect signs of degeneration or connective tissue disease. Computerized tomography (CT) scanning is rarely required in the hand

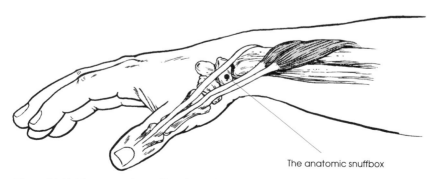

The anatomic snuffbox

**Figure 16-10.** The anatomic snuffbox, bounded by the extensor pollicis brevis and abductor pollicis longus on the volar side and the extensor pollicis longus on the dorsal side. The navicular bone lies between the tendons at the wrist.

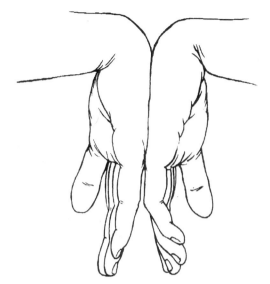

**Phalen's Test to reproduce symptoms of carpal tunnel syndrome.**

**Figure 16-11.** Phalen's test. The hands are held for 1 minute as shown. Pain or abnormal sensation in the hand is a positive finding.

and wrist and is used mainly to detect bony abnormalities. Magnetic resonance imaging (MRI) is sometimes useful in detecting tendonitis in the deep tendons of the wrist. Bone scans are used to detect stress fractures and avascular necrosis of bone. Laboratory tests are commonly used to help diagnose connective tissue disease, which may first become manifest as hand disorders.

Electromyography (EMG) is one of the most useful diagnostic procedures to be used as an extension of the clinical examination of the hand and wrist. It primarily is used to help diagnose carpal tunnel syndrome or other nerve compression, peripheral neuropathy, or radiculopathy.

## Diagnosis and Treatment of Specific Disorders

### Carpal Tunnel Syndrome

Carpal tunnel syndrome (CTS) is a compression neuropathy of the median nerve as it passes under the transverse carpal ligament of the wrist. The ligament is relatively unyielding and any condition that causes increased pressure within the space of the carpal tunnel can damage the median nerve.

Patients with CTS have been shown to have greater pressures within their carpal tunnels than do asymptomatic individuals.[9] The increased pressure can occur in metabolic conditions such as diabetes mellitus and hypothyroidism and in pregnancy. It can also occur as an overuse syndrome in jobs that stress the wrist with repetitive motion (e.g., secretary, computer work), awkward posture (dental hygienist), or vibration. Manual wheelchair users, weight lifters, meat cutters, secretaries, and computer workers, among others, may develop CTS. It can also be caused by trauma to the wrist or by synovitis such as in rheumatoid arthritis. Often the etiology is unknown.

### Diagnosis

Patients with CTS commonly present complaining of pain, numbness, tingling, or paresthesias in the median nerve sensory distribution. This may initially occur at night and wakes the patient from sleep. It is often relieved by "shaking it out" of the hand. It can also occur with activity or certain hand postures such as those used during driving. Weakness and atrophy may eventually occur in the thenar muscles, and this weakness allows the thumb to rotate radially to give the hand a flat appearance ("simian" or "ape" hand). Occasionally, pain and other symptoms are felt in the arm proximal to the wrist, even as high as the elbow or shoulder.[10]

The diagnosis of CTS is made with the help of the characteristic history previously described and by a positive Phalen's test. Tinel's sign may be positive as well. Patients may also have reduced two-point discrimination and can have decreased light touch sensation as well. To make the definitive diagnosis, an EMG should be performed. It reveals slowing of nerve conduction across the wrist or signs of axonal damage or thenar muscle denervation. Occasionally, patients with intermittent symptoms may not have objective EMG abnormalities.[10]

When patients present with signs and symptoms of CTS, other conditions, such as diabetes mellitus, hypothyroidism, peripheral neuropathy, more proximal median neuropathy, radiculopathy, and rheumatoid arthritis should be ruled out, if indicated.

## Treatment

The treatment of CTS is controversial. Some argue that surgical resection of the transverse carpal ligament is the best treatment. Others feel that a trial of conservative care is indicated before considering surgery. The best course is to make the treatment plan on a case by case basis. A patient with severe symptoms and marked EMG abnormalities should probably be treated with surgery as soon as possible. Surgery is relatively simple, safe, and effective.

Patients with intermittent symptoms, mild EMG changes, and a clear cause of the condition might be treated conservatively. This should consist of avoiding the exacerbating activity, nonsteroidal antiinflammatory drugs (NSAIDs), and wearing a wrist splint at night. The splint should keep the wrist out of extreme flexion or extension, as these positions increase the pressure within the carpal tunnel. Splints may need to be worn during the day as well. If symptoms progress or persist more than 4 to 6 weeks, the EMG should be repeated. If it does not show improvement of the condition, surgery should be considered. It is important not to avoid surgery too long, as permanent nerve damage may result. In severe cases, surgery may not improve symptoms because irreversible damage has already occurred. It may, however, prevent further worsening of symptoms.

Pregnant patients, or those with temporary causes of CTS, can usually be treated conservatively.

Some physicians inject the carpal tunnel with steroid solution to treat CTS. This is not without risk, as the injection itself increases pressure on the nerve, and it is not often required.

Patients treated successfully with conservative management should have appropriate workplace or activity modifications made, in order not to exacerbate the condition. In general, there is a poor prognosis for conservative management in patients over 50 years, those who have had symptoms for more than 10 months, those with constant paresthesias, those with stenosing flexor tenosynovitis, and those with a Phalen's test in less than 30 seconds.[7]

## Ulnar Neuropathy at the Wrist

This condition is less common than CTS but involves similar mechanisms. The ulnar nerve can become entrapped and compressed as it enters the wrist medial to the pisiform bone in what is called Guyon's canal. This may occur in bicyclists, weight lifters, in persons who work with vibrating tools, or in others who stress the extended wrist. It can also occur with trauma.

## Diagnosis

Presentation is similar to CTS except that sensory changes, paresthesias, and pain involve the ulnar nerve sensory distribution. Motor weakness affects the hypothenar muscles, the intrinsic hand muscles (thus causing weak finger abduction/adduction), and the thumb adductors (therefore Froment's sign is positive). In advanced cases, the hand is flat and atrophic. Intrinsic hand muscle weakness also results in a "claw-hand" deformity.

Electrodiagnostic testing is the best way to confirm an ulnar neuropathy at the wrist and rules out more proximal nerve damage such as at the elbow or neck.

## Treatment

Frequently the symptoms of ulnar compression at Guyon's canal resolve with removal of the offensive activity. With bicyclists, recommendations for padding the handlebars and frequent changes of position should be made. In the workplace, grips can be modified with larger handles to reduce the compressive forces of a power grip. A period of rest from exacerbating activities is indicated, and occasionally occupational or recreational activity must be modified.

Other treatment options include NSAIDs and rarely oral or injected steroid medication.

In refractory or recurrent cases, surgical decompression may be necessary. Surgery may also be considered early in the course of the disease if the condition is felt to be due to a mass or trauma.

## Rheumatoid Arthritis Involvement of the Hand and Wrist

Rheumatoid arthritis (RA) and other connective tissue diseases are systemic processes, and for a more in-depth discussion of these conditions the reader is referred elsewhere.[11] They often present

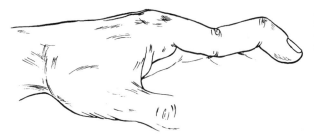

**Figure 16-12.** Swan-neck deformity of the finger. Intrinsic hand muscle tightness causes metacarpophalangeal flexion, proximal interphalangeal hyperextension, and distal interphalangeal flexion.

initially with complaints in the hand. The extensive inflammatory changes and bony erosions that lead to mechanical instabilities of the hand have given RA the distinction of being the "crippling arthritis."

The joints that are likely to be involved are the MCP, PIP, and the joints of the wrist. When the PIP joints are swollen they are sometimes called Bouchard's nodes. When joints are affected, they often cause an inflammation of the adjacent tendons. The extensor tendon sheaths are more frequently involved than the flexor tendons and may lead to tendon rupture.[12]

*Diagnosis*

Acutely inflamed joints are boggy and warm to the touch. Late manifestations of the disease result in deformity. There is an "ulnar drift" of the digits at the MCP joints. This is actually due to tendon imbalances at the wrist.[13]

Swan-neck deformity (Figure 16-12) is a term describing hyperextension of the PIP joint and flexion of the DIP joint. It is due to a contracture of the intrinsic hand muscles due to chronic inflammation.

The boutonnière deformity (Figure 16-13) is characterized by flexion of the PIP joint with extension of the DIP joint. It is due to a rupture of the central extensor tendon, which allows the PIP joint to slip dorsally between the two peripheral extensor tendon branches.

*Treatment*

Medical management of RA consists of medications to reduce inflammation. This includes the use of NSAIDs, oral steroids, gold salts, and chemotherapeutic agents.

Rehabilitation begins with patient education on joint protection and energy conservation techniques to reduce inflammation and fatigue. Often a few visits with an occupational therapist help patients and their families to structure their activities to place less stress on the joints. Assessment of daily activities is important with the goal of reducing excessive flexor forces. The patient may be instructed in the use of large handled tools, cooking utensils, and doorknobs.

During acute flare-ups resting hand and wrist splints may be used to reduce joint stress and inflammation. Passive and active range of motion exercises are avoided in acutely inflamed joints, as they increase the inflammation. Isometric exercise is acceptable to maintain strength.[14]

Splinting of the hand and wrist may help to provide a more functional position and to prevent joint subluxation. In particular, splints are used to correct swan-neck and boutonnière deformity.

Maintaining joint range of motion should be a goal in managing these patients. They should do a daily or twice daily stretching routine (as long as their joints are not acutely inflamed).

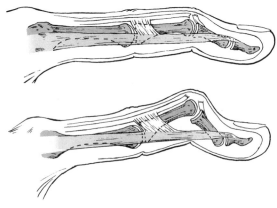

**Figure 16-13.** Boutonnière deformity of the finger, caused by rupture of the central slip of the extensor tendon. This allows the proximal interphalangeal joint to migrate between the lateral slips of the tendon.

## Degenerative Joint Disease

Degenerative joint disease (DJD), also known as osteoarthritis, affects many joints in the body, including those of the hand. The condition involves a degeneration of the joint with a loss of joint cartilage and a compensatory proliferation of subchondral bone. Bony spurs form around the joint. Typically, the joints in the hand most affected by this phenomenon are the DIP and PIP joints as well as the first carpometacarpal (CMC) joint. The affected joints of the digits appear hard and swollen. The DIP joints with this appearance are known as Heberden's nodes.

### Diagnosis

The primary complaints in DJD are pain and joint stiffness. This is often relieved by moderate activity. The involved joints are hard and enlarged. X-ray studies help to confirm the joint degeneration.

### Treatment

DJD is managed by focusing on the maintenance of function with protection against further stressors. Patients should be educated about joint protection and energy conservation techniques. Heating modalities provide symptomatic relief; cold may worsen symptoms. NSAIDs are used to control pain and inflammation as needed, but prolonged periods of using these drugs are to be avoided due to their side effects, especially in the older population more likely to suffer from DJD. Occasionally, steroid medication injection into the painful joints is used to provide temporary pain relief.[15] Such injections may ultimately hasten joint deterioration, but can postpone functional losses. They are performed a maximum of two to four times a year and should be separated by at least a few months.

### DeQuervain's Tenosynovitis

A stenosing tenosynovitis of the abductor pollicis longus and extensor pollicis brevis tendon sheath causes wrist and hand pain and may cause severe limitation of function. It is usually an overuse syndrome and has been called "washerwoman's sprain" in the past. It can be diagnosed by Finkelstein's test and the presence of local tenderness, crepitus, and swelling of the tendon sheath at the distal radius (the tendons form the volar border of the anatomic snuffbox (Figure 16-10). Treatment can initially be with a resting wrist/hand splint, NSAIDs, ice, and refraining from exacerbating activity. If this is not successful, a local tendon sheath injection with steroid-anesthetic solution may be therapeutic, and in refractory cases a surgical release may be necessary.

### Tendonitis

With so many tendons crossing the wrist into the hand there is ample opportunity to develop tendonitis. Almost any tendon can be afflicted if it is overused. Diagnosis is made by identifying the local area of tenderness and swelling and by noting which activity exacerbates the symptoms. Occasionally MRI may help to make the diagnosis. Treatment is with rest, ice, NSAIDs, and modification of activity.

### Ganglion Cysts

Ganglion cysts appear to be local mucoid outpouchings of joints. Most occur on the dorsal wrist at the scapholunate joint.[16] They appear to be caused by a one-way valve type structure which allows fluid to be pumped from the joint into the cyst. Most dorsal ganglion cysts are located between the extensor pollicis longus and the extensor digitorum, but occasionally the cystic mass may extend to surface at other sites on the wrist.[16]

These cysts can be tender, and may interfere with hand and wrist function by pressing on the surrounding structures. They are a response to overuse. They are diagnosed by their characteristic feel and appearance. Occasionally they regress spontaneously, but they often recur. If they are present for a long time they become hard and fibrotic.

Asymptomatic ganglion cysts require no treatment except for cosmetic reasons. They may respond to a period of rest. Early treatment of the cysts may be given by applying forceful pressure over the swelling to cause the cyst to rupture. (In the past they were called "bible bumps" because hitting them with a bible would make them disappear.) Other treatment may include rest, NSAIDs, wrist splints,[17] needle aspiration/steroid injection, or surgical resection.

### Trigger Finger

Tendons normally glide freely through their tendon sheaths, but if a local nodular swelling on the tendon develops, it disrupts this smooth motion. The swelling gets caught on the entrance to the sheath and has trouble moving through the sheath.[18] The condition usually affects the finger flexors and appears to be an overuse reaction. It usually occurs in otherwise healthy persons, often middle-aged women, but may be seen in connective tissue disease states as well. It can cause a painful locking of the digit in flexion once the nodule is lodged within the tendon sheath. This is what is known as the "trigger finger." The nodule can be palpated and is felt to move with passive finger flexion and extension. The condition is treated with rest, NSAIDs, local steroid injections into the tendon sheath, local heat, stretching, and in refractory cases, surgery. X-ray studies should be obtained to rule out a bony block to movement. There may be a variant of the trigger finger, with development of diffuse swelling rather than a nodular swelling. This condition may respond less favorably to injection and conservative care and may be better treated with surgery.[18]

### Dupuytren's Contracture

This is a progressive contracture of the palmar aponeurosis, the transverse fascia lying between the skin and the flexor tendons. It results in the formation of nodules and thickened skin cords which limit finger motion. It primarily affects white males of northern European descent.[19]

The pathogenesis of Dupuytren's contracture is poorly understood. It is often painful early on, but later, pain is not usually a problem. It primarily affects the motion of the fourth digit with lesser involvement of the fifth digit and then the third digit.

When assessing this disorder, the hand and finger joints must be examined to rule out synovitis as a cause of loss of range of motion. Treatment in-

cludes patient education and reassurance. This is not a life-threatening disorder. The patient should be instructed in a home stretching program and may use heating modalities as needed. One simple stretch is to encourage the habit of "sitting on one's hands." In severe cases, surgical release of the contracture is indicated, but since the digital collateral ligaments may have become contracted by the time this is undertaken, the results may be suboptimal.

### Raynaud's Disease

Raynaud's disease involves a painful vasoconstriction of the arteries of the digits. Usually the vasoconstriction occurs in response to environmental stimuli such as cold and repetitive trauma, or central factors such as emotions and nicotine use.

Raynaud's disease may be seen in association with connective tissue diseases such as rheumatoid arthritis and scleroderma. It may even be the first sign of such a disorder. It can also occur as a less severe form of painless vasoconstriction called Raynaud's phenomenon.

Patients with this disorder complain of painful pale digits shortly after they are exposed to cold temperatures. The normal skin color does not return for some time, even after reentering a warm environment.

These patients should be evaluated with Allen's test to rule out arterial abnormality. In selected cases, a connective tissue examination may be indicated as well. The symptoms can sometimes be reproduced by placing the extremity in iced water. This may actually cause vasoconstriction in the digits of the contralateral extremity as well.

Treatment includes patient education about the need to keep the hands warm and protected. In severe cases calcium channel blockers may be used to control the condition. Biofeedback may also be useful to help regulate blood flow.

### Reflex Sympathetic Dystrophy

Also known as traumatic dystrophy, causalgia, and shoulder-hand syndrome (in stroke patients), among others, reflex sympathetic dystrophy (RSD) is a condition of abnormal unrestrained sympathetic nervous system outflow to the limb. It can cause early symptoms of hand swelling and excessive warmth. Later the skin becomes shiny and atrophic. There is abnormal sweating, skin is tender to the touch, and joint range of motion causes pain. The condition is often caused by nerve injury or trauma, sometimes seemingly minor trauma.

This condition can become chronic and debilitating and must be treated aggressively as soon as possible. Treatment may consist of NSAIDs, heat and cold modalities, gentle range of motion, transcutaneous electrical nerve stimulation, biofeedback, Coban wrap, elastic gloves, desensitization, and contrast baths. In addition, pharmacologic treatment may be undertaken with alpha-adrenergic blockers, sympathetic (stellate) ganglion blocks, or a short course of high-dose oral steroids. It is important to avoid causing pain with the treatment. Pain increases the sympathetic nerve response and worsens the condition. Therefore it is important to be gentle in treating this condition, especially with passive range of motion therapy. Unless the clinician is an expert at treating RSD, patients should be referred to someone who is. Delayed proper treatment can leave the patient with severe pain for life.

### Ulnar Artery Thrombosis

Thrombosis of the ulnar artery is usually due to repetitive trauma such as from recoiling power tools. It most commonly occurs in men in their fifties. The patient complains of pain, cold intolerance, and numbness. On examination, the ulnar side of the hand is cool. The patient may have signs of arterial insufficiency and Allen's test is positive. There may also be numbness, and sometimes a palpable mass is noted at Guyon's canal. Treatment is by discontinuing the aggravating activity, refraining from smoking, and biofeedback. If this does not relieve the symptoms, surgical release or grafting is considered.[20]

### Trauma

Traumatic injuries such as fractures, dislocations, and tendon ruptures are beyond the scope of this chapter. Nevertheless, nearly every clinician will be exposed to some of them, so a rudimentary understanding of the more common injuries is important.

Ulnar collateral ligament injuries of the MCP of the thumb are fairly common. In the past they were called "gamekeeper's thumb" because they occurred from trained birds taking off from and landing on the thumb. Today such injuries are seen primarily in skiers, wrestlers, and football players. They are due to forceful abduction of the thumb. Patients present with pain, tenderness, swelling, and a weak thumb pinch. The joint should be examined for stability in flexion and extension and should be compared with the uninjured side. X-ray films should be obtained to rule out fracture. Stress radiographs are sometimes useful in assessing the degree of joint laxity. Treatment is with casting, splinting, or possibly surgery, depending on the severity of the injury.

The collateral ligaments of the PIP joints are also frequently injured, especially in sports trauma. Such injury is again diagnosed by history and the location of pain and swelling. In complete ruptures there is joint instability. Treatment for partial tears usually consists of immobilizing the joint in extension for 3 weeks followed by "buddy taping," or taping the injured finger to the adjacent uninjured one. Unstable joints require surgical correction.

The finger extensor mechanism can be injured at either the middle or distal phalanx. If rupture of the central slip of the tendon occurs at the middle phalanx it can eventually lead to a boutonnière deformity. This can be prevented by treatment with splinting in extension to allow healing. If the insertion of the extensor tendon is ruptured at the DIP, it leads to a mallet-finger deformity. The distal phalanx is fixed in flexion and can be passively, but not actively, extended. Treatment is with 6 to 8 weeks of splinting in extension. This injury is commonly caused by sports injuries, such as when a ball hits the extended finger and forces it into flexion.

If the flexor digitorum profundus or flexor digitorum superficialis is ruptured, the finger loses its ability to actively flex at the appropriate joints. This can occur with forced extension of the finger. "Jersey finger" is caused in football when a player holds an opposing team member by the jersey. The other player pulls away and causes rupture of the

FDP. The patient is not able to make a proper fist because the DIP cannot be flexed. Treatment of flexor tendon rupture is usually with surgery.

Hyperextension sprains of the digits are common. Mild cases are called a "jammed" finger. Treatment includes NSAIDs, edema control, "buddy taping" to the adjacent finger, range of motion exercise, and healing with time. If there is an associated complete ligamentous rupture, surgical repair may be needed.

Fractures of the wrist and hand are fairly common. Colles' fracture is caused by a fall on the outstretched arm, and involves a disruption of the distal radius. Navicular fractures can be refractory to treatment and may evolve into an aseptic necrosis of the bone due to poor blood supply. This fracture causes tenderness to palpation in the anatomic snuffbox. Bennett fractures are located at the base of the first metacarpal. Boxer's fractures involve the distal fifth metacarpal. The hook of the hamate bone can be injured in golf or baseball.

X-ray studies are important in hand and wrist trauma to rule out avulsion fractures. In adolescents they may also detect epiphyseal injury.

The triangular fibrocartilaginous complex is sometimes torn in acute injury; this may cause lasting impairment and pain.

Other injuries may involve fracture of any bone, dislocation of any joint, or sprain of any ligament. The muscles of the hand can be contused, and vasculature, nerves, and tendons may be lacerated.

## Case Report

A 24-year-old man reports numbness and tingling of the ulnar two digits of the right hand. Symptoms wake him at night and also occur during other activities. He has recently taken up bicycling and is riding every day. On physical examination he has a mild decrease in sensation over the fifth digit and mild weakness in finger abduction/adduction compared with his other (nondominant) side. A presumptive diagnosis of ulnar compressive neuropathy at Guyon's canal of the wrist is made. This is confirmed by EMG, which reveals moderate slowing of nerve conduction across the canal but no evidence of axonal nerve damage.

Treatment includes education about the nature of his condition. He is told to refrain from bicycling until symptoms resolve. He is prescribed a course of NSAIDs and is given a cock-up wrist splint to be worn at night. His symptoms resolve within 3 weeks. He subsequently returns to bicycling but uses padded gloves and modified handlebars to decrease the pressure on his wrist. He changes position often while riding and only gradually increases his mileage. Symptoms have not recurred.

## Points of Summary

1. Collateral MCP ligaments are lax when the fingers are extended, and taut when flexed. They are prone to contracture if immobilized in an extended position.
2. The carpal tunnel is a fixed space that contains the median nerve. The nerve is susceptible to pressure damage within this structure.
3. Phalen's test is the most valuable clinical examination in diagnosing carpal tunnel syndrome.
4. Patients with carpal tunnel syndrome have increased pressure within the carpal tunnel.
5. Desensitization techniques are useful in conditions of cutaneous hypersensitivity.
6. Compression neuropathy can be diagnosed with the help of EMG.
7. DeQuervain's tenosynovitis is usually diagnosed with the help of a positive Finkelstein's test.
8. Hand and wrist joint problems may be the first signs of connective tissue disease.
9. Reflex sympathetic dystrophy requires prompt proper treatment by an expert.

## References

1. Elkins EC, Herrick JF, Grindlay JH, et al.: Effect of various procedures on the flow of lymph. *Arch Phys Med* 1953;34:31–39.
2. Bender LF: Upper extremity orthotics. In Kottke FJ, Lehmann JF (eds): *Krusen's Handbook of Physical Medicine and Rehabilitation*, 4th ed. Philadelphia: WB Saunders, 1990:580–592.
3. Ragnarsson KT: Orthotics and shoes. In DeLisa JA: *Rehabilitation Medicine: Principles and Practice*. Philadelphia: JB Lippincott, 1988:307–330.
4. McCue FC, Mayer V: Rehabilitation of common athletic injuries of the hand and wrist. *Clin Sports Med* 1989;8:731–775.

5. American Medical Association: *Guides to the Evaluation of Permanent Impairment*, 3rd ed, revised. Chicago: AMA, 1990:16–17.

6. Seror P: Phalen's test in the diagnosis of carpal tunnel syndrome. *J Hand Surg* 1988;13B:383–385.

7. Kaplan SJ, Glickel SZ, Eaton RG: Predictive factors in the non-surgical treatment of carpal tunnel syndrome. *J Hand Surg* 1990;15B:106–108.

8. Gellman H, Gelberman RH, Tan AM, et al.: Carpal tunnel syndrome: An evaluation of the provocative diagnostic tests. *J Bone Joint Surg* 1986;68A:735–737.

9. Gelberman RH, Hergenroeder PT, Hargens AR, et al.: The carpal tunnel syndrome: A study of carpal canal pressures. *J Bone Joint Surg* 1981;63A(3):380–383.

10. Grundberg AB: Carpal tunnel decompression in spite of normal electromyography. *J Hand Surg* 1983;8:348–349.

11. Schumacher HR (ed): *Primer on the Rheumatic Diseases*, 9th ed. Atlanta: Arthritis Foundation, 1988.

12. Moore JR, Weiland AJ, Valdata L: Tendon ruptures in the rheumatic hand: Analysis of treatment and functional results in 60 patients. *J Hand Surg* 1987;12A:9–14.

13. Shapiro JS: A new factor in the etiology of ulnar drift. *Clin Orthop* 1970;68:32–43.

14. Merritt JL, Hunder GG: Passive range of motion, not isometric exercise, amplifies acute urate synovitis. *Arch Phys Med Rehabil* 1983;64:130–131.

15. Swanson AB, Swanson G: Osteoarthritis in the hand. *J Hand Surg* 1983;8:669–675.

16. Angelides AC, Wallace PF: The dorsal ganglion of the wrist: Its pathogenesis, gross and microscopic anatomy, and surgical treatment. *J Hand Surg* 1976;1:228–235.

17. Richman JA, Gelberman RH, Engber WD, et al.: Ganglions of the wrist: Results of treatment by aspiration and cyst wall puncture. *J Hand Surg* 1987;12A:1041–1043.

18. Freiberg A, Mulholland RS, Levine R: Nonoperative treatment of trigger fingers and thumbs. *J Hand Surg* 1989;14A:553–558.

19. Early PF: Population studies in Dupuytren's contracture. *J Bone Joint Surg* 1962;44B:602–613.

20. Koman LA, Urbaniak JR: Ulnar artery thrombosis. *Hand Clin* 1985;1:311–325.

## Suggested Readings

Cailliet R: *Hand Pain and Management*, 3rd ed. Philadelphia: FA Davis, 1982.

Culver JA (ed): Injuries of the hand and wrist. *Clin Sports Med* 1992;11(1).

Rider BA: Carpal tunnel syndrome rehabilitation. *Critical Reviews in Physical and Rehabilitation Medicine* 1991;3(1):27–57.

Terrono AL, Millender LH: Evaluation and management of occupational wrist disorders. In Millender LH, Louis DS, Simmons BP (eds): *Occupational Disorders of the Upper Extremity*. New York: Churchill Livingstone, 1992:117–143.

# Chapter 17
# Hips and Pelvis

ANDREA CONTI

The hip joints and pelvis act to transfer forces across the pelvic girdle and thus provide a smooth transfer of kinetic energy. Dysfunction within the pelvic girdle can be the cause of significant pain in any generalized motion of the trunk or the lower extremities. Exacerbation of this pain by normal motion interrupts the synchronous action of the musculoskeletal system and interferes with daily life activities.

## Anatomy

The bony pelvis is a ring formed by two os coxae which connect to each other at the pubis anteriorly and which are joined to the sacrum and coccyx posteriorly. The os coxae consists of three parts which fuse during development: the ilium, ischium, and pubis. The acetabulum is the meeting place for the three parts, which form this cup-shaped cavity to articulate with the head of the femur. The hips and pelvis have a number of bony landmarks including the anterior superior iliac spine, posterior superior iliac spine, ischial tuberosity, and the greater trochanter (Figure 17-1).

There are four articulations within the pelvic girdle. They are the sacroiliac (SI) joints, the pubic symphysis, and the sacrococcygeal joint.

The ligaments of the pelvis are dense and strong (Figure 17-2). The iliolumbar ligaments connect the transverse processes of L5 to the iliac crests bilaterally. These ligaments may assist in preventing L5 from sliding forward on the sacrum.

The sacrotuberous ligament passes from the sacrum to the ischium, as does the sacrospinous ligament. These ligaments act together to hold the sacrum in position and resist posterior rotation of the inferior sacrum. The interosseous and sacroiliac ligaments are composed of very strong short fibers that unite the sacrum and ilium.

The musculature of the pelvis (see Figure 17-1) includes several large, strong muscles which act as prime movers for the lower extremities during ambulation. The iliacus and psoas muscles are the chief flexors of the leg. Posteriorly, the pelvis is covered by several layers of muscles. The superficial gluteus maximus extends the leg, while the deeper gluteus medius and minimus act to abduct and rotate the thigh. When the foot is planted on the ground these muscles exert their forces to control the trunk and pelvis.

The piriformis muscle originates on the anterior surface of the sacrum and passes through the greater sciatic notch to insert onto the greater trochanter of the femur. It acts as an abductor of the leg when the hip is flexed. The belly of this muscle lies over the sciatic nerve and in some people the sciatic nerve actually passes through the muscle. Because of the anatomic relationship between the nerve and muscle, sciatic-type referral symptoms may be present with dysfunction in the pelvis or piriformis (Figure 17-3).[1]

Other muscles important to the function of the hip and pelvis are the hamstring group made up of the semitendinosus, semimembranosus, and

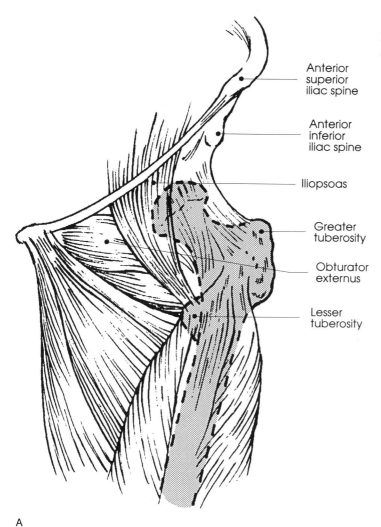

Anterior
superior
iliac spine

Anterior
inferior
iliac spine

Iliopsoas

Greater
tuberosity

Obturator
externus

Lesser
tuberosity

A

**Figure 17-1.** The hips and pelvis. *A*, Anterior view (deep muscles).

biceps femoris. The hamstrings have a common origin from the ischial tuberosity. In addition there are numerous smaller muscles that act around the hip.

### Rehabilitative Approach

As in other parts of the body, rehabilitation of pelvic and hip problems should emphasize a patient-active approach with early mobilization, minimal rest, and proper exercise.

Various therapeutic modalities may be useful as well. Bursitis may respond to ultrasound or ice treatment. Myofascial pain may be treated with cold in the acute stage and later on by heat or cold. Ice massage is sometimes helpful as well (see Chapter 12, section on ice massage). Transcutane-ous electrical nerve stimulation (TENS) units may provide temporary pain relief.

Nonsteroidal antiinflammatory drugs (NSAIDs) are commonly prescribed to ameliorate pain and inflammation. Oral, or more commonly, injectable steroids are often useful as well, especially in conditions of sacroiliitis or bursitis. Care must be taken not to inject any medication into the nerves of the pelvis and legs as this may cause nerve damage and possibly prolonged pain.

### Examination and Testing Techniques

#### History and Physical Examination

Obtaining a clear and thorough history from a patient with musculoskeletal problems is of primary

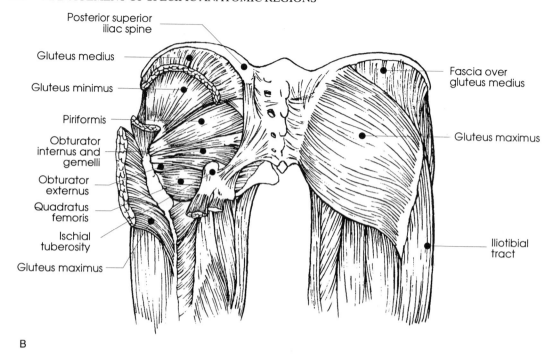

**Figure 17-1.** *Continued. B,* Posterior view (*left:* deep; *right:* superficial).

importance (this is described in greater detail in Chapter 11). Musculoskeletal pain often stems from traumatic or overuse injury, and the specific nature of the motions involved is important in making the diagnosis. It is valuable to ask the patient complaining of "hip pain" to point to the site of pain. Patients generally call the posterior or lateral buttock, the "hip." True hip joint pain is usually felt in the anterior groin at the inguinal ligament.

General assessment begins with the static examination to compare the heights of the iliac crests, greater trochanters, and medial malleoli with the patient standing and supine. The posterior superior iliac spine dimples should be observed to make sure they are level. Muscle mass and posture should be assessed as well.

The bony landmarks and soft tissues should be palpated. The areas of the greater trochanter or

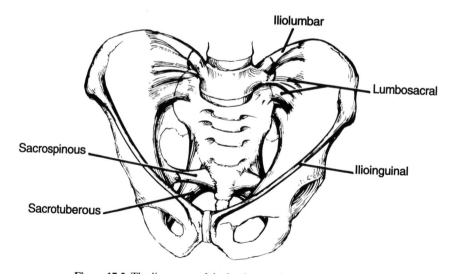

**Figure 17-2.** The ligaments of the lumbosacral and pelvic region.

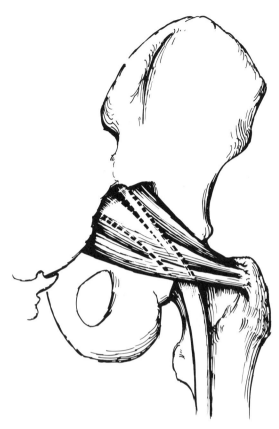

**Figure 17-3.** The intimate relationship between the piriformis muscle and the sciatic nerve, which runs directly below the muscle.

ischial tuberosity are tender in bursitis of these locations. The iliac crest is tender in apophysitis or avulsion fracture. The coccyx is tender in coccydynia. In conditions of sacroiliitis, the ligaments overlying this joint are often tender and their palpation may cause pain to radiate down the leg. The piriformis muscle is also often tender in sacroiliitis as well as in piriformis syndrome. The gluteus medius and minimus sometimes have tender areas or trigger points (see Chapter 20) which cause pain to radiate down the leg. In conditions of sciatica the sciatic nerve is tender. It can be palpated halfway between the ischial tuberosity and the greater trochanter, especially when the hip is flexed.

Range of motion of the low back, pelvis, and legs should be assessed, as should muscle strength (see the suggested readings at the end of this chapter). A complete neurologic examination must be performed as well. It is important to realize that low back disease can cause pelvic, buttock, and hip pain, and thus the lower back should routinely be evaluated also. The reader is encouraged to study Chapter 13 for additional, complementary information. A few special tests to help assess flexibility and strength, as well as other components of the examination, are described in more detail below.

**Measuring Leg Length.**    A crude measure of leg length is to estimate the height of both the left and the right iliac crest of the standing patient. When the pelvis is tilted—a so-called pelvic obliquity (which can be due to muscle splinting or poor posture)—the leg lengths can seem to be unequal when in fact they are not. True leg length is measured (with the patient supine) from the anterior superior iliac spine to the medial malleolus. An apparent (false) leg length discrepancy can be detected by measuring from the left and right medial malleoli to the umbilicus. In a pelvic obliquity this distance is unequal, even though true leg length is the same on both sides. Leg length may also be measured radiographically.[2] Pelvic obliquity may cause the posterior superior iliac spine dimples to be at different heights when standing.

**Hip Internal and External Rotation.**    Flexing the hip and knee to 90 degrees while in the supine position allows the examiner to assess internal and external rotation. These movements are often restricted in degenerative joint disease (DJD) of the hips. Applying downward pressure while rotating the leg causes pain in hip DJD.

**Thomas Test.**    This is a test to assess hip flexion contracture. The patient is asked to lie supine and with his or her hands to pull one knee to the chest to stabilize the pelvis. The other leg can normally be laid flat on the table. Patients with hip flexion contracture cannot lower their leg all the way to the table.

**Patrick's Test** (Figure 17-4).    The supine patient crosses the foot over the opposite knee (a figure-4 position). The knee of the upper leg is then gently pushed toward the table. Pain radiating from the hip to the groin is indicative of hip joint pathology, while pain at the sacroiliac joint is a sign of dysfunction of this joint. This test is also called the Faber test, which stands for *f*lexion, *ab*duction, and *ex*ternal *r*otation.

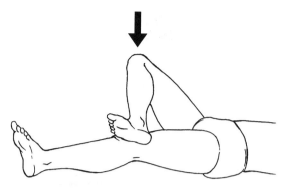

**Figure 17-4.** Patrick's test (also known as the Faber test, which stands for *f*lexion, *ab*duction, *e*xternal *r*otation).

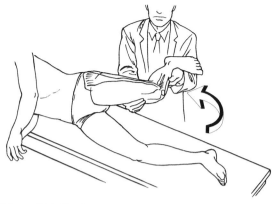

**Figure 17-6.** Ober's test.

**Piriformis Stretching and Test** (Figure 17-5).   To assess piriformis flexibility the patient lies supine while the examiner flexes the hip and knee. The examiner adducts the leg (pushes it to the opposite side) to gauge flexibility on each side. If the patient is asked to resist this motion (the piriformis test) he or she stresses the piriformis muscle. Pain in the buttock is a positive sign. It may radiate into the leg and is indicative of piriformis syndrome.

**Ober's Test** (Figure 17-6).   With the patient in a side-lying position, the upper leg is passively abducted. The knee is flexed to 90 degrees. When the leg is released it should drop to the lower leg.[3] If the iliotibial tract or the tensor fascia lata are excessively tight, the leg remains in the abducted position. The hip may be extended slightly (by the examiner) during this test.

**Gaenslen's Test** (Figure 17-7).   The patient again assumes a side-lying position and pulls the lower leg to the chest. The examiner passively ex-

tends the upper thigh at the hip. Pain in the sacroiliac area is indicative of sacroiliac joint dysfunction. A variation of this test is performed with the patient prone. The examiner passively extends the thigh with the knee bent. Pain in the sacroiliac joint is again a positive finding.

**Standing Gillette (Stork) Test** (Figure 17-8).   The patient stands and raises one knee and then the other toward the ceiling. Self-steadying with a hand against a wall or other object is permissible, but he or she should not support any weight on this hand. The examiner sits behind the patient and palpates the motion at the sacroiliac joint. Asymmetric motion is indicative of sacroiliac joint dysfunction.

**Trendelenburg Test.**   The patient stands on one leg. If the pelvis tilts downward excessively it indicates that the gluteus medius and minimus on the supporting side are weak.

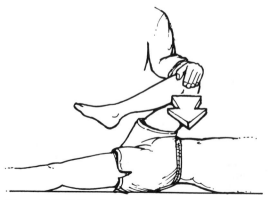

**Figure 17-5.** Piriformis stretching.

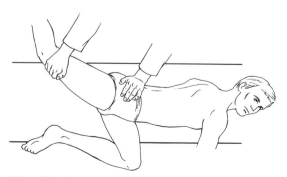

**Figure 17-7.** Gaenslen's test.

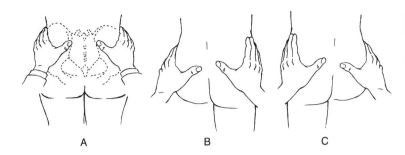

A    B    C

**Figure 17-8.** The standing Gillette test. As the patient raises the leg, downward motion is felt over the posterior superior iliac spine (PSIS). Asymmetry of motion is a sign of sacroiliac joint dysfunction.

**Abdominal Strength Testing.**    One simple way of assessing abdominal strength is to have the supine patient bring the knees to the chest, then straighten the knees, and slowly lower the legs to the examination table. Inability to slowly lower the legs is a sign of abdominal muscle weakness.

**Rectal Examination.**    This test should usually be performed in patients with back or pelvic pain of insidious onset. It may identify tumors or an enlarged prostate in some cases. It also allows palpation of the undersurface of the piriformis muscle.

*Ancillary Testing*

Plain x-ray studies may be needed to look for signs of DJD, fractures, chondrocalcinosis, congenital bony anomalies, or a displacement of the pelvic structures. Computerized tomography (CT) helps to diagnose bony pathology as well. It may reveal occult fractures, herniated lumbar disks, or tumors, and is a good way to visualize the sacroiliac joint. Magnetic resonance imaging (MRI) is used to assess the soft tissues and may also reveal tumors, herniated disks, and inflamed tendons. Bone scans help to detect stress fractures.

**Diagnosis and Treatment
of Specific Disorders**

*Sacroiliac Joint Dysfunction*

This is a controversial condition and many deny that it even exists. In the author's opinion, however, it is a common condition and is probably greatly underdiagnosed.[4,5]

The sacroiliac joint is often said to be immobile. Motion at the joint does, however, occur.[6] (Persons doubting this should palpate their own sacroiliac joints while sitting and alternately raising the left and right foot off the ground.) With age the joint degenerates and may develop a bony bridging-type fusion.

Sacroiliac joint dysfunction is not well understood. It may be caused by a hypertonicity of the muscles overlying the joint which prevents the joint from moving properly. Then again, joint dysfunction may cause the overlying muscles to become hypertonic. In any case, both the joint itself and the overlying ligaments and muscles seem to be causes of pain.

Pain from the sacroiliac joint may be local or radiating. The radiating type of pain may be felt in the groin, laterally, and most commonly in the buttock. It does not usually radiate below the knee.

Sacroiliitis may be caused by trauma (rarely), and may also be due to leg length discrepancy, muscle strength imbalance, or poor athletic or work technique.[7] Often the cause is unknown. It often recurs unless the patient maintains proper flexibility and conditioning.

Since the sacroiliac joint is intimately associated with the piriformis muscle, sacroiliitis often occurs along with piriformis syndrome.

The sacroiliac joint may be involved in connective tissue diseases such as ankylosing spondylitis and Reiter's disease. When there is an insidious onset of joint pain in persons (usually males) less than 40 years of age which persists for more than 3 months, is associated with morning stiffness, and improves with exercise, ankylosing spondylytis should be suspected[8] and appropriate x-ray studies and laboratory tests obtained. Reiter's syndrome is usually associated with other lower extremity joint involvement as well. When sacroiliitis appears in children, especially if the condition is unilateral, an infected joint should be suspected.[9] This usually is associated with fever, chills, and signs of infection.

### Diagnosis

The patient with sacroiliitis complains of back or buttock pain, often localized over the joints and often radiating down the posterior thigh. Pain is worse with rotational movements, when climbing stairs, or when bending forward and to the side.

Examination of the sacroiliac joint involves motion testing while palpating over the joint. The palpatory fingers perceive reflected motion through the posterior ligaments, subcutaneous tissue, and skin. With the patient standing, the Gillette test may detect asymmetry of motion of the left versus the right joint. Palpating both joints while having the patient bend forward may also reveal such motion asymmetry.

Other provocative tests for sacroiliac joint dysfunction include Patrick's test, Gaenslen's test, and passive hip extension. In addition, direct pressure on the sacrum, squeezing the iliac crests together (Eriksen's test), or pushing the anterior superior iliac spines apart may cause local sacroiliac joint pain. Direct palpation of the joint often causes pain to radiate into the buttock and thigh.

### Treatment

Many times patients with acute sacroiliac joint dysfunction respond to a short period of rest, local heat, and NSAIDs.

Because the piriformis attaches to the sacrum it is often involved in sacroiliac joint dysfunction. A hypertonic or contracted piriformis may even be the cause of the dysfunction. Thus, stretching of the piriformis is one of the keystones to treating sacroiliac joint problems. The joint must also be mobilized to restore normal movement.

In addition to attaining proper flexibility, a number of other techniques can be used to treat the sacroiliac joint. In acute dysfunction the patient may be taught to abduct the knees against resistance (while sitting) and then immediately adduct them against resistance (adductor squeeze technique.) Often a pop is felt or heard and symptoms are lessened. Various other muscle energy techniques (see Chapter 9) may also be used to mobilize the joint. A complete discussion of these maneuvers is beyond the scope of this text. Patients should be referred to a physician or spine therapist trained in providing such treatment. Ultimately, the goal of treatment is to restore normal flexibility and sacroiliac joint biomechanics through a series of stabilization and strengthening exercises. These should be made a part of the patient's daily routine to prevent recurrence of the condition.

In addition to therapy and exercises, the treatment of sacroiliitis is occasionally augmented by steroid-anesthetic joint injections. Ultrasound and other heating or cooling modalities are also helpful, and sometimes a pelvic belt (sacroiliac belt) provides comfort as well.

### Piriformis Syndrome

As described earlier, the piriformis muscle is closely associated with the sacroiliac joint and also with the sciatic nerve. With spasm or inflammation of the piriformis a pain referral pattern of sciatica is common, as are symptoms of sacroiliitis.[1] Only rarely does piriformis syndrome present as an isolated entity.

### Diagnosis

Patients with piriformis syndrome complain of pain with walking, when climbing stairs, and when twisting their bodies. On examination the muscle is exquisitely tender to palpation. Piriformis testing reveals weakness and inflexibility of the muscle and reproduces the patient's pain. The tender muscle may be palpated on rectal examination.

### Treatment

This condition is managed by relaxing the overstressed and inflamed muscle. Treatment includes rest, NSAIDs, ice massage, ultrasound, and a stretching program. Surgical sectioning of the muscle has been recommended by some,[1] but is almost never necessary.

## Trochanteric Bursitis

The greater trochanter is a relatively superficial structure. Direct trauma, prolonged pressure, or a tight iliotibial tract can be sources of irritation to the bursa. It can become inflamed.

### Diagnosis

Patients often complain of pain "in the hip." When asked to point to the site of pain they place a finger right behind or on the greater trochanter. The area of the trochanter is very tender, and in some cases pain is referred down the leg with palpation.

### Treatment

As in any bursitis, treatment consists of removing irritating pressure, rest, ice massage, and NSAIDs. Later, ultrasound and stretching of the iliotibial tract and hamstrings are helpful. The bursa may also respond well to steroid-anesthetic injection.

## Degenerative Joint Disease of the Hip

The most common painful condition of the hip joint is osteoarthritis, or DJD. It involves a deterioration of the articular cartilage, subchondral bony sclerosis, and osteophyte formation. The cause is not known, but it is associated with aging.

### Diagnosis

Patients complain of pain in the groin area. The pain is often relieved by mild activity and worsens with inactivity. Range of motion in the hip is often restricted, especially in rotation (mainly internal rotation). X-ray findings confirm the bony changes of the condition, but severity of the disease on x-ray films correlates poorly with symptom magnitude.

### Treatment

Conservative rehabilitative care includes maintaining joint range of motion without placing excessive stress on the joint. Non-weight-bearing activities such as swimming and bicycling may be most beneficial as aerobic exercise in these pa-tients. They should be taught a program of energy conservation techniques so that they can better pace themselves. Frequent rest periods (two to four times a day) with no weight bearing at all may help in controlling symptoms and slowing the progression of the degeneration.[10] Weight loss may also be advised in overweight persons. NSAIDs are used judiciously. Rarely, surgical treatment with total joint replacement is necessary.

In conditions of hip pain the patient often walks with the leg externally rotated and shifts weight toward the affected side while walking. External rotation tends to "unwind" the ligaments of the joint thus relieving pressure and pain. It may eventually cause knee and foot pain, however, due to poor gait biomechanics. The shift in weight to the affected side during gait may seem paradoxical at first. However, it makes sense when one realizes that the action of the gluteus medius and minimus in holding the pelvis level during stance, plus body weight, produces a compressive force on the hip joint that is four times body weight. This is due to the short lever arm of the hip abductors relative to the center of the body. Listing of the body toward the painful side helps reduce the compressive force on the joint by reducing the lever arm of the center of the body relative to the abductors (see Chapter 11). A cane on the unaffected side, by utilizing an effectively even longer lever arm, can help decrease the compressive force many times more than the weight it actually carries. This is depicted in Figure 17-9.

## Myofascial Pain

Leg length discrepancies, abnormal gait, or overuse can cause myofascial pain of the muscles of the hips and pelvis. The most common muscles involved are the hip abductors, the gluteus medius and minimus, and the tensor fascia lata. Having legs of unequal length may create a condition of muscle overwork. The patient has characteristic trigger points (or sometimes tender points) which cause pain to radiate into the leg.

Treatment, as outlined in Chapter 20, is through rest, orthotic shoe inserts if necessary, ice massage, and possibly trigger point injection, as well as stretching and strengthening exercises.

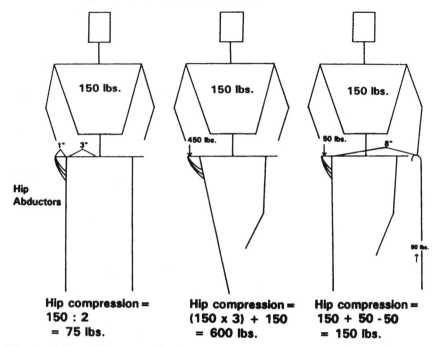

**Figure 17-9.** Normal hip compression force is a function of both body weight and muscular action. When standing on one leg, the hip abductors produce a compressive force of three times body weight (due to leverage effects). A cane held on the opposite side has great leverage and reduces joint compressive force many times more than the actual weight being carried on the cane.

### Coccydynia

Pain in the coccygeal region may be a result of direct trauma with displacement of the coccyx. Referred pain from internal organs should also be considered as causes of pain in this region. Treatment of acute coccydynia includes ice, pressure relief, relaxation training, proper sitting (on the ischial tuberosities, not on the sacrum and coccyx), and NSAIDs. In addition, ultrasound treatment may be useful. A program of steroid-anesthetic injection combined with coccygeal manipulation has been reported to be successful in approximately 85% of patients.[11]

### Osteoporosis/Hip Fractures

As described in more detail in Chapters 22 and 23, osteoporosis can cause painful fractures. This can lead to vertebral compression fractures with back and buttock pain. Hip fractures are common and can be devastating. They should be suspected in an elderly patient who has fallen and who presents with an inability to bear weight on the extremity and with a shortened, externally rotated leg. Osteoporotic fractures may also occur in other bones of the pelvis, for instance in the pubis.[12]

### Connective Tissue Disease

A discussion of these diseases is beyond the scope of this chapter, but such conditions are always in the differential diagnosis of hip, back, and sacroiliac joint dysfunction. Laboratory (see Chapter 8) and x-ray testing help in making the diagnosis.

### Groin/Pelvic Pain

There are many other less common causes of groin and pelvic pain which can only be mentioned briefly here.

Meralgia paresthetica is a condition of compression of the lateral femoral cutaneous nerve at or near the inguinal ligament. It can cause pain and sensory loss in the anterolateral thigh. It can be due to trauma, tight clothing, or pressure during surgery. Diagnosis is confirmed electromyographically. Often the nerve can be palpated as a swollen mass.[13]

Tendonitis or strained adductor muscles are other causes of groin pain. In addition, nonmusculoskeletal conditions such as abdominal hernias and torsion testes may cause groin pain.

Pubic and sacroiliac joint pain may be caused by stress fractures, pubic instability,[14] or osteitis pubis. Pelvic floor pain may be myofascial in nature.[15,16]

Other conditions to include in the differential diagnosis of pelvic and hip pain include intraabdominal or intrapelvic pathology, aseptic necrosis of the hip joint, lesser trochanteric avulsion fractures, iliac crest avulsion or contusion (hip pointer), ischial bursitis, and congenital abnormalities such as a sacralization of the lumbar vertebrae or vertebralization of sacral segments.

## Case Report

A 56-year-old woman with left hemiparesis due to a stroke 2 years earlier was referred for evaluation of low back pain. She had had a herniated disk at the left L4 level which was surgically removed. Prior to surgery she had had several weeks of low back pain and intermittent left leg pain. These symptoms were completely relieved for a few days after back surgery, but soon she started having back pain radiating from the buttock to the left leg.

On examination her left sacroiliac joint was tender, the left piriformis was less flexible than the right, she had evidence of left sacroiliac joint hypomobility on standing Gillette testing, and she had a reproduction of her pain with passive hip extension.

Her left sacroiliac joint was injected with a steroid-anesthetic solution, and she was started on a program of physical therapy mobilization and piriformis stretching.

One month later she was completely pain free. Her sacroiliitis was most likely due to hemiparesis and improper back biomechanics following disk surgery. The disk surgery was a confounding element since it caused the referring physician to assume that her pain "recurrence" was due to radiculopathy.

## Points of Summary

1. The sacroiliac joint is a mobile joint.
2. Sacroiliac disease is a common cause of low back and buttock pain.
3. The piriformis muscle is often involved in sacroiliac joint dysfunction.
4. Trochanteric bursitis is a common cause of "hip" pain.
5. Degenerative joint disease of the hip is often effectively treated with a cane, which by virtue of the leverage it provides, relieves the hip joint of much more force than the weight it actually supports.

## References

1. Solheim LF, Siewers P, Paus B: The piriformis muscle syndrome. *Acta Orthop Scand* 1981;52:73–75.
2. Giles LGF, Taylor JR: Low back pain associated with leg length inequality. *Spine* 1981;6:510–521.
3. Hoppenfeld S: Physical examination of the hip and pelvis. In Hoppenfeld S (ed): *Physical Examination of the Spine and Extremities*. Norwalk, CT: Appeton-Century-Crofts, 1976:143–169.
4. Kirkaldy-Willis WH, Hill RJ: A more precise diagnosis for low-back pain. *Spine* 1979;4:102–109.
5. Bernard TN, Kirkaldy-Willis WH: Recognizing specific characteristics of nonspecific low back pain. *Clin Orthop* 1987;217:266–280.
6. Bowen V, Cassidy JD: Macroscopic and microscopic anatomy of the sacroiliac joint from embryonic life until the eighth decade. *Spine* 1981;6:620–628.
7. Marymont JV, Lynch MA, Henning CE: Exercise-related stress reaction of the sacroiliac joint. *Am J Sports Med* 1986;14:320–323.
8. Calin A: Ankylosing spondylitis. In Schumacher HR Jr (ed): *Primer on the Rheumatic Diseases*, 9th ed. Atlanta: Arthritis Foundation, 1988:145–146.
9. Reilly JP, Gross RH, Emans JB, et al.: Disorders of the sacroiliac joint in children. *J Bone Joint Surg* 1988;70A:31–40.
10. McKeag DB: The relationship of osteoarthritis and exercise. *Clin Sports Med* 1992;11:471–488.
11. Wray CC, Easom S, Hoskinson J: Coccydynia: Aetiology and treatment. *J Bone Joint Surg* 1991;73B:335–338.
12. Nicholas JJ, Haidet E, Helfrich D, et al.: Groin and hip pain due to fractures at or near the pubic symphysis. *Arch Phys Med Rehabil* 1989;70:696–698.
13. Williams PH, Trzil KP: Management of meralgia paresthetica. *J Neurosurg* 1991;74:76–80.
14. LaBan MM, Meerschaert JR, Taylor RS, et al.: Symphyseal and sacroiliac joint pain associated with pubic

symphysis instability. *Arch Phys Med Rehabil* 1978;59:470–477.

15. Slocumb JC: Neurological factors in chronic pelvic pain: Trigger points and the abdominal pelvic pain syndrome. *Am J Obstet Gynecol* 1984;149:536–543.

16. Sinaki M, Merritt JL, Stillwell GK: Tension myalgia of the pelvic floor. *Mayo Clin Proc* 1977;52:717–722.

## Suggested Readings

Bernard TN, Kirkaldy-Willis WH: Recognizing specific characteristics of nonspecific low back pain. *Clin Orthop* 1987;217:266–280.

Davis RW: Pelvic pain. *Physical Medicine and Rehabilitation: State of the Art Reviews* 1991;5(3):609–621.

Hoppenfeld S: *Physical Examination of the Spine and Extremities.* Norwalk, CT: Appleton-Century-Crofts, 1976: 143–169.

Kirkaldy-Willis WH: *Managing Low Back Pain,* 2nd ed. New York: Churchill Livingstone, 1988.

# Chapter 18
# Thigh and Knee

JOE H. GIECK,
SUSAN A. FOREMAN,
ETHAN N. SALIBA,
RALPH BUSCHBACHER

The knee is a complex joint. It is structured to provide both mobility and stability, and this dual role is often challenged by movements which can impose great stresses on the knee. The asymmetric articular interfaces of the knee place an extreme burden on the muscles and ligaments, which must statically and dynamically stabilize an intrinsically unstable structure. As a result the knee is susceptible to a wide array of pathologies, either traumatic or overuse in nature.

The biomechanical demands of the knee joint are affected by the hip and ankle. Therefore, in evaluating disorders of the knee it is essential to possess a thorough knowledge of the anatomy and injury mechanisms of the entire lower extremity. The thigh, being the origin of the major muscles which control the knee, must be understood especially well.

## Anatomy

The knee (Figure 18-1) is comprised of two joints, the tibiofemoral and the patellofemoral joints. The tibiofemoral joint is the articulation of the distal end of the femur with the proximal aspect of

Acknowledgement: The authors would like to thank Kevin Cross for his assistance in the preparation and development of this chapter.

the tibia. The femur's articular surfaces are the medial and lateral condyles which are convex and asymmetric. The medial and lateral tibial plateaus serve as the concave housing for the femoral condyles, and are asymmetric as well. They are also shallow. The incongruity of the articular surfaces causes the femur and tibia to move on each other in several planes. In addition to flexion and extension, the joint surfaces also glide on each other and during the final degrees of knee extension they rotate as well. This rotation increases the stability of the joint.

Placed between the bony prominences of the femur and the tibia are two fibrocartilaginous disks called the medial and lateral menisci. They serve to deepen the interface between the two bones to enhance stability and act as shock absorbers during weight-bearing activities. The medial meniscus is held rigidly in place by means of its attachments to the deep medial joint capsule, the tibial collateral ligament, and the semimembranosus muscle. The lateral meniscus is more mobile. The menisci are vascularized only on their periphery.[1]

The patellofemoral joint is the articulation between the sesamoid patella and the intercondylar groove of the femur. The patella moves superiorly and inferiorly within the intercondylar groove as the knee extends and flexes. It is connected to the fascia surrounding the knee by the medial and

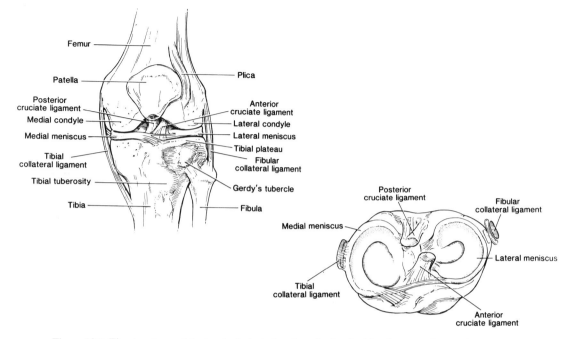

**Figure 18-1.** The structures of the knee. *A*, Anterior view; *B*, view looking down on the proximal tibia.

lateral retinacula, which are fibrous sheets of connective tissue (Figure 18-2).

There are several key supporting ligamentous structures which, in addition to the joint capsule, reinforce the stability of the knee. The medial knee is protected by the tibial collateral (also called medial collateral) ligament. A segment of this ligament blends with the joint capsule and attaches to the medial meniscus, thereby associating these structures with similar mechanisms of injury. The tibial collateral ligament protects the knee against valgus forces such as a blow to the outside of the knee.

The lateral knee is reinforced by the fibular collateral ligament, also known as the lateral collateral ligament. Unlike its medial counterpart, the fibular collateral ligament has little association with injuries to the lateral meniscus. It aids in stabilization against varus forces to the knee.

There are two crossed intraarticular ligaments of the knee, called the cruciate ligaments. The anterior cruciate ligament runs from the anteromedial tibia to the posterolateral femur. This ligament prevents excessive anterior translation of the tibia on the femur as well as hyperextension and excessive rotation of the knee. The posterior cruciate ligament extends from the posterolateral tibia to the anteromedial femur. It prevents excessive posterior movement and rotation of the tibia.

The muscles of the thigh also contribute to the stability of the knee joint. They are depicted in Figure 18-2. The main anterior muscles, known as the quadriceps, extend the knee. The posterior muscles, known collectively as the hamstrings, flex the knee. The medial thigh muscles belong to the hip adductor group. Posteriorly, the knee joint is also crossed by the gastrocnemius and popliteus calf muscles.

The iliotibial band extends from the tensor fascia lata and gluteus maximus muscles to insert onto Gerdy's tubercle, located lateral to the tibial tuberosity. It provides the knee with lateral support and is often associated with overuse injuries.

Medially is a structure known as the pes anserinus ("goose's foot"). It is the combined tendinous insertion of the sartorius, gracilis, and semitendinosus muscles. It is located on the medial aspect of the knee at the level of the tibial tuberosity.

## Rehabilitative Approach

Rehabilitation should begin the day after injury to help prevent the deleterious effects of disuse.

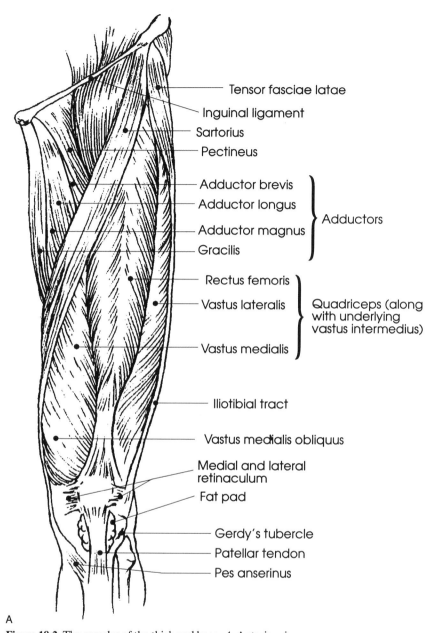

**Figure 18-2.** The muscles of the thigh and knee. *A*, Anterior view.

Typically muscles, tendons, and ligaments shorten and atrophy during the inflammatory process of healing, and the restoration of function as quickly as possible is the primary goal of rehabilitation. Early mobilization facilitates proper collagen orientation during healing.[2–4]

In early rehabilitation it is important to establish goals with the patient. The goals must be accepted by the patient for rehabilitation to be successful.

*Acute Injury Treatment Principles*

Immediate treatment of traumatic injuries begins with the application of ice, compression in the form of an elastic wrap, and elevation of the lower extremity for 20 minutes each hour during waking hours. If ice is not available, a quick method of rapid application of cold is to use a large bag of frozen vegetables that can be returned to the

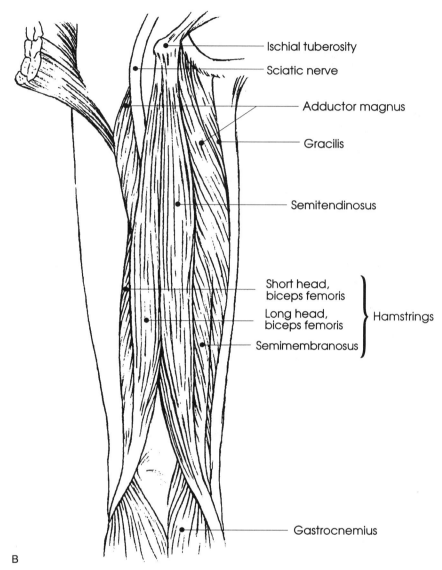

B

**Figure 18-2.** *(Continued)* B, *Posterior view.*

freezer after treatment. The injured area should be wrapped with an elastic bandage to prevent the formation of edema. The wrap can be applied over the ice to provide the most effective cooling. If the wrap is applied under the ice bag, it should be wet to allow proper conduction of cold to the area. Caution is in order when applying the ice near the fibular head. The common peroneal nerve passes over the fibula just below this point and can be damaged by cold injury.

If the patient has a limp in the acute phase, he or she should be taught to use crutches or a cane. Partial weight bearing with crutches simulates nor-mal gait. Limping only stresses the injured and inflamed tissues and delays their healing.

After 24 hours, the patient begins the ISE (*ice, stretch, exercise*) routine (Figure 18-3).[5] The pa-tient places ice on the injured area for 20 minutes while attempting to stretch or move the part through a full range of motion. At the end of this session, resistive exercise is performed in three sets of ten repetitions. The weight or resistance used should be low enough to be tolerated throughout a full pain-free range of motion.

Following this routine the area is wrapped in an elastic bandage. Ideally the ISE treatment is

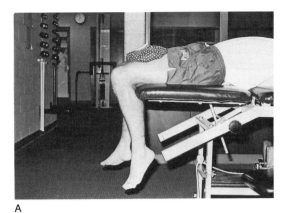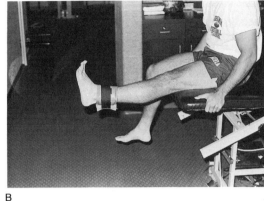

**Figure 18-3.** The ISE protocol. *A*, *I*ce and *s*tretch; *B*, *e*xercise.

performed twice a day. When the patient has full pain-free range of motion, when there is no excessive warmth in the body part, when edema has stabilized, and when the patient is making no further progress with the use of ISE then the treatment can be modified to replace the ice with moist heat during the protocol. Ice may still be applied following exercise to diminish postexercise inflammation.

When the knee is injured, flexion is the most commonly lost motion. Therefore, this is the motion that should be emphasized in the ISE protocol. The quadriceps (especially the vastus medialis) are particularly prone to atrophy after knee injury and begin to lose function almost immediately following such injury. Extension exercise of the ISE program helps to retard their atrophy. If a knee effusion is present after injury, then full range of motion exercise is contraindicated and quadriceps exercise should be limited to straight leg raising.

### Overuse Injury Treatment Principles

The most important phase of management for overuse injuries is counseling the patient to reduce or eliminate the activity causing the problem. No treatment of overuse injuries is successful without modification of the causative activity.

Prolonged overuse problems often result in weakness and loss of flexibility. Therefore, manual muscle testing and flexibility assessment of the entire lower extremity should be performed. Postural assessment and observation during activity should also be included in the evaluation.

### Pain-Free Exercise

Pain-free exercise is the gauge that the patient should use as a guide in advancing exercise. The exercise intensity level should be just below the level that causes pain. While some temporary discomfort is inevitable, rehabilitation should not be painful, especially the day after exercise. If the exercise causes pain the intensity should be reduced. If there is no discomfort the next day, then the exercise intensity may gradually be increased.

### Proprioceptive Exercise

Proprioception is affected by injury.[6] Therefore, balance exercises should begin as soon as the patient can bear weight comfortably. The patient may be asked to balance on one extremity for 30 seconds. This activity is repeated twice and the routine is practiced multiple times daily. To increase the difficulty of the exercise, the patient may lean forward, backward, sideways, and finally pick up small objects off the floor, all while standing on one leg. After this is mastered, the patient may perform the same activities with eyes closed to remove visual cues that make balancing easier.

Other proprioceptive exercises such as using a balance board or a tilt board may also be used.

### Quadriceps Strengthening Exercise

The patella is situated to act as a lever for the quadriceps to increase their force of pull on the tibia. As it slides down into the intercondylar groove of the femur during knee flexion the forces acting to compress the patellofemoral joint increase.[7] Thus patellofemoral joint dysfunctions are aggravated by greater knee flexion. When the knee is held in greater extension, the patellofemoral joint compressive force is less. The vastus medialis obliquus is also preferentially exercised in this position. These principles provide the basis for most quadriceps strengthening exercises.

**Quadriceps Setting.** This isometric exercise is performed to strengthen the muscles without irritating the joint structures. The patient lies supine with the knee extended. He or she slowly contracts the quadriceps, holds this position for 10 seconds, relaxes, and finally repeats the sequence for eight sets of ten repetitions. This exercise can be performed as often as possible during the day and in positions other than being supine, and with the knee at various angles.

**Straight Leg Raising** (Figure 18-4). When quadriceps setting has been mastered, the patient may progress to straight leg raises. In this exercise the patient should lie supine with the opposite leg flexed. The quadriceps should be contracted as when doing the quadriceps setting exercise and the foot should be dorsiflexed. The injured leg is then lifted to the height of the opposite leg, slowly lowered, and then the muscles are relaxed. The sequence is again repeated for eight sets of ten repetitions and is followed by quadriceps exercise with weights and stretching. Ankle weights may be added as tolerated. The patient should be able to perform the exercise at up to 5% of body weight before progressing to full-arc isotonic exercise.

**Terminal Extension Exercise.** This is an isotonic exercise. The patient performs active exercise over the final 30 degrees of extension only. This can be performed with special weight machines found at many health clubs or can be done by rolling a blanket under the knee to allow the foot to be lifted. It can be performed with ankle weights. This exercise (as well as the straight leg raise) may be performed with the lower extremity in slight external rotation to preferentially strengthen the vastus medialis obliquus.

**Exercise Bicycle.** Bicycling with the knee in excessive flexion aggravates patellofemoral dysfunction. Therefore the bicycle seat should be kept a bit high to keep the knees relatively extended during this exercise.

### Endurance Exercise

After strength, flexibility, and proprioception are regained, an endurance program may be initiated. This should begin with walking, if tolerated, without limping.

When patients can walk slowly for 30 minutes (uninterrupted) a day, they progress to a more rapid pace. Later a walk/jog program with 50 steps of walking alternated with 50 steps of jogging may be initiated. At first this is done only every other day for 30 minutes. Gradually the walking phase is reduced and the jogging increased until the patient is jogging 30 minutes every other day. Swimming and bicycling are also forms of acceptable endurance exercise.

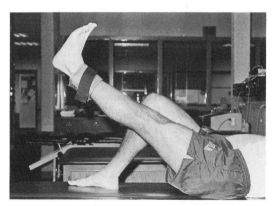

**Figure 18-4.** Quadriceps straight leg raising exercise. The leg is held in extension throughout the leg raise.

## Examination and Testing Techniques

### History

The most important aspect of injury evaluation is the history. If the patient can describe the mechanism of injury in a traumatic situation, the clinician can speculate on the structure that was injured. In overuse injuries patients should be questioned about any potential causative factors. For example, changes in training duration or intensity, or changing running shoes can cause knee pain. Even consistent running on one side of the road can cause injury because most roads are crowned for drainage, and the lower (outside) leg absorbs different forces than the inside leg. A number of other issues are also important in taking the history, which are discussed in the following sections.

**Swelling.**    Rapid swelling of the knee, usually within a few hours after injury, is indicative of hemorrhage into the joint.[8] If it occurs very rapidly it is often a sign of anterior cruciate ligament tear. Osteochondral fractures also cause rapid swelling. More gradual swelling may be a sign of meniscal tear.

**Knee Catching and Locking.**    The patient may report that the knee catches or locks in certain positions. Such catching may be seen in meniscus tears, osteochondral fractures, patellofemoral dysfunction, or plica syndrome, among others. True locking with a complete inability to move the knee usually occurs only in meniscal tears or in osteochondral fractures associated with the presence of loose bodies of bone in the joint.

**History of a "Pop."**    If the patient reports hearing or feeling a pop in the knee during some maneuver, it is suggestive of a cruciate ligament tear. Osteochondral fractures, meniscal tears, and patellofemoral subluxation are also possible.

**Subluxating Patella.**    If the patient reports that the kneecap jumped out of place, this may be indicative of a dislocating or subluxating patella.

**Location of the Pain.**    The exact location of the pain is important. Obviously, medial or lateral pain helps determine which side of the knee is involved. Pain along the joint line is indicative of possible meniscal or capsular damage. Pain on the patella or behind the patella may be indicative of patellofemoral disturbance, and pain below the patella may be indicative of patellar tendon inflammation.

### Observation

Observation of the injured area should include careful study of the patient walking. The knees and thighs can be compared for size, alignment, discoloration, and swelling. The quadriceps should be observed to evaluate the bulk and tone of the muscle. The position of the patella should be noted. Either a high-riding or low-riding patella, called patella alta or patella baja respectively, are associated with some types of knee disorders. The high-riding patella is subject to developing patellar instability since it is less well stabilized in the intercondylar groove of the femur. Since it provides less leverage in knee extension than a normally situated patella it makes the quadriceps more susceptible to overuse as they compensate for this deficit. A patella baja, due to greater forces being exerted on the patella, is involved in more degenerative problems. In addition, a laterally positioned patella is important, as it may be associated with patellofemoral tracking abnormalities. The patella should be observed with the patient sitting and the knee flexed to 90 degrees. The patellar surface should normally face straight forward with an upward angle.

### Palpation

Palpation of the injured area should begin with structures least likely to have been injured. Once patients feel pain during the examination, they become apprehensive, and it is difficult to continue palpation. Palpation can help determine the exact location of pain and can reveal defects in some extraarticular soft tissues. The clinician should also palpate for crepitus and swelling.

The medial part of the vastus medialis, also called the vastus medialis obliquus, should be palpated during active muscle contraction to assess its muscle mass, especially in relation to the opposite side. Often weakness of this part of the muscle results in abnormal patellar tracking.

The patellofemoral joint can be assessed by placing the knee in extension and passively moving the patella medially and laterally. This allows one to slip a finger underneath the edges of the patella to determine whether there is tenderness here. If so, it is an indication of patellofemoral dysfunction. The fibular collateral ligament can best be palpated by having the patient cross the leg, the figure-4 position.

### Range of Motion and Muscular Strength

Joint range of motion and muscular strength should be assessed. The uninvolved side of the body can be used as a control to determine normal range and strength. To evaluate the knee for abnormal hyperextension the patient can be asked to lie supine while the examiner lifts both feet. If the thigh muscles are relaxed, an abnormally lax knee hyperextends.

Active, pain-free range of motion can be an effective indicator of the severity of knee and thigh injuries. The clinician should determine whether pain, spasm, or obstruction limits range of motion. Squatting can be used to assess knee flexion range as a screening technique.

### Stability Testing

Varus and valgus stress testing should be performed with the knee fully extended and in 30 degrees of flexion (Figure 18-5). During full extension the anterior and posterior cruciate ligaments as well as the medial and lateral joint structures are taut. Thus if valgus or varus stress at full extension reveals abnormal laxity in any direction it is indicative of very significant soft tissue damage. When valgus and varus stress is applied at 30 degrees of knee flexion, the cruciate ligaments become lax and the medial and lateral stabilizing structures are tested in isolation. Thus if the collateral ligaments are damaged, varus and valgus stress testing is more likely to reveal this at 30 degrees of flexion.

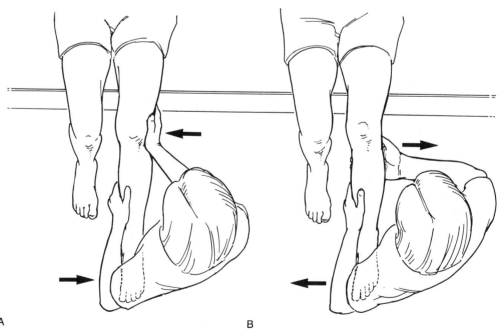

A                                               B

**Figure 18-5.** Valgus (A) and varus (B) stress testing at the knee. This should be performed with the knee fully extended and in 30 degrees of flexion.

*Special Tests*

A number of special tests for various knee structures exist, and a full discussion of all of these is beyond the scope of this chapter. The reader is referred to the suggested readings at the end of the chapter for more information. However, a few of these tests deserve special mention.

**Anterior and Posterior Drawer Tests** (Figure 18-6A). These tests are performed at 90 degrees of knee flexion. The patient is usually supine, and the examiner may sit on the patient's foot to stabilize the lower leg. In this position either an anterior or posterior force is applied to the proximal tibia. Excessive anterior movement is indicative of a deficient anterior cruciate ligament. Excessive posterior movement is indicative of a torn posterior cruciate ligament. When the patient is in this position with the quadriceps relaxed, a sagging of the proximal tibia may be present and is also indicative of a posterior cruciate ligament tear.

**Lachman Test** (Figure 18-6B). This is a test of the anterior cruciate ligament and is more sensitive than the anterior drawer test. The posterior tibia has a lip that projects upward. This, as well as the meniscus, creates a wedge that may stabilize the knee during anterior drawer testing (see insert on Figure 18-6A). The Lachman test removes this wedge by placing the knee in 30 degrees of flexion. The lower leg is again stabilized and an anterior force is directed on the proximal tibia. Excessive

anterior translation is indicative of an anterior cruciate ligament tear.

**McMurray's Test** (Figure 18-7). A torn meniscus often produces a click or a catch in the knee during flexion and extension. McMurray's test is designed to elicit this click or catch more readily during the physical examination. The patient is supine. The examiner passively flexes the knee while holding the knee in one hand and the foot in the other. The lower leg is externally rotated while applying a valgus stress. The leg is slowly extended, and a palpable or audible click is indicative of a probable meniscal tear. The test is also performed with a varus stress and internal rotation to the knee. When the click occurs on internal rotation and varus stressing it is indicative of a lateral meniscus tear, while the opposite maneuver causes clicking in a medial meniscus tear. It is important to realize that not all meniscus tears elicit a positive McMurray's test. A negative test does not rule out such a tear.

**Apley's Test** (Figure 18-8). This is also a test of meniscus tears. The patient is prone with the knee flexed to 90 degrees. The examiner applies a downward force on the lower leg to push it in toward the femur. In this position the lower leg is internally and externally rotated. Pain is indicative of a meniscus tear.

**Patellar Apprehension Test.** This is similar to the apprehension sign in the shoulder and is indicative of a subluxating or dislocating patella. The

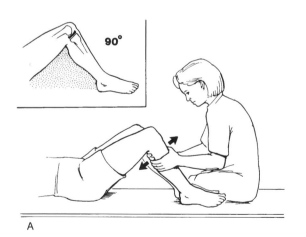

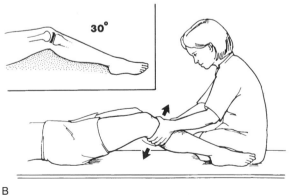

A

B

**Figure 18-6.** *A*, Anterior and posterior drawer testing. *B*, The Lachman test.

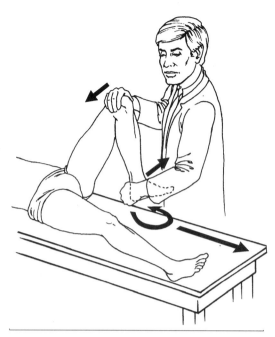

**Figure 18-7.** McMurray's test for meniscus tears. The examiner passively flexes the patient's knee, applies valgus stress to the knee, and externally rotates the lower leg. The leg is then slowly extended. The same procedure is repeated with the lower leg internally rotated while applying varus stress.

patient is asked to lie supine with the quadriceps relaxed. The examiner manually pushes the patella laterally. The patient who has had instability of the patella becomes apprehensive and contracts the quadriceps on this maneuver.

**Patellofemoral Grinding Test.** The patient again is supine with the quadriceps relaxed. The examiner pushes the patella distally and applies pressure downward on the patella to compress the patellofemoral joint. The patient is then asked to pull the patella proximally by contracting the quadriceps. In patellofemoral joint dysfunction this elicits pain and roughness as the patella moves proximally. This test is often uncomfortable even in asymptomatic patients and is therefore relatively nonspecific.

**Q-Angle Measurements** (Figure 18-9). The Q-angle (quadriceps angle) is the angle formed between the quadriceps (measured to the anterior superior iliac spine) and the patellar tendon. An excessive Q-angle is felt to predispose individuals

to patellofemoral joint dysfunction because the quadriceps tend to pull the patella laterally. A normal Q-angle is 10 degrees or less in males and 15 degrees or less in females.[9] A Q-angle greater than 20 degrees is considered abnormal.

**Thigh Measurement.** Measuring the circumference of the thigh approximately 10 cm proximal to the superior pole of the patella (or 10 cm proximal to the medial joint line) gives an idea of quadriceps mass and can be compared from side to side. Knee disorders often cause a reflexive type of inhibition of the quadriceps which leads to rapid atrophy. Serial thigh measurements are important in following the progression and recovery of such atrophy.

**Functional Tests.** A number of functional tests can be performed to assess knee and thigh function. They include tests such as squatting, one legged squatting, hopping on one or both feet with the foot externally or internally rotated, running in place, or running in figure-eight patterns.

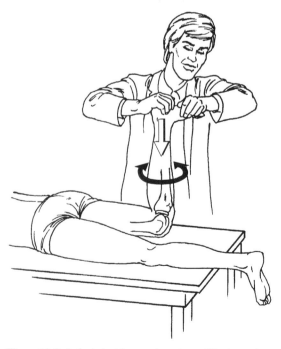

**Figure 18-8.** Apley's test for meniscus tears. The lower leg is pushed downward and is rotated from side to side.

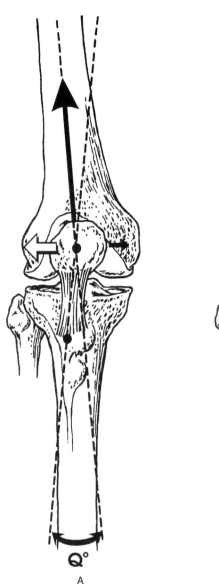

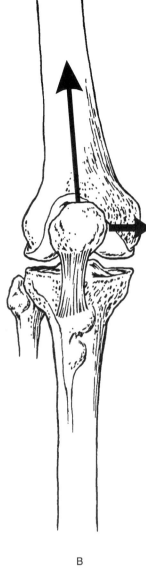

**Figure 18-9.** The Q-angle and the muscular forces acting on the patella. Since the bulk of the quadriceps pulls along the line of the femur (*long black arrow*), it tends to pull the patella laterally out of place (*open arrow*). This is counteracted by the fibers of the vastus medialis, especially the vastus medialis obliquus (*small black arrow*). In (*A*) a weak vastus medialis obliquus cannot counteract the stronger bulk of the quadriceps. This results in a net lateral force vector (*open arrow*). In (*B*) the vastus medialis obliquus is strong and counteracts the lateral force to achieve neutral patellar tracking.

**Q°**

A

B

*Ancillary Diagnostic Testing*

**X-Ray Studies.** The standard x-ray views that should be obtained in knee disorders are antero-posterior, lateral, and sunrise views (Figure 18-10). Another possible view is the tunnel view (also known as the notch view) which is made to view the intercondylar notch (Figure 18-10). A narrow intercondylar notch is associated with cruciate ligament damage in some kicking sports.

**Joint Aspiration.** In conditions of effusion or suspected hemorrhage into the joint, a joint aspiration is often helpful. Obviously, bloody fluid helps to make a diagnosis. If there is fat within this fluid it may be indicative of an osteochondral fracture. Analysis of joint fluid may also reveal signs of chronic inflammation or infection as well as many metabolic diseases.

**Magnetic Resonance Imaging (MRI) and Computerized Tomography (CT).** MRI is useful in assessing the soft tissues of the knee and can be

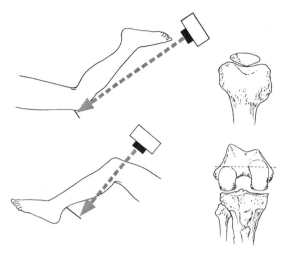

**Figure 18-10.** Sunrise (*top*) and tunnel (*bottom*) x-ray views. Figures on the right demonstrate the positions of the bones from the x-ray's point of view.

used to detect some meniscal and ligament tears and cartilage damage. CT is used to detect fractures.

**Arthrography.** This test involves injection of radiopaque dye into the knee joint and can be used to detect ligamentous or meniscal tears.

**Arthroscopy.** This involves the direct insertion of a fiberoptic viewing scope into the knee. It can be used diagnostically to detect ligament damage or meniscus tears and is also used therapeutically to débride some meniscal tears as well as degenerative tissue or an inflamed plica. It should be performed whenever hemarthrosis is present, even in the face of an otherwise nonspecific examination. In such cases, intraarticular damage has most likely occurred.[10]

## Diagnosis and Treatment of Specific Disorders of the Knee

### Ligamentous Injury

Injuries to the ligaments of the knee especially those incurred in athletic events are usually caused by trauma. They may involve the anterior or posterior cruciate ligaments or the tibial or fibular collateral ligaments, or any combination of these.

Anterior cruciate ligament injuries commonly occur when an athlete stops abruptly or changes running direction with the foot firmly planted on the ground. They are often associated with medial ligament and meniscus damage. Posterior cruciate ligament injury, less common than anterior cruciate damage, occurs when the proximal tibia is pushed posteriorly. This can happen in a fall on the knee, during auto accidents, and sometimes during knee hyperextension.

Tibial and fibular collateral ligament injuries occur from the application of valgus or varus force to the knee. The tibial collateral ligament is more commonly affected. Due to the relationship between the tibial collateral ligament and the medial meniscus, more complex injuries such as the "unhappy triad of O'Donoghue" can result. This triad includes tibial collateral ligament sprain, anterior cruciate sprain, and medial meniscus lesion. Ligamentous injury can be graded from I (sprain with no laxity), II (sprain with some laxity), to III (complete rupture).

### Diagnosis

The history usually guides in determining which ligament, if any, is injured. Which direction the knee was stressed provides an idea of which ligament bore the brunt of the stress. Often the patient will have heard a "pop." In anterior cruciate ligament injury, anterior drawer testing may be positive and the Lachman test is usually positive. These tests must be performed as soon as possible after injury. Effusions develop within hours, and once effusion has formed, it is difficult to evaluate ligamentous integrity on physical examination. MRI, arthrography, or arthroscopy can help make the diagnosis.

In posterior cruciate ligament damage there may be posterior sagging of the proximal tibia, and posterior drawer testing should be positive. Again MRI, arthrography, or arthroscopy confirms the tear of the ligaments.

Collateral ligament injuries do not result in a tense joint effusion unless the capsular structures are damaged as well. The patient, however, experiences pain and tenderness along the joint line and along the affected ligament. Complete active and passive range of motion of the knee may be possible, but the injury causes stiffness with all motions. Depending on the severity of the injury, ligamentous stress tests may reveal laxity of the joint. All stress testing must be done bilaterally to determine if a difference in laxity exists.

## Treatment

Treatment for anterior and posterior cruciate ligament injuries is controversial and such injuries should be evaluated by an orthopedic surgeon. Acute injury, especially in a young or active patient, is usually treated surgically. When nonsurgical treatment is pursued it involves strengthening of the muscles surrounding the knee.

Treatment of collateral ligament injury depends on the severity of the ligament injury. In mild (grade I) injury, treatment may consist of ice, compression, elevation, and possibly antiinflammatory medications followed by an isometric strengthening program, isotonic exercise, and exercise bicycle riding. Resumption of normal activity, especially athletic activity, should begin only when normal strength and range of motion are regained.

Grade II sprains can be treated similarly to grade I except, of course, that the recovery time is prolonged. In some cases, a knee brace may be selected to help support the knee and prevent valgus forces during the early recovery period.

Grade III sprains, which involve complete disruption of the ligament, are treated either with a cast brace or by surgical repair followed by a strengthening program of the quadriceps and hamstrings.

One helpful hint to patients with any of these ligament injuries is not to tuck in their bedsheets when sleeping. When turning in one's sleep it is easy to get the foot caught in a tight bedsheet. This can be very painful. For the more severe injuries a period of limited weight bearing is often necessary. The injured knee should never be allowed to dangle, with the weight of the lower leg pulling on the remaining ligamentous fibers. This can worsen an injury.

## Meniscus Tears

Injury to the meniscus generally involves a twisting movement with the knees bent. Since the medial meniscus is less mobile than the lateral meniscus (due to its attachment to the joint capsule and tibial collateral ligament), it is damaged more often than the lateral meniscus. Injury to the medial meniscus is often associated with tibial collateral damage. Tears of the meniscus are often traumatic, but repetitive trauma, such as from running, may

also cause a gradual separation of collagen fibers resulting in a tear. Tears may result from rotatory forces being superimposed on weight bearing.

In older patients, degenerative meniscal tears may develop. These cannot usually be attributed to any specific traumatic event.

## Diagnosis

In an acute meniscus injury there may be an audible pop. Patients usually complain of pain on one side of the knee or the other. This is worsened by twisting and squatting activities. Occasionally, there can be locking of the knee in one position. Effusions tend to be mild to moderate and develop gradually (8 to 12 hours).[8] McMurray's test and Apley's test may be positive, and the joint line is generally tender. There may be pain on passive forced knee flexion. Knee extension is often incomplete. The diagnosis can be confirmed by MRI, arthroscopy, or arthrography. Overuse type tears may be associated with intermittent pain and mild swelling.

## Treatment

Because the meniscus has only a tenuous blood supply around its periphery, it tends not to heal very well. Small peripheral tears may sometimes heal if the knee is protected after injury with rest accompanied by ice and nonsteroidal antiinflammatory drugs (NSAIDs). This early treatment is followed by a strengthening and functional progression program. Positions of extreme knee flexion are avoided.

In the past, meniscus tears were often treated with total meniscectomy, which is a complete removal of the meniscus. This usually resulted in surprisingly little functional disability, but often led to degenerative osteoarthritis of the knee joint over a period of years.

Currently, as much of the meniscus is left in place as is feasible. Small asymptomatic tears are generally treated conservatively with NSAIDs as needed, ice, and a strengthening program. If they become symptomatic, a partial arthroscopic meniscectomy can be done. Occasionally, total meniscectomy for large tears is still required.

Degenerative meniscus tears can generally be treated conservatively with a period of rest, ice, NSAIDs, and when symptoms are stabilized, a strengthening program. This is usually successful, and surgical débridement is rarely necessary.

### Patellar Instability

The patella connects the quadriceps tendon to the patellar tendon to provide greater leverage in extension. It rides in the intercondylar groove of the patella. In patients who have a greater than normal Q-angle, patella alta, or a shallow intercondylar groove, the patella may slip out of the groove laterally. This is normally prevented by the vastus medialis obliquus (see Figure 18-9).[11] In patients with a weak vastus medialis obliquus, it is felt that lateral subluxation or dislocation is more likely to occur. Other factors that may predispose an individual to lateral displacement of the patella include external tibial torsion, a lax medial retinaculum, a tight lateral retinaculum, an excessively strong vastus lateralis, excessive foot pronation, and pes planus.

Instability of the patella can result in acute dislocation, acute subluxation, or chronic dislocation and subluxation.

### Diagnosis

An acutely dislocated patella can usually be detected by observation or palpation. The athlete or the patient has a feeling that the knee went "out of joint" and has marked pain and decreased range of motion. There is usually a history of the patient feeling that something popped and gave way in the knee. This is often associated with muscle exertion, especially when turning away from the side of the dislocation.

When the patella has subluxated, the patient may again report that the knee went out of joint. Knee locking, catching, and a feeling of weakness at the knee are also common. Examination of the knee may reveal swelling and tenderness along the medial patella and the medial retinaculum. There may be lateral hypermobility of the patella, and passive movement of the patella in this direction may cause acute pain and apprehension.

### Treatment

Acute dislocation of the patella should be reduced with gentle straightening of the leg. Occasionally,

medial pressure must be applied to reduce the joint. This is followed by splinting, ice, and follow-up x-ray films, as osteochondral fractures or other fractures may be associated with this condition. After an initial acute dislocation, the leg can be held extended (the position of least pressure on the patella) in a knee immobilizer (with crutch walking and partial weight bearing) for several weeks to facilitate healing. In recurrent dislocations, the patient may be put in a knee immobilizer until symptoms resolve. Both of these conditions are followed by a strengthening program. A brace may be worn in this early period. Special knee braces, such as the Palumbo brace, may help to hold the patella in place by providing pressure with a lateral pad and strapping.[12] They also probably provide proprioceptive feedback. In cases refractory to conservative care, the lateral retinaculum may need to be released and the tibial tubercle may be surgically shifted medially to reduce the Q-angle.

### Patellofemoral Dysfunction (Chondromalacia)

Chondromalacia is a term which has been used and abused widely in the past. It implies that there is a degeneration of the patellofemoral joint and is actually not a clinical but rather a pathologic diagnosis. Patients with patellofemoral joint pain may have chondromalacia. However, many patients with obvious degeneration noted by arthroscopy or x-ray studies have no joint pain. Consequently, the cause of the pain is not clear. Most patellofemoral dysfunction occurs because of muscular imbalance in the quadriceps.[11] This may be associated with some of the patellar abnormalities described earlier for patellar subluxation. There may be a patella alta, an increase in the Q-angle, pes planus, and external tibial torsion as well as inflexibility of the hamstrings, gastrocnemius, and iliotibial tract. Patients suffering from patellofemoral dysfunction are often young women in their teens or twenties and are usually active.

### Diagnosis

Patellofemoral dysfunction generally has an insidious onset. Pain and discomfort first appear after activity such as climbing stairs. Later there are characteristic complains of knee pain, especially during running up or down hills, aching of the knees after sitting for long periods of time, or occasional painful catching or locking of the knee. Physical examination reveals tenderness of the medial patella, pain on patellar compression, a positive apprehension sign, and often joint crepitus. A thickened plica is sometimes felt. These patients may have less than normal knee valgus, and the vastus medialis obliquus may be poorly developed.

### Treatment

Treatment involves strengthening of the quadriceps as outlined earlier, especially of the vastus medialis obliquus. In addition, hamstring and gastrocnemius flexibility, NSAIDs, ice, shoe orthotics, and avoidance of exacerbating activities are important. A patellar sleeve, which prevents excessive lateral movement of the patella, is also sometimes useful,[13] and as noted above may possibly exert its action mainly through proprioceptive feedback. Manual stretching of the lateral retinaculum or taping of the patella may be attempted in conjunction with strengthening.[14,15] Conservative care is usually successful. Only rarely is a lateral retinacular release necessary to improve patellar tracking.[16]

### Osgood-Schlatter Disease

This is a condition of tibial apophysitis. The apophysis is the area of tendon attachment to the bone. During growth, the apophysis grows to accommodate the increasing size of the tendon. In cases of overuse or excessive stress on the patellar tendon, the apophysis may become inflamed, and there can be a partial avulsion of the tibial tubercle. This occurs in teenagers, mainly boys at ages 11 to 15. Patella alta and tight hamstrings may predispose to this condition. The patient complains of pain during running, jumping, and kneeling. The tibial tubercle becomes prominent.[17]

### Diagnosis

Diagnosis is made from a history of activity-related anterior knee pain aggravated by running, jumping, and kneeling, and by a palpable tenderness over the prominent tibial tubercle.

### Treatment

Treatment is usually conservative and involves reducing aggravating activities, stretching the hamstrings, and progressive strengthening of the quadriceps. Occasionally, short periods of immobilization or rest are required to reduce the inflammatory process, and NSAIDs may be prescribed. The injury generally resolves as the apophysis matures; however, the patient is left with a prominent tibial tubercle. This condition is similar to Sinding-Larsen-Johansson syndrome, which is an apophysitis of the patellar tendon attachment to the patella.[18] Treatment for this syndrome is generally the same for Osgood-Schlatter disease.

### Patellar Tendonitis

Patellar tendonitis, known as jumper's knee, is an overuse syndrome of the patellar tendon. It is seen in running, jumping, climbing, and kicking activities.[19] Generally, examination of the knee yields point tenderness along the patellar tendon and at the inferior pole of the patella. The patient may complain of the knee becoming stiff and sore with prolonged periods of sitting. If the tendonitis persists without treatment, the tendon may rupture.

### Diagnosis

History and location of the pain are clues to this disorder and there may be tenderness and minor swelling around the patellar tendon. The patient often describes pain during the landing phase of jumping.

### Treatment

Treatment consists of rest, ice, and NSAIDs followed by hamstring and gastrocnemius stretching, heat, and a strengthening program emphasizing the vastus medialis obliquus. Eccentric exercise may be valuable.[20,21]

### Bursitis

There are numerous bursae distributed throughout the knee between tissue interfaces to reduce frictional irritation. These fluid filled sacs can become inflamed following direct impact or overuse.

The most prevalent site of bursitis in the knee is the prepatellar bursa on the surface of the patella. This injury is caused by a fall directly onto the knee or by persistent kneeling, and is often referred to as housemaid's knee. Prepatellar bursitis is common in wrestlers. Inflammation in the bursa can be treated with ice, compression, and NSAIDs.

Occasionally, aspiration of the bursa is necessary to rule out infection. However, it must also be appreciated that introduction of a needle into the bursa can itself cause infection. Thus, special care should be taken, especially when injecting steroidal antiinflammatory medications into the bursa.

### Iliotibial Tract Inflammation

This condition, also known as runner's knee, involves irritation and inflammation of the iliotibial band. The iliotibial tract is a thick band of fascia that extends from the tensor fascia lata and gluteus maximus muscles to Gerdy's tubercle. It rubs over the lateral femoral condyle as the knee is flexed to approximately 30 degrees. When this flexion is performed repeatedly, especially in distance runners, it can develop into a friction syndrome. This may be more common in runners who supinate their feet excessively.

### Diagnosis

When the knee is slowly flexed, the iliotibial band can be felt to slip over the femoral condyle. Pain and tenderness of the tract as it slips over the condyle are indicative of inflammation of this structure. Occasionally, the tensor fascia lata is inflexible, and stretching it may reproduce the symptoms of knee pain (see Ober's test in Chapter 17).

### Treatment

Treatment consists of ice, stretching the tensor fascia lata, NSAIDs, and rest. Avoiding running on hills and slopes, not wearing new shoes, and possibly corrective shoe orthotics may be helpful as well.

### Inflamed Plica

The medial plica is a redundant fold of synovial membrane situated in the medial knee (See Figure 18-1). It is present in some persons as a vestigial embryonic fold of the membrane.[22] Because it can be entrapped in the patellofemoral joint, the plica is sometimes inflamed and produces anterior knee pain. This can occur due to trauma or to overuse.

### Diagnosis

Patients complain of anterior or anteromedial knee pain. This is exacerbated by running, especially running on hills, and is worsened by prolonged sitting. Characteristically the patient reports that knee pain occurs with prolonged sitting, and after getting up and taking a few steps it resolves. This is most likely because the plica slips back out of the patellofemoral joint. An inflamed plica may cause knee clicking, swelling, catching, and weakness. It is sometimes confused with meniscal tears or patellofemoral dysfunction. It can sometimes be differentiated from these conditions if the inflamed plica is palpable at the anteromedial knee.

### Treatment

Treatment consists of rest, NSAIDs, and strengthening of the quadriceps. A small muscle called the articularis genu pulls the synovial membrane out of the joint during knee extension, and quadriceps strengthening exercises may help develop this muscle to pull the plica out of the area where it is being compressed. Conservative care usually gives good results,[22] although occasionally arthroscopic resection of the plica is necessary.

### Degenerative Joint Disease

Degenerative joint disease occurs in the knee, as in many other joints of the body. It is associated with aging, although it is probably not caused solely by aging. There is some element of "wear and tear" involved in its progression.

## Diagnosis

This condition is characterized by a history of pain in the knee which may be relieved with gentle activity. The pain can occur at night and after rest. There is also joint crepitus and prominent bony spurs (both palpable and revealed by x-ray study). There may be intermittent mild joint effusion.

## Treatment

Treatment is with rest, ice, and NSAIDs, followed by a strengthening program. Regular exercise of moderate intensity may help to decrease the symptoms or prevent their progression. In severe cases, surgical treatment with cartilage débridement by arthroscopy, or even a total joint replacement, may be necessary. Patients should be told to avoid squatting or sitting on low chairs.

### Osteochondritis Dissecans

This is a condition of ischemic injury to the cartilage and subchondral bone. It occurs mainly in boys of ages 10 to 14 and is most likely due to trauma and possibly a predisposing anatomy. Symptoms may consist of joint catching, swelling, and decreased range of motion. The physical examination is similar to that for meniscal tears. The patient often walks with the leg externally rotated for comfort. When a piece of damaged bone dislodges, a loose body is formed. X-ray findings can help make the diagnosis by demonstrating the characteristic bony changes. Management varies from rest to surgery, depending on the severity of the disorder.

## Diagnosis and Treatment of Specific Disorders of the Thigh

### Quadriceps Contusion

Quadriceps contusion is a frequently encountered athletic injury. Its severity is often underestimated early on while the athlete is active and the muscle is warmed up by sports activity. After a brief rest,

however, the symptoms worsen. Any continued activity may exacerbate the injury and result in more significant hemorrhage.[23]

## Diagnosis

This condition is diagnosed mainly by a history of trauma, thigh pain and swelling, and decreased range of motion, especially of knee flexion.

## Treatment

Early treatment for a quadriceps contusion is essential. This includes protection from further aggravation or injury. Crutches may be necessary if walking is painful. Ice should be applied for 20 to 30 minutes while a comfortable stretch is applied. No assistive stretching should be attempted. Compression in the form of a foam pad and elastic wrap is then applied. The patient is encouraged to minimize activity and to maintain lower extremity elevation whenever possible. NSAIDs can also be helpful in reducing the amount of edema in the injury site.

Heat modalities including hot whirlpools and ultrasound are not indicated until the individual starts to show good progress in knee range of motion. Massage is also contraindicated in the acute and subacute stages of the quadriceps contusion. Only active stretching exercises should be done by the patient—no assistance should be attempted.

A serious complication of a severe or repeated contusion to the anterior thigh is myositis ossificans, a form of heterotopic ossification. In this condition the hemorrhagic tissue is gradually replaced by an island of bone. This complication may severely limit an athlete's sports participation.

### Quadriceps Strain

Delayed-onset muscle soreness occurs frequently in the quadriceps when a new activity is initiated, especially if it is an eccentric activity.[20] Soreness progressively worsens over a 24- to 48-hour period and then begins to resolve. A strain is suspected if pain, stiffness, and spasm continue beyond this time. Muscle injuries in the anterior thigh occur most commonly in the rectus femoris muscle, which crosses two joints.

*Diagnosis*

The symptoms associated with a muscle strain can range from a perception of tightness to generalized pain radiating down the anterior thigh. Localized tenderness is usually palpable at the site of injury. Manual muscle tests can help isolate the injured structure. The degree of injury is best determined by the amount of functional restriction the athlete has and by the limitation in knee range of motion.

*Treatment*

Ice and *gentle* stretching in the pain-free ranges are recommended initially. This is followed by progressive strengthening. Bilaterally equal strength and flexibility along with a gradual progression back to activity are essential to avoid reinjury, which frequently occurs. Because of the potential complications that exist with a thigh contusion, any strain which presents with a significant hematoma should be treated very conservatively.

### Hamstring Strain

Injuries to the hamstrings have been categorized into two types: acute and insidious onset. The acute-onset hamstring injury is commonly associated with a sprinting effort, while insidious-onset strains are associated with a progressive lack of flexibility of the hamstrings.[24]

*Diagnosis*

In an acute strain the athlete experiences a sudden severe pain which results in marked functional restriction. A pop or tearing sensation is often described during the history. Generalized pain occurs, but typically localized tenderness can be palpated. Swelling can occur and may make the palpation of any defects difficult to appreciate. Insidious-onset strains are associated with less well localized hamstring pain. These muscles are usually lacking in normal flexibility.

*Treatment*

Hamstring strains are often debilitating injuries because they seem to recur when a rehabilitation program is not followed. Acute strains should be treated with ice, gentle stretching, and the gradual addition of strengthening exercise. Functional activities should be added cautiously and should include walking backward, climbing, and running (to emphasize hamstring activity.)

Treatment of insidious-onset hamstring injury includes taking the same considerations as with acute injury. It should include physical therapy modalities such as ultrasound, massage, lumbosacral mobilization, and flexibility and strengthening of the hamstrings, quadriceps, and hip extensors. Shoe orthotics are indicated if biomechanical factors of the feet are implicated.

### Other Conditions of the Thigh

Other conditions which can cause thigh problems include metabolic or connective tissue disease, quadriceps rupture, hernias, nerve compression, infection, and tumors, among many others.

### Case Report

A 24-year-old woman presented with an episode of painful knee catching and popping. She had never experienced such symptoms in the past. Examination revealed a poorly developed vastus medialis obliquus, painful patellofemoral joint crepitus, and an otherwise normal examination. She was taught a program of quadriceps setting exercise, leg lifts, and terminal extension exercise with weights. She subsequently exercised regularly on a stationary bicycle and has been symptom free for several years.

### Points of Summary

1. Most knee injuries can be treated conservatively using the ISE protocol.
2. Radiographic testing should be performed to rule out associated fractures.

3. In injuries to the knee where major ligament damage or meniscal tears are suspected or if there is a rapid onset of effusion or hemarthrosis, orthopedic surgery consultation should be obtained.
4. Overuse injuries can be caused by postural and strength imbalances, and evaluation should include all aspects of the kinetic chain from the foot to the hip.
5. Eliminating the source of overuse injuries rather than just treating the symptoms is imperative for long-term success.
6. Thigh injuries are commonly perceived as being insignificant. However, they can result in serious sequelae and must be properly addressed.

## References

1. Arnoczky SP, Warren RF: Microvasculature of the human meniscus. *Am J Sports Med* 1982;10:90–95.
2. Buck RC: Regeneration of tendon. *J Pathol Bacteriol* 1953;66:1–18.
3. Tipton CM, Matthes RD, Maynard JA, et al.: The influence of physical activity on ligaments and tendons. *Med Sci Sports Exerc* 1975;7:165–175.
4. Vailas AC, Tipton CM, Matthes RD: Physical activity and the influence on the repair process of medial collateral ligaments. *Connect Tissue Res* 1981;9:25–32.
5. Kuland D: *The Injured Athlete*. 2nd ed. Philadelphia: JB Lippincott, 1988.
6. Freeman MAR, Dean MRE, Hanham IWF: The etiology and prevention of functional instability of the foot. *J Bone Joint Surg* 1965;47B:678–685.
7. Hungerford DS, Lennox DW: Rehabilitation of the knee in disorders of the patellofemoral joint: Relevant biomechanics. *Orthop Clin North Am* 1983;14:397–402.
8. Roy S, Irvin R: *Sports Medicine: Prevention, Evaluation, Management, and Rehabilitation*. Englewood Cliffs, NJ: Prentice-Hall, 1983:293–368.
9. Hughston JC, Walsh WM, Puddu G: *Patellar Subluxation and Dislocation*. Philadelphia: WB Saunders, 1984.
10. Noyes FR, Bassett RW, Grood ES, et al.: Arthroscopy in acute traumatic hemarthrosis of the knee. *J Bone Joint Surg* 1980;62A:687–695.
11. Eisele SA: A precise approach to anterior knee pain. *Physician Sports Med* 1990;19:127–139.
12. Palumbo PM Jr: Dynamic patellar brace: A new orthosis in the management of patellofemoral disorders. *Am J Sports Med* 1981;9:45–49.
13. Garrick JG: Anterior knee pain (chondromalacia). *Phys Sports Med* 1989;17:75–84.
14. Walsh WM, Helzer-Julin M: Patellar tracking problems in athletes. *Primary Care* 1992;19:303–330.
15. Shelton GL: Conservative management of patellofemoral dysfunction. *Prim Care* 1992;19:331–349.
16. Campbell ED, Collins HR, Mattalino AJ: Patellofemoral problems of the knee. *Surg Rounds Orthop* 1989;6:40–45.
17. Kujala UM, Kvist M, Heinonen O: Osgood-Schlatter's disease in adolescent athletes: Retrospective study of incidence and duration. *Am J Sports Med* 1985;13:236–241.
18. Medlar RC, Lyne ED: Sinding-Larsen-Johansson disease: Its etiology and natural history. *J Bone Joint Surg* 1978;60A:1113–1116.
19. Blazina ME, Kerlan RK, Jobe FW, et al.: Jumper's knee. *Orthop Clin North Am* 1973;4:665–678.
20. Curwin S, Stanish WD: *Tendinitis: Its Etiology and Treatment*. Lexington, MA: The Collamore Press, 1984.
21. Fyfe I, Stanish WD: The use of eccentric training and stretching in treatment and prevention of tendon injuries. *Clin Sports Med* 1992;11:601–624.
22. Calvo RD, Steadman JR, Sterling JC: Managing plica syndrome of the knee. *Phys Sports Med* 1990;18:64–74.
23. Bull CR: Soft tissue injuries to the hip and thigh, in Torg JS, Welsh RP, Shephard RJ (eds): *Current Therapy in Sports Medicine--2*, Toronto, BC Decker, 1990.
24. Garrett WE, Rich FR, Nikolau PK, Vogler JB: Computed tomography of hamstring muscle strains. *Med Sci Sports Exerc* 1989;21:506–514.

## Suggested Readings

Anderson SJ: Overuse knee injuries in young athletes. *Phys Sports Med* 1991;19:69–80.
Calvo RD, Steadman JR, Sterling JC: Managing plica syndrome of the knee. *Phys Sports Med* 1990;18:64–74.
Hoppenfeld S: *Physical Examination of the Spine and Extremities*. Norwalk, CT: Appleton-Century-Crofts, 1976.
Walsh WM, Helzer-Julin M: Patellar tracking problems in athletes. *Prim Care* 1992;19:303–330.

# Chapter 19

# Lower Leg, Ankle, and Foot

JOHN LEARD,
DENISE L. MASSIE,
JACK BRAUTIGAM,
RALPH BUSCHBACHER

Complaints of lower leg, ankle, and foot problems are common, but because of the complexity of this region, they are often misunderstood. This chapter attempts to shed some light on the fundamentals of diagnosing and treating this important anatomic region. The interested reader is referred to the suggested readings at the end of the chapter for further study.

## Anatomy

Only the major structures that are pertinent to the discussion of pathologies later in the chapter are presented in this section.

### Bony Anatomy

The lower leg bones, the tibia and fibula, are depicted in Figure 19-1. Only the larger and medial tibia articulates proximally with the femur in the knee joint. Distally, both the tibia and the fibula contribute to form the ankle mortise, which along with the talus forms the talocrural (ankle) joint.

The bones of the foot and ankle are divided into four groups (Figure 19-2): the tarsals, metatarsals, phalanges, and sesamoids. The sesamoid bones are small, rounded masses of bone found within the tendon of the flexor hallucis brevis. They are located on the weight-bearing surface of the first metatarsophalangeal joint.

### Articulations *(Figures 19-1 through 19-3)*

There are two tibiofibular joints, one proximal and the other distal. The distal tibiofibular joint contributes to form the ankle mortise of the talocrural joint.

The talocrural joint (TCJ) is typically thought of as the "ankle joint." This joint is located between the superior, medial, and lateral articular surfaces of the talus and the distal articulating surfaces of the tibia and fibula. It mainly allows dorsiflexion and plantarflexion motion to occur. The talus is wider anteriorly than posteriorly and dorsiflexion brings the wider part of the bone into the ankle mortise. This "wedging" effect makes the ankle more stable and less prone to injury in dorsiflexion than in plantarflexion.

The subtalar joint (STJ) is the articulation formed by the inferior talus and the superior calcaneus. Motion at the STJ occurs in the three cardinal planes of flexion/extension, abduction/adduction, and inversion/eversion.

**Figure 19-1.** The bones of the lower leg.

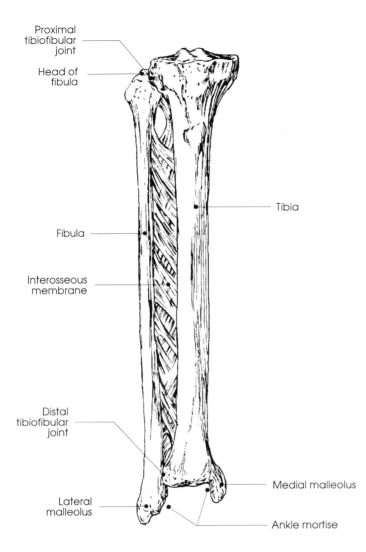

Proximal
tibiofibular
joint

Head of
fibula

Fibula

Interosseous
membrane

Distal
tibiofibular
joint

Lateral
malleolus

Tibia

Medial malleolus

Ankle mortise

The midtarsal (transverse tarsal) joint (MTJ) is comprised of two joints, the talonavicular and calcaneocuboid joints. Motion at the MTJ joint occurs on the longitudinal axis and on the oblique axis, allowing for movement in all three planes as well.

In addition, there are joints between all the adjacent tarsals, between the tarsals and metatarsals, and in the phalanges. Of these, the first metatarsophalangeal (MTP) joint is most often involved in foot dysfunction.

### Ligaments *(Figure 19-3)*

The tibia and fibula are connected along their shafts by an interosseous membrane which helps to stabilize the TCJ and which also serves as a place of origin for several muscles in the leg. The proximal and distal tibiofibular joints are supported by anterior and posterior ligaments which allow some gliding and longitudinal rotation of the fibula to occur. The distal ligaments play an important role in the stability of the TCJ.

Other ligamentous structures which provide stability to the TCJ include the medial deltoid ligament and the lateral ankle ligaments (the anterior talofibular, calcaneofibular, and posterior talofibular ligaments). The anterior talofibular (ATF) ligament passes from the anterior fibula to the lateral talus. Its fibers are horizontal when the ankle is dorsiflexed but become vertically oriented when the ankle is plantarflexed. This ligament prevents

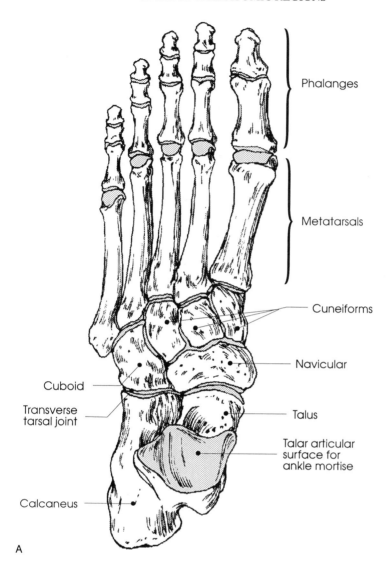

Phalanges

Metatarsals

Cuneiforms

Navicular

Cuboid

Transverse
tarsal joint

Talus

Talar articular
surface for
ankle mortise

Calcaneus

A

**Figure 19-2.** The bones of the foot: *A*, Dorsal view.

excessive inversion and anterior translation of the talus on the fibula and is often sprained. The calcaneofibular (CF) ligament passes from the inferior lateral malleolus to the lateral calcaneus. It prevents excessive inversion, particularly when the ankle is dorsiflexed. The posterior talofibular (PTF) ligament is located on the posterior aspect of both the talus and the fibula. It prevents excessive inversion of the rearfoot complex.

The deltoid ligament lies over the medial TCJ joint. This broad ligament is typically divided into four parts (tibionavicular, tibiocalcaneal, anterior tibiotalar, and posterior tibiotalar) which prevent excessive eversion of the ankle

and which support the medial longitudinal arch of the foot.

The MTJ is supported from below by the plantar calcaneonavicular ("spring") ligament, a thick band of fibers whose primary function is to maintain the medial longitudinal arch

### Compartments and Muscles of the Lower Leg
*(Figure 19-4)*

There are three main lower leg compartments, the anterior, posterior, and the lateral. The anterior compartment contains the muscles which dorsiflex

**Figure 19-2.** *(Continued) B*, Plantar view.

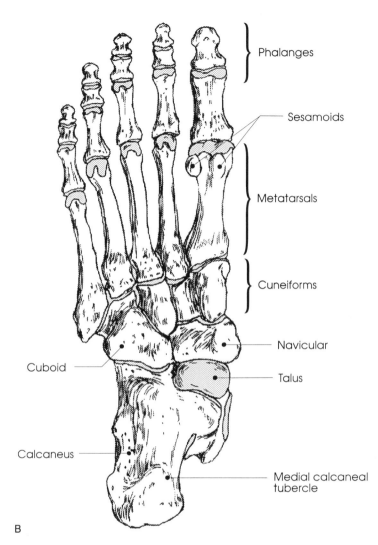

Phalanges

Sesamoids

Metatarsals

Cuneiforms

Navicular

Cuboid

Talus

Calcaneus

Medial calcaneal tubercle

B

the foot and extend the toes. The posterior compartment contains the calf muscles which plantarflex the foot and flex the toes. The lateral compartment muscles evert the foot. Inversion is accomplished by some of the muscles of the anterior and posterior compartments working together.

### Fascia

The plantar fascia originates from the calcaneus and inserts onto the five heads of the metatarsal bones. It supports the longitudinal arch of the foot. Fascial bands also separate the muscles of the leg compartments, and some (the retinacula) anchor the tendons of the leg muscles where they pass by the ankle to the foot.

### Normal Gait

The foot plays an important and complex role in gait (see also Chapter 11). While it is being planted onto the ground it must be flexible to provide stability, yet during push-off it must be rigid to act as a lever.

During normal gait, initial heel contact is on the lateral aspect of the calcaneus with the foot in a slightly supinated (adducted, inverted) position.

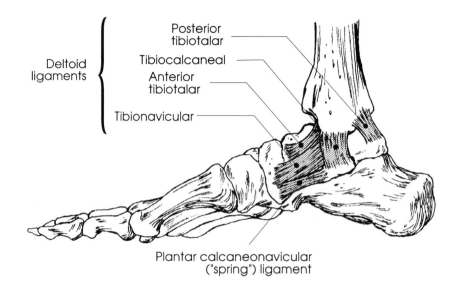

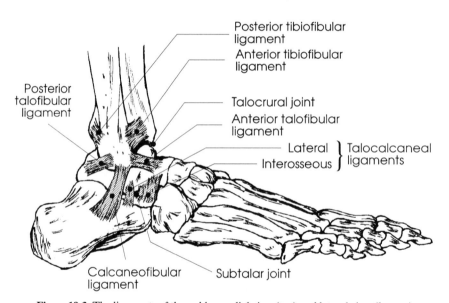

**Figure 19-3.** The ligaments of the ankle: medial view (*top*) and lateral view (*bottom*).

The contact phase is characterized by pronation (abduction, eversion). Pronation is an important component of the contact phase for two reasons. First, it allows the foot to become a loose adapter to uneven terrain, and second, it assists in shock absorption.[1] Since the foot pronates during the contact phase, the lower extremity rotates internally.

The midstance period is characterized by the foot being in full ground contact and beginning to

supinate. This motion continues throughout the midstance and propulsive phases. The initiation of supination allows the foot to become a rigid lever in preparation for propulsion.[2] Additionally, since the midstance phase is characterized by the onset of supination, the lower extremity begins to rotate externally.

During the midstance period of the gait cycle, the tibia migrates anteriorly over the talar dome by approximately 10 degrees. Therefore, this amount

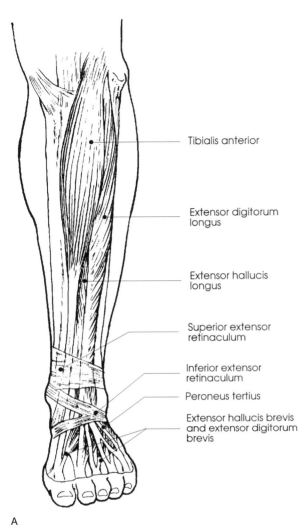

**Figure 19-4.** The muscles of the lower leg and foot: *A*, Anterior view.

Tibialis anterior

Extensor digitorum longus

Extensor hallucis longus

Superior extensor retinaculum

Inferior extensor retinaculum

Peroneus tertius

Extensor hallucis brevis and extensor digitorum brevis

A

of motion must be present in the talocrural joint to allow for normal gait.[3] If this 10 degrees is not present, whether due to a tight gastrocnemius-soleus complex or osseous deformity, the foot must compensate for the deficit.

During the push-off (propulsion) phase of gait increased tension is developed in the plantar aponeurosis. This helps to elevate the medial longitudinal arch, which in turn facilitates supination and stabilizes the foot.[4] At the same time, the sesamoid bones allow the first metatarsal head to glide posteriorly, which makes propulsion more efficient by providing proper MTP extension.

**Rehabilitative Approach**

As with all areas of the body, rehabilitation of leg, ankle, and foot problems begins at the time of injury or onset of symptoms. Early intervention in the appropriate form promotes healing of the affected structures and limits the area of insult and tissue inflammation. The sports medicine approach to rehabilitation may be applied to all types of patients for timely, cost-effective rehabilitation. This approach is described in more detail in Chapter 4. It is divided into four overlapping phases: (1) control of inflammation; (2) attaining adequate flexibility;

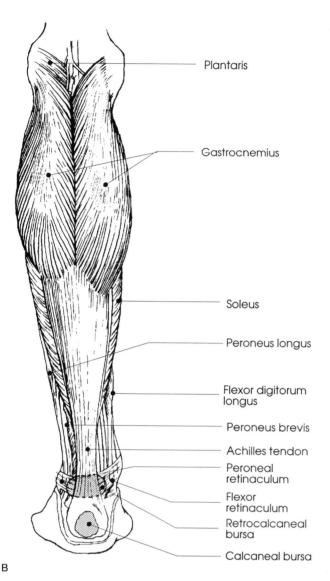

Figure 19-4. *(Continued) B*, Posterior (superficial) view,

Plantaris

Gastrocnemius

Soleus

Peroneus longus

Flexor digitorum longus

Peroneus brevis

Achilles tendon

Peroneal retinaculum

Flexor retinaculum

Retrocalcaneal bursa

Calcaneal bursa

B

(3) strengthening the injured area; and (4) promotion of functional progression to return to normal activity (Table 19-1). In addition, a number of therapeutic techniques may help to speed recovery.

### Therapeutic Modalities

The modalities and therapies used in lower leg, ankle, and foot injuries are similar to those used in other disorders and include heat, cold, flexibility, and strengthening exercises. A few of these of special interest in the lower extremity are described below in greater detail.

**Whirlpool.**    This modality can be used as either a form of convective heating or cooling. For injuries, cold water is generally preferred over a warm whirlpool, as the latter may increase soft tissue inflammation and swelling. The size of the whirlpool generally allows for range of motion exercises to be performed in conjunction with cold application.

**Ankle Bracing and Taping.**    In acute ankle sprain injury the joint may be taped (open Gibney basketweave technique) to provide support and compression. Another alternative is to apply an air stirrup splint (Figure 19-5) to provide support and

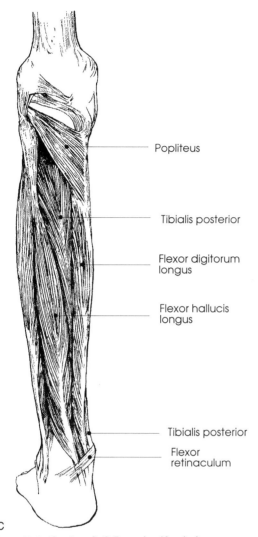

C

**Figure 19-4.** *(Continued) C*, Posterior (deep) view.

Popliteus

Tibialis posterior

Flexor digitorum longus

Flexor hallucis longus

Tibialis posterior

Flexor retinaculum

**Therapeutic Exercise.**    The use of exercise modalities should address any deficiencies that the patient may have. Quality as opposed to quantity of exercise should be stressed. Hence, a cookbook approach to exercise is not appropriate.

Weight-bearing status must be determined initially and should progress as healing proceeds. The appropriate assistive devices should be utilized depending on the amount of weight that can safely be placed on the lower extremity. Early weight bearing may aid the healing process as the injured tissue adapts to imposed stresses.[6] In order to prevent improper gait from becoming a habit, it is recommended that patients continue with crutch or walker use as long as they walk with a limp. Canes should be employed as balance aids only. When the patient is in a non-weight-bearing status, the use of a three-point crutch or walker gait with emphasis on normal hip swing and upright trunk posture helps to deter the development of muscle imbalances of the proximal lower extremity.

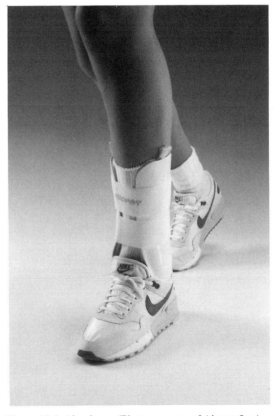

**Figure 19-5.** Air stirrup. (Photo courtesy of Aircast, Inc.)

compression. As the acute inflammation subsides, patients may be treated with lace-up ankle supports for a brief period of time to provide extra support. In athletes, either taping or lace-up bracing may be helpful in preventing reinjury. Proper technique in applying tape is essential. The reader is referred elsewhere[5] for more information on ankle bracing and taping.

**Low Dye Strapping.**    This is a taping technique to support the arch of the foot. It is helpful in treating plantar fasciitis, arch sprains, metatarsalgia, or other conditions related to excessive foot pronation.

**Table 19-1.** General Outline of Functional Progression After Ankle Sprain

| | DATE |
|---|---|
| 1. Partial weight bearing | _____ |
| 2. Weight shifting (double leg stance) | _____ |
| 3. Heel raises (assisted) | _____ |
| 4. Full weight bearing | _____ |
| 5. Proprioception drills (single leg stance) | _____ |
| 6. Heel raises (single leg) | _____ |
| 7. Step-ups: 1 inch (3 × 10) | _____ |
|     4 inch (3 × 10) | _____ |
| 8. Walk (¼ mile briskly; no limp) | _____ |
| 9. Walk–jog progression (level surface) | _____ |
| 10. Jumping (both feet): | _____ |
|     Side to side | _____ |
| 11. Hop (one foot): | |
|     Side to side | _____ |
| 12. Half-speed to full-speed sprint | |
|     progression | |
|     (forward; backward) | _____ |
| 13. Jog (uneven surface) | _____ |
| 14. Figure 8's: 20 yd @ ½ speed | _____ |
|     ¾ speed | _____ |
|     full speed | |
|     • 10 yd @ ½ speed | _____ |
|     ¾ speed | _____ |
|     full speed | _____ |
|     • 5 yd @ ½ speed | _____ |
|     ¾ speed | _____ |
|     full speed | _____ |
| 15. Concentric circles: 10 yd @ ½ speed | _____ |
|     ¾ speed | _____ |
|     full speed | _____ |
|     • 5 yd @ ½ speed | _____ |
|     ¾ speed | _____ |
|     full speed | _____ |
| 16. Cross over/carioca | _____ |
| 17. Cutting (spot/command): 45° @ ½ speed | _____ |
|     ¾ speed | _____ |
|     full speed | _____ |
|     • 90° @ ½ speed | _____ |
|     ¾ speed | _____ |
|     full speed | _____ |
| 18. Activities specific to sport: | _____ |
| | |
| | |
| 19. Return to drills only: Noncontact | _____ |
|     Practice | _____ |
|     Competition | _____ |

Neuromuscular control, strength, and muscular endurance may be increased by a variety of methods. The use of manual resistance and pro-prioceptive neuromuscular facilitation (PNF) (see Chapter 7) may be performed in the clinic. The use of rubber tubing or straps is useful in the clinic and at home. Isometric exercise may be used initially on a submaximal basis to begin PNF. It is also useful in avoiding painful positions in the range of motion, when there is restricted motion, or when other exercise devices cannot be employed. Towel curls (Figure 19-6), towel gathering, and "windshield wiper" exercises are isotonic exercises used with minimal equipment to build foot and ankle neuromuscular control. Seated and standing toe raises may be used for strengthening the calf musculature. Partial squats (against the wall) and step-ups can be utilized to strengthen the quadriceps and gluteal muscles. Weight machines and stair climbing machines are also useful for low-impact strengthening of the lower extremity.

**Pool.**   Pool therapy may be beneficial for range of motion exercises, progression of weight-bearing and gait activities, resistive exercise, and cardiovascular exercise. This may be incorporated in the clinic program or be performed by the patient independently at a local fitness facility or at home. Specific instructions must be given to the patient regarding the level of activity, duration, and frequency of treatment.

**Proprioceptive Exercise.**   Proprioceptive loss occurs after injuries to the ankle (see Chapter 4) and is felt to impair the return to normal activity.[7] Exercises for proprioception, balance, and agility

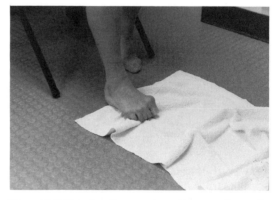

**Figure 19-6.** Towel curling exercises to improve foot and ankle neuromuscular control. A weight may be placed on the towel to increase the difficulty of the exercise.

may include balance board activities (Figure 19-7A), slide board exercises (Figure 19-7B), mini-trampoline exercises, single leg stance exercises, and single leg stance exercises with rubber tubing on the nonaffected limb or around the trunk (Figure 19-7C).

## Examination and Testing Techniques

### *History and Physical Examination*

The history should include questions regarding the mechanism of injury, past medical history, whether the onset was sudden or gradual, ability to continue sports participation after the injury occurred, the duration of symptoms, and the patient's general health status. Inquiring about training errors, equipment (especially shoes), and changes in training surfaces helps identify causes of an overuse related injury.

The biomechanical examination begins after the onset of injury or as the patient enters the room. Observing for a limp, limited motion, or any gait deviations serves as the basis of the examination.

Observation should include looking for signs of edema, ecchymosis, deformities, scars, or abnormal biomechanics. Clinical signs of hyperpronation include callus formations, clawing or splaying of the toes, and hallux valgus deformities. Retrocalcaneal exostoses ("pump bumps") are signs of abnormal shearing forces occurring at the calcaneus due to hyperpronation.[3] The alignment of the calcaneus with respect to the lower leg should be evaluated to detect varus or valgus deformity of the hindfoot.

Palpation of the injury should begin away from the injured site or on the uninvolved extremity. Initial palpations which are not pain producing improve the patient's relaxation and trust.

Since all parts of the lower extremity are components of a "kinetic linkage system," it is important

**Figure 19-7.** Proprioceptive exercises: *A*, Balance board; *B*, slide board; and *C*, rubber tubing resisted exercise. The patient is weight bearing on the involved extremity with the tubing around the unbalanced leg. This strengthens the involved extremity and stimulates proprioception.

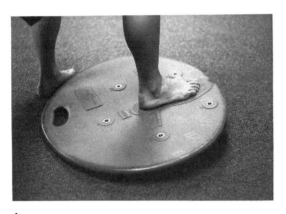

A

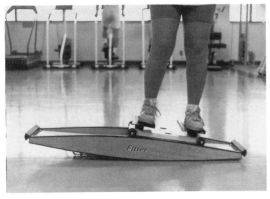

B

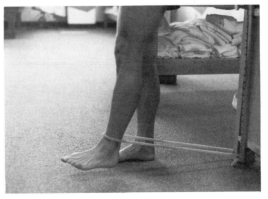

C

to examine the joint above and below the injured area. A thorough examination helps to differentiate between musculoskeletal and referred pain.

Range of motion and muscle strength testing are also important in evaluating the foot and ankle. Appropriate normal ranges of motion are described elsewhere.[8,9] Pain or laxity on inversion and eversion range of motion stress testing are signs of ankle ligament sprain. A number of specific examination techniques are also helpful and are described in the following text. In addition to these tests it is helpful to observe the patient's gait and examine the shoes to detect abnormal patterns of wear.

**Subtalar Neutral Foot Positioning.** The alignment of the foot and ankle is best evaluated with the subtalar joint in the neutral position. This position is located by the examiner passively inverting and everting the foot, finding that position in which the talus is equally palpable, or not palpable at all, on each side of the ankle. Slight dorsiflexion "locks" the foot in this position (Figure 19-8). Once neutral alignment is attained, the foot and ankle can be assessed for the presence of varus or valgus deformity. The calcaneus is compared with the lower leg and the forefoot is compared with the calcaneus.

TCJ motion is examined by placing the STJ in the neutral position and passively dorsiflexing the foot. A minimum of 10 degrees' dorsiflexion is required for normal gait. If this amount of motion is absent, the knee is flexed to eliminate the influence of possible gastrocnemius contracture. An increase in dorsiflexion after flexing the knee is indicative of a tight gastrocnemius muscle. However, no change in joint motion might be indicative of either a congenitally short gastroc-soleus complex or an abnormal osseous "block" at the ankle.[1]

**First MTP Joint Motion.** Passive motion of the first MTP joint is affected by the position of the first metatarsal. If the metatarsal is allowed to move freely, the joint should extend 60 to 70 degrees to allow for normal gait.[1] If the examiner stabilizes the first metatarsal, the amount of motion obtained by passively extending the great toe is less, approximately 30 degrees.

**Alignment of the First Ray.** The examiner grasps the first metatarsal head between the index finger and thumb of one hand, while holding the

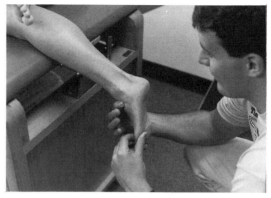

**Figure 19-8.** Locating the neutral position of the subtalar joint. The foot is inverted and everted until the talus is equally prominent on either side of the ankle. Passive dorsiflexion "locks" the foot in this position.

remaining metatarsal heads with the other hand. The thumbs located on the plantar surface should be level. If the thumb holding the first metatarsal head rests below (caudal to) the other thumb, the first ray is in an abnormal plantarflexed position. Passive dorsiflexion and plantarflexion of this bone should be equal in both directions.

**Thompson's Test.** A special test to detect a rupture of the Achilles tendon, Thompson's test is performed with the patient lying prone and feet resting over the edge of the table. Gently squeezing the calf musculature normally causes the foot to plantarflex. The absence of plantarflexion is considered a positive test.

**Anterior Drawer Test** (Figure 19-9). The anterior drawer test is used to detect laxity of the anterior talofibular ligament. The distal tibia and fibula are stabilized with one hand while the other cups the heel and exerts pressure anteriorly. The foot is placed in approximately 20 degrees of plantarflexion. Excessive anterior translation of the talus is indicative of compromise of the ATF ligament.

**Inversion/Eversion Stress Test.** The patient lies supine with feet over the edge of the table (or remains sitting), then, the lower leg is stabilized while the talus is tilted from side to side, applying inversion and eversion stress. This tests the integrity of the lateral (mainly calcaneofibular) and deltoid ligaments.

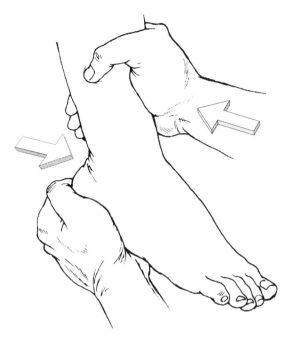

**Figure 19-9.** The anterior drawer test. The foot is in 20 degrees of plantarflexion. The examiner pulls the foot anteriorly to test the integrity of the anterior talofibular ligament.

### Ancillary Diagnostic Testing

Plain radiographs are commonly used to evaluate bony alignment, joint condition, and to detect fractures. They are indicated in all but the most simple ankle sprains to rule out associated fractures. Occasionally, they are supplemented by arthrography to help diagnose ligamentous injury. Bone scans are useful to detect stress fractures. Magnetic resonance imaging (MRI) and computerized tomography (CT) are rarely necessary.

## Diagnosis and Treatment of Specific Disorders

### Ankle Sprains

There are many different ankle ligaments that can be damaged, and the exact ligament which is torn or stretched is dependent on the mechanism of the injury. Typically, three mechanisms cause ankle sprains: inversion, eversion, or rotation. These can occur in combination with one another or in isolation. The following descriptions of the three ankle

sprains assume that isolated injury mechanisms have occurred. Combinations of injury mechanisms add to the damage and symptoms described. In all ankle sprains it is important to perform the physical examination as early as possible. Edema forms rapidly and hampers the exact localization of the site of injury. Also, pulses and sensation in the foot should be checked in all ankle sprains to rule out associated neurovascular compromise. Radiographic studies should be obtained to rule out fracture.

**Inversion Ankle Sprains.**    This is by far the most common type of ankle sprain. It may involve damage to any of the three lateral ligaments, but most sprains are to the ATF ligament. The CF ligament is often injured as well, but usually is damaged along with the anterior ligament. With the ankle in the plantarflexed position, the ATF ligament is stretched and the talocrural joint is at its least stable position. Thus this ligament is at risk of injury. With the ankle in the neutral position (90-degree angle formed by the fibula and foot), the CF and PTF ligaments are more likely to be damaged.

DIAGNOSIS.    The ankle may be forcefully inverted by running on uneven surfaces, by landing on someone's foot while jumping, or by having the foot stabilized and forced into inversion. Upon inspection immediately after injury, there may be swelling over the lateral ligament which is injured. If not treated immediately with ice, compression, and elevation, diffuse forefoot and ankle swelling develop. Palpation elicits point tenderness over the injured ligament. Since an inversion ankle sprain may occur in combination with a fracture of the fibula or the base of the fifth metatarsal (Jones fracture), these structures must be palpated as well.

Range of motion and strength may be limited by pain, swelling, and possible injury to the peroneal muscles.

Special tests to evaluate the ligamentous structures include the anterior drawer test, plantarflexed inversion, and neutral inversion. Rarely arthrography is necessary to help diagnose ligamentous tearing.

**Eversion Ankle Sprains.**    The eversion ankle sprain causes damage to the deltoid ligament. Eversion sprains often occur in combination with a rotational mechanism of injury.

DIAGNOSIS. The history may be of forced eversion caused by an uneven surface or from another person falling on the lateral leg while the foot is stabilized. Inspection and palpation reveal swelling and point tenderness over the injured medial ligament. Range of motion and strength are limited due to pain, swelling, and possible muscular injury to the inverters of the ankle. Special tests should include passive eversion and examining the integrity of the medial longitudinal arch. This is important since the deltoid ligament provides stability to the arch of the foot as well as to the talocrural joint.

**Rotational Ankle Sprains.** With a rotational ankle sprain, the talus is rotated within the ankle mortise, causing the tibia and fibula to separate and damage the distal tibiofibular ligament. This torsion may also be accompanied by a spiral fibular fracture.

DIAGNOSIS. The common history includes a twisting of the body while the foot is planted and stabilized. Inspection and palpation reveal minimal swelling and point tenderness over the distal tibiofibular ligament. Weight bearing increases symptoms over the torn ligaments, and dorsiflexion is limited and painful. Strength loss is due mainly to the pain and swelling that are present. Special tests should include rotational stress testing and passive dorsiflexion, which will stress the distal tibiofibular joint.

TREATMENT. As previously stated, the immediate treatment for all ankle sprains is ice, compression, and elevation. Regardless of the mechanism of injury, these steps help control secondary damage caused by swelling and bleeding into the soft tissue. Elastic wrap or tape application may help to provide compression. Air stirrups are also useful and may provide enough stabilization to allow the patient to ambulate within a day or two (or immediately in some cases) of injury. Intermittent compression may also help to reduce edema formation.

Rehabilitation begins with relative rest to control swelling and encourage healing. For most patients, controlled ambulation is allowed as long as it does not stress the damaged ligaments. During the subacute period, gentle non-weight-bearing exercises in an elevated position maintain joint range of motion, and nonsteroidal antiinflammatory drugs (NSAIDs) reduce inflammation and pain. Gentle exercises to improve plantarflexion and dorsiflexion without stressing the injured structures are indicated. Those exercises include passive heelcord stretching with a towel, isometric exercises for dorsiflexion/plantarflexion, seated multidirectional tilt board range of motion exercise, and elevated active range of motion. The period of rest is kept to a minimum to eliminate the deleterious effects of immobilization. Forced dorsiflexion exercises, particularly weight bearing, should be avoided in an ankle sprain which may have a rotational component. Such dorsiflexion causes the tibia and fibula to separate and prevents proper healing.

Crutches may be used early on for a partial weight-bearing gait. In some cases a neutral foot orthotic device similar to a UCBL shoe insert (see Chapter 24) is effective at enabling patients to progress to weight-bearing status more comfortably and at a faster rate of return. The orthotic device holds the subtalar joint in its neutral position, the optimal position for function, and eliminates any extra stress to the healing tissue. Lace-up braces, continued taping, or an air stirrup application may also be used to provide support during early return to activity. Isometrics should begin as tolerated to promote strengthening of the ankle musculature.

Proprioception has been shown to be impaired following an injury to the ankle.[7] It is theorized that joint nerve receptors are damaged and must be retrained before one may safely return to activity. Exercises to improve proprioception begin with balancing on one foot, multidirectional board balancing, and eventually progress to tubing-resisted hip motions while bearing weight on the involved ankle (see Figure 19-7C). Functional activity is added when tolerated. Long-term bracing or taping is rarely necessary but may be considered in some athletes. Rarely, patients with complete ligamentous rupture and unstable joints require surgical treatment.

### Achilles Tendonitis, Achilles Tendon Rupture, and Retrocalcaneal Bursitis

The Achilles tendon is the common tendon of the gastrocnemius and soleus muscles which insert onto the posterior calcaneus. This tendon serves as a primary plantarflexor and secondary supinator. Located between the tendon and the calcaneus is the retrocalcaneal bursa.

The Achilles tendon possesses a "zone of avascularity" which is the most common site of tendon microtrauma or rupture. Located 2 to 6 cm above the tendon insertion, this avascular zone is also an area where the collagen fibers of the tendon tend to rotate and are more prone to overuse and injury.[10]

Common etiologic factors of Achilles tendonitis and rupture are overuse, excessive forced dorsiflexion, an inflexible gastroc-soleus complex, and hyperpronation[10] (which may be caused by tibia varum or varus foot deformity). Curwin states that the Achilles tendon is most stressed during eccentric contractions, such as with sudden dorsiflexion.[11] Achilles tendonitis is fairly common. A rupture of the tendon is less common.

The retrocalcaneal bursae may become inflamed as the result of direct trauma, compressive forces (caused by poor fitting footwear), or abnormal biomechanical stresses, and this condition may initially be confused with tendonitis.

Some patients also get bursitis between the tendon and the skin, a so-called "pump bump" because it is often caused by shoe irritation.

### Diagnosis

Evaluation of an inflamed Achilles tendon reveals swelling, point tenderness, and discomfort with passive dorsiflexion or active plantarflexion. A thorough biomechanical examination should be conducted to identify any rearfoot/forefoot abnormalities.

If the retrocalcaneal bursae are inflamed, the examiner may elicit point tenderness by palpating anterior to the distal tendon, directly superior to the calcaneus. This area is localized by pinching just anterior to the tendon.

With an Achilles tendon rupture, the patient often reports experiencing a sensation similar to being shot or kicked in the calf. Palpation reveals a defect at the rupture site and Thompson's test is positive. These patients cannot walk "on their toes."

### Treatment

The treatment program for tendonitis should address any biomechanical abnormalities while pursuing antiinflammatory management. Ice, antiinflammatory medications, and cold whirlpools are all indicated treatments for acute tendonitis. The patient may also find that a heel lift shortens the injured structure enough to allow ambulation with reduced discomfort. A medial heel wedge or temporary orthotic device may help to control excessive pronation.

Long-term treatment focuses on restoring proper flexibility to the gastroc-soleus structure and to the first MTP joint. This is followed by strengthening exercise, including eccentric training. Curwin outlines a program consisting of a rapid concentric contraction followed by an eccentric loading of the tendon.[11] The speed of contraction, number of repetitions, and single versus double leg support vary depending on the symptoms of the athlete.

Patients with a retrocalcaneal bursitis are treated with NSAIDs, ice, heelcord stretching, rest, and proper footwear. The bursa may in some cases be injected with a steroid-anesthetic solution. Extreme care must be taken not to inject the tendon itself or to overstress the tendon for up to 6 weeks after the injection, as the tendon may be more prone to rupture during this time. Rarely, excision of the bursa is necessary.

Partial tears of the tendon are treated with a period of enforced rest, usually with casting, followed by further rest and the use of a heel lift. Surgical repair may achieve equivalent long-term results more quickly. In complete tears of the tendon surgical repair is performed.

### Plantar Fasciitis

Common etiologic factors of plantar fasciitis include pes cavus/pes planus, training errors, repetitive trauma, and biomechanical factors (i.e., hyperpronation).[12] Typically, this problem is an overuse injury, and it may be aggravated by an increase in body weight, poor shoe support, or a change in running surface. In chronic cases, the insertion of the fascia may form a heel spur which can be seen radiographically.

### Diagnosis

Signs and symptoms of plantar fasciitis generally evolve with the insidious onset of heel pain which is worse in the morning and which improves as the day progresses. Typically, the patient reports pain with passive dorsiflexion and great toe extension. Palpation reveals tenderness over the narrow origin of the fascia at the medial calcaneal tubercle.

### Treatment

Treatment and rehabilitation of plantar fasciitis should focus on reducing inflammation and controlling exacerbating forces. Ice immersion or ice massage, performed three to four times per day, especially after exercise, helps reduce the inflammation. Since the plantar fascia is part of the lower extremity kinetic linkage system, flexibility exercises of the calf and foot musculature and the first MTP joint should be performed three to four times per day. When tolerated, strengthening exercises for the gastrocnemius and arch musculature, such as towel curls, marble pick-ups, and towel gathering exercises, must also be incorporated into the rehabilitation program. NSAIDs help reduce pain and inflammation and occasionally steroid-anesthetic injections are necessary. These injections are, however, extremely painful.

Comprehensive management should also address proper footwear and possibly the implementation of an orthotic device. An in-shoe heel cup, to provide a slight lift to the heel, is often beneficial in the early treatment. If pes cavus/planus or other biomechanical factors are considered etiologic factors, these abnormalities may be addressed with a temporary or permanent orthotic device to help control abnormal stresses and encourage proper stress distribution. Treatment for heel spurs often includes injections and orthotic devices to help resolve the problem. Rarely surgical removal of the spur is necessary. The spur will, however, recur if the underlying etiologic factors are not addressed.

### Shin Splints

The term *shin splints* has long been identified as a catch-all term for any pain which occurs below the knee and above the foot. The list of differential diagnoses includes tibialis posterior tendonitis, tibialis anterior tendonitis, anterior compartment syndrome, medial tibial stress syndrome, tibial stress microfractures, chronic periostalgia, and chronic posterior compartment ischemia.[13] These conditions are the result of cumulative trauma and are considered overuse injuries.[6] Clinically, the authors find that the tibialis posterior tendon is the most commonly injured structure in patients complaining of shin splint symptoms.

The tibialis posterior muscle provides arch support to the foot. Abnormalities such as a forefoot varus, which lead to compensatory STJ pronation, increase the stress placed on the muscle. It contracts eccentrically in an effort to slow the compensatory pronation, thereby placing its tendon under additional stress.[14]

### Diagnosis

With irritation of the tibialis posterior tendon, the patient reports discomfort along the medial border of the tibia, and palpation reveals point tenderness along the middle and distal thirds of the tibia.[15] Manual muscle testing by resisting plantarflexion and inversion may elicit a report of pain or weakness. The evaluation should also include looking for possible hyperpronation.

Symptoms occurring in the leg are typically related to overuse (i.e., performing too much, too soon, too fast). Other etiologic factors include a change in running terrain, poor flexibility, and biomechanical abnormalities.

### Treatment

A management program for tibialis posterior tendonitis should focus on controlling inflammation, improving flexibility of the heelcord and first MTP joint, strength training, and reducing excessive pronatatory forces. Strengthening exercises, such as toe raises with tubing resistance and towel gathering exercises, strengthen the plantarflexors and inverters of the foot. Foot abnormalities and training errors should be addressed if they are a problem.

### Stress Fractures

Stress fractures of the foot or lower leg are frequently seen as a result of training errors or improper lower extremity biomechanics. The training errors include improper footwear, running surface, and ballistic training techniques. An excessively rapid progression of training intensity or duration may lead to stress fractures as well. In addition, excessive pronation is a biomechanical factor which can lead to increased torsion stress on the tibia.

*Diagnosis*

Diagnosis is made through palpation, plain radiographic studies, or bone scans. Palpation may reveal local tenderness. Percussion of the bone, even at sites distant from the stress fracture, may cause pain to be felt at the fracture site. Plain x-ray studies may not detect the stress fracture in its early stages. A bone scan makes the definitive diagnosis.

*Treatment*

Stress fractures are managed with a period of prolonged rest to allow adequate healing of the defect to occur. If activity is resumed too early, the fracture will recur.

### Anterior Compartment Syndrome

Acute injury to the anterior compartment of the leg is caused by direct trauma and may be a medical emergency. Such injury causes bleeding and swelling to occur within the compartment. Because the compartment borders are relatively unyielding, this causes an increase in intracompartmental pressure. This pressure may increase to a point where the anterior tibial artery and deep peroneal nerve are compromised. If not treated, permanent nerve damage and muscle necrosis may ensure. Some patients develop chronic compartment syndrome; they have symptoms mainly during exercise when increased blood flow to the muscles increases intracompartmental pressure.

*Diagnosis*

Upon inspection of an acute compartment syndrome the skin appears taut and shiny from distention. Ecchymosis may or may not be present. Palpation reveals that the anterior compartment is harder and warmer than the uninvolved side. Sensation may be diminished at the web space of the first and second toes. The dorasalis pedis pulse may be absent. The patient has difficulty with the function of the muscles in the anterior compartment (toe extension, inversion, and dorsiflexion), possibly presenting with a "dropfoot" posture. In addition, range of motion may be limited due to pain. The definitive test for this condition is a compartmental pressure examination.

*Treatment*

Treatment of severe acute compartment syndrome is by surgical release. In the chronic condition treatment may range from avoiding exacerbating exercise to surgical release of the fascia.

### Metatarsalgia

Metatarsalgia is a catch-all term for foot pain in the proximity of the metatarsal heads. It is most commonly caused by abnormal foot biomechanics and repetitive forces which cause increased stress to the transverse metatarsal arch. It is more common in the pes cavus foot.

*Diagnosis*

Palpation reveals point tenderness over the metatarsal heads, most commonly the second and third. Compression of the metatarsal heads elicits pain. Differential diagnoses include a metatarsal stress fracture or a neuroma.

*Treatment*

This condition is treated with correction of abnormal biomechanics. Metatarsal arch pads, orthotics, change in training techniques, strengthening and flexibility exercises, and local ice application are helpful. The metatarsal pads or "bar" can be inserted in the patient's shoes just proximal to the metatarsal heads to relieve some of the weight from the painful area. If needed, such a support can be built into a custom-made shoe as well.

### Morton's Neuroma

This is a swelling of the distal nerves of the foot, usually between the third and fourth metatarsals, and may be caused by narrow shoes.

*Diagnosis*

The patient may complain of a shooting pain in the forefoot which worsens with activity. Forefoot compression or palpation between the metatarsals elicits pain if a neuroma is present.

*Treatment*

Treatment consists of NSAIDs, modalities to control pain and inflammation, and flexibility exercises. Steroid-anesthetic injection around the neuroma may help relieve the inflammation. Adequate shoe fitting should be stressed.

### Hallux Valgus

Hallux valgus is a progressive deformity of the great toe. It may cause a bunion to form along the medial surface of the first metatarsal head.

*Diagnosis*

Hallux valgus is considered abnormal if the first metatarsal–hallux angle is greater than 15 degrees. Observation reveals apparent abduction of the hallux.

*Treatment*

Several etiologic factors may lead to hallux valgus, so the treatment program should focus on the cause of the deformity. In most cases, abnormal biomechanics are the contributing factor. Therefore, a treatment program which addresses any flexibility, strength, or biomechanical deficits is helpful. Wide shoes with orthotic supports, local ice application, NSAIDs, and taping also decrease symptoms. In many cases surgical correction of the deformity is required.

### Hallux Rigidus

Hallux rigidus, as its name implies, involves a loss of range of motion of the first MTP joint. It is caused by trauma, varus or valgus stress, and degenerative joint disease. There are often bony spurs adjacent to the joint. The result is pain and restricted first MTP motion. It is more common in persons, such as dancers, who stress their toes.

*Diagnosis*

Pain and limited motion of the first MTP joint should prompt an x-ray evaluation to assess osteoarthritic changes. Roentgenographic studies may reveal the formation of osteophytes on the dorsal aspect of the first metatarsal head and at the base of the proximal phalanx.[16] There is a decrease in range of motion, especially of extension, at the joint.

*Treatment*

Conservative management includes NSAIDs, ice, taping, and shoe protection to decrease symptoms acutely. Later mobilization of the joint may be helpful. In addition, orthoses with a first metatarsal extension may help to decrease the stress on the joint. In some cases joint injection with steroid-anesthetic solution is required to decrease the inflammation. Surgical fusion is rarely necessary.

### Turf Toe

Turf toe is an injury of the first MTP joint typically caused by acute or chronic forced extension of the joint. This condition involves joint capsule irritation with secondary trauma to the musculotendinous structures. Differential diagnoses include a flexion sprain of the first MTP joint and sesamoiditis.

*Diagnosis*

Evaluation reveals point tenderness and limited MTP motion due to pain and joint swelling. Gait analysis reveals an inability to perform the push-off motion efficiently during gait.

*Treatment*

Treatment consists of controlling the pain and swelling. In addition, there are three methods the authors have found successful in allowing patients to continue pain-free ambulation throughout the healing process. The first is a taping of the joint to decrease the motion at the MTP joint and provide stability during the propulsive period of gait. The second is to have the patient wear stiff-soled shoes. In athletics, a thin piece of steel is cut and inserted under the entire sole of the shoe to stiffen the shoe and limit the motion at the first MTP joint. The other method successfully used is an orthotic device that has a first ray (first metatarsal) cutout. This modification allows the first ray to plantarflex further than normal so that the first MTP joint does not extend as far during push-off. These methods may be used individually or in combination to allow pain-free functional activities while the soft tissue is healing.

### Sesamoiditis

Located on the inferior aspect of the first MTP joint, the sesamoid bones are located within the flexor hallucis brevis tendon. Sesamoiditis is an inflammation of the tissues which surround the sesamoid bones.

#### Diagnosis

The patient reports discomfort during gait, especially with propulsion. Palpation reveals point tenderness over the sesamoid bones. Passive great toe extension coupled with palpation over the plantar aspect of the MTP joint elicits pain. In some cases the sesamoids may fracture and x-ray study or bone scan (for stress fractures) may help to make this diagnosis.

#### Treatment

The treatment may include metatarsal pads or a metatarsal bar placed proximal to the metatarsal heads to relieve pressure on the sesamoids. An orthotic insert with metatarsal extension relieves the stress on the bones. Flexibility exercises for the first MTP joint and heelcord, as well as NSAIDs and modalities to control pain and inflammation promote tissue healing.

### Pes Planus

Pes planus is often referred to as a pronated foot or flatfoot. The cause may be congenital or due to muscle weakness, ligamentous laxity, trauma, paralysis, or postural deformity.

#### Diagnosis

Examination may reveal that the pes planus foot is either rigid or flexible. Depending on the severity of the deformity, there may be an associated calcaneus valgus or foot varus deformity.[3]

#### Treatment

Strengthening exercises for the intrinsic muscles of the foot, as well as flexibility exercises for the calf musculature, are indicated. The patient with a pes planus deformity may benefit from a semirigid orthotic device to provide arch support and calcaneal control. Patients with a flexible flatfoot are more likely to benefit from an arch support. A rigid pes planus cannot be corrected by an orthosis.

### Pes Cavus

The cavus foot may also be either rigid (maintaining a high arch on weight bearing) or flexible (arch height decreases on weight bearing). This foot type may predispose the individual to problems caused by a lack of shock absorption (i.e., stress fractures).

#### Diagnosis

Depending on the severity of the deformity, biomechanical analysis may reveal clawing of the toes, a rearfoot varus, and/or a forefoot valgus deformity.

#### Treatment

Patients with pes cavus should tolerate a rigid orthotic device with a forefoot valgus post. In addition they should be placed on a thorough flexibility program of the lower extremity.

### Tarsal Tunnel Syndrome

The lower extremity counterpart of carpal tunnel syndrome, tarsal tunnel syndrome is an entrapment neuropathy of the posterior tibial nerve as it passes beneath the lacinate ligament behind the medial malleolus. It is extremely rare, and most cases are caused by posttraumatic deformity. Diagnosis is made electromyographically.

### Other Disorders

Other conditions that cause foot, ankle, and lower extremity dysfunction and pain are plantar warts, calluses, an ingrown toenail, hammer toe/claw toe deformity, reflex sympathetic dystrophy, posterior compartment syndrome, subluxating peroneal tendons, tendonitis of virtually any tendon, rupture of the proximal gastrocnemius muscle, and tibialis posterior tendon rupture, among many others.

## Case Report

A 40-year-old runner complained of left Achilles tendon pain which started after he stepped in a hole during a race. He was able to complete the race. He had been treating himself for several weeks with calf stretching, ice, and bilateral heel lifts. On examination he had a swollen tender Achilles tendon, decreased great toe extension, and excessive pronation bilaterally. His examination was otherwise normal. He was diagnosed as having Achilles tendonitis which was triggered by an acute strain. He was instructed in further heelcord stretching, ice application, and was given an in-shoe orthosis with a first ray cutout to provide additional great toe mobility. He was told to continue to use a quarter-inch heel lift with the orthosis for running activities only. The orthosis alone was used otherwise.

Several weeks later he reported that his symptoms were much improved but still present. He was started on a program of preexercise moist heat application and passive great toe extension stretching. One month later he was symptom free.

This case demonstrates the importance of the kinetic linkage system, in which the Achilles tendon is viewed as a part of the continuum of connective tissue from the great toe to the calf muscles. The whole system must be evaluated and treated to be successful.

## Points of Summary

1. Ankle inversion sprains are more common when the foot is plantarflexed. This is due to the loosening of the talar "wedge" in the ankle mortise.
2. Inversion sprains are by far the most common ankle sprains.
3. Proprioception is impaired after ankle sprain. Proper treatment should include proprioceptive exercise.
4. Anterior drawer testing isolates the ATF ligament.
5. Great toe abnormalities are often treated with in-shoe orthoses with first metatarsal extensions to provide support.
6. Plantar fasciitis usually responds to local ice, stretching of the fascia and gastroc-soleus complex, and an orthotic device.
7. Acute anterior compartment syndrome is a medical emergency. It is diagnosed with intra-compartmental pressure measurement and is treated with surgical decompression.
8. Thompson's test detects a ruptured Achilles tendon.
9. Stress fractures are detected early with a bone scan.
10. A complete examination should focus on the joints above and below the area of injury.

## References

1. Root ML, Orien WP, Weed JH: *Normal and Abnormal Function of the Foot*, vol 2. Los Angeles: Clinical Biomechanics, 1977:5–59.
2. McPoil TG, Brocato RS: The foot and ankle: Biomechanical evaluation and tretment. In Gould JA, Davies GJ (eds): *Orthopaedic and Sports Physical Therapy*. St. Louis: CV Mosby, 1985:317.
3. Subotnick SI: *Podiatric Sports Medicine*. Mt. Kisco, NY: Futura Publishing, 1975:37, 42, 60.
4. Franco AH: Pes cavus and pes planus: Analyses and treatment. *Phys Ther* 1987;67:688–694.
5. Buschbacher R: Ankle bracing. *Physical Medicine and Rehabilitation: State of the Art Reviews* (in press).
6. Frank CB, Hart DA: Cellular response to loading. In Leadbetter WB, Buckwalter JA, Gordon SL (eds): *Sports-Induced Inflammation*. Park Ridge, IL: American Academy Orthopaedic Surgeons, 1990:560–562.

7. Freeman MAR, Dean MRE, Hanham IWF: The etiology and prevention of functional instability of the foot. *J Bone and Joint Surgery* 1965;47B:678–685.

8. Magee DJ: *Orthopedic Physical Assessment*, 2nd ed. Philadelphia: WB Saunders, 1992:468–472.

9. Hoppenfeld S: *Physical Examination of the Spine and Extremities*. Norwalk, CT: Appleton-Century-Crofts, 1976:223–226.

10. Clement DB, Taunton JE, Smart GW: Achilles tendinitis and peritendinitis: Etiology and treatment. *Am J Sports Med* 1984;12:179–184.

11. Curwin S: Eccentric exercise for chronic tendinitis. In D'Ambrosia RD, Drez D (eds): *Prevention and Treatment of Running Injuries*, 2nd ed. Thorofare, NJ: Slack, 1989:240–241.

12. Roy S: How I manage plantar fasciitis. *Phys Sports Med* 1983;11:127–131.

13. Jenkins W: Pathomechanical considerations in the treatment of inflammatory conditions of the lower leg. Presented at the *National Athletic Trainers Association Annual Meeting and Clinical Symposium* June 5, 1992, Denver, CO.

14. Delacerda FG: A study of anatomical factors involved in shinsplints. *J Orthop Sports Phys Ther* 1980;2:55–59.

15. Scheuch PA: Tibialis posterior shin splint: Diagnosis and treatment. *Athletic Training* 1984;19:271–274.

16. Donatelli R: *The Biomechanics of the Foot and Ankle*. Philadelphia: FA Davis, 1990:258–259.

## Suggested Readings

D'Ambrosia RD, Drez D: *Prevention and Treatment of Running Injuries*, 2nd ed. Thorofare, NJ: Slack, 1989.

Leadbetter WB, Buckwalter JA, Gordon SL (eds): *Sports-Induced Inflammation*. Park Ridge, IL: American Academy of Orthopaedic Surgeons. 1990.

Subotnick SI: A biomechanical approach to running injuries. *Ann NY Acad Sci* 1977;301:888–889.

Vogelbach WB, Combs LC: A biomechanical approach to the management of chronic lower extremity pathologies as they relate to excessive pronation. *Athletic Training* 1987;22:6–18.

# PART THREE
## Special Issues

# Chapter 20

# Fibromyalgia and Myofascial Pain Syndrome

LESLIE SCHUTZ

Musculoskeletal pain, stiffness, achiness, fatigue, and disturbed sleep are common complaints that have been documented for centuries in medical and literary circles. Nearly as numerous as the variety of complaints are the terms used to describe the syndromes with which they are associated. Nonarticular rheumatism, tension rheumatism, myalgia, lumbago, myositis, myofasciitis, fibromyositis, and fibrositis are just a few of these terms. Today we recognize two distinct clinical entities of muscular pain. They are fibromyalgia (FM) and myofascial pain syndrome (MPS) (Table 20-1).

## Fibromyalgia

This nonarticular rheumatic disorder is characterized by chronic, diffuse musculoskeletal pain, aching, stiffness, fatigue, and disturbed sleep. It is also associated with exaggerated tenderness at specific reproducible locations. These are known as tender points (Figure 20-1). Symptoms of FM are typically aggravated by cold, humid weather, tension, fatigue, inactivity, and overactivity and are decreased by heat, moderate physical activity, stretching, massage, and restful sleep. This entity is reportedly five to ten times more common in females than in males, and it can cause painful menstruation. It may also be associated with irritable bowel syndrome.[1]

Laboratory, x-ray, and electromyographic studies are normal in FM, and other conditions that cause similar symptoms such as hypothyroidism and connective tissue diseases must be ruled out before the diagnosis can be made. Muscle biopsies have been reported to be abnormal in some studies, but there is no conclusive evidence of abnormalities strictly characteristic of the disease. The criteria for diagnosing the condition, as developed by the American College of Rheumatology,[2] are listed in Table 20-2.

### Etiology

FM may be associated with a primary or secondary sleep disturbance. It has been demonstrated that patients with FM have a lack of stage IV non-REM sleep.[3] This stage of sleep plays a role in restorative functions.

FM may also be related to psychological and personality characteristics. There is research support for such a relationship;[4,5] however, it is not a factor in all cases,[6] and the strength of the relationship varies widely among individual patients. Patients with FM appear to have a generalized amplification of pain sensitivity.[7]

FM does not appear to be caused by muscle spasm. In fact, painful muscles in FM patients may be electrically silent.

**Table 20-1.** Similarities and Differences Between Primary Fibromyalgia Syndrome (PFS) and Myofascial Pain Syndrome (MPS) Due to Trigger Points

| PFS | MPS |
|---|---|
| **Similarities** | |
| Muscle pain present | Muscle pain present |
| Muscle tenderness on palpation | Muscle tenderness on palpation |
| Very common | Very common |
| **Differences** | |
| *Symptoms* | |
| Diffuse pain involving many muscles, ligaments, and bones | Referred pain pattern specific to each muscle; pain is usually local or regional |
| Pain is chronic. | Pain may be acute or chronic. |
| Trauma may perpetuate local symptoms, but is not a cause. | Physical stress to muscle, including obvious trauma, is the cause. |
| Nonmusculoskeletal symptoms, e.g., fatigue, poor sleep, chronic headaches, are common. | Nonmusculoskeletal symptoms are unusual. |
| *Signs* | |
| Tender points (TPs)* are present in muscles and other tissues, including tendon insertions and bones; radiation of pain, twitch response, and surrounding taut band in a TP are unusual, but have not been well studied. TPs are usually more than 4 among the 14 specified sites. | Myofascial trigger point(s) are limited to muscle(s) with radiation of pain to a referred zone, twitch response, and accompanying taut band. Number of trigger points may be 1 or more. |
| Skin roll tenderness and cutaneous hyperemia are frequent. | Skin signs are not common. |
| *Laboratory Tests* | |
| Usual laboratory tests are normal; nonspecific pathologic changes are seen by muscle biopsy. | Laboratory tests are usually normal, but not contributory to diagnosis; differences in muscle pathology not clear at this time. |
| *Theory and Concept* | |
| Pathogenesis not well understood; disturbed sleep is a factor in most cases; psychologic factors important in about 25% of patients. | Pathogenesis is acute or chronic muscle stress. Poor sleep may result from pain; psychological status usually not a factor. |

*American College of Rheumatology criteria describe pain in 11 of 18 tender points.
(Yunus MB, et al.: Primary fibromyalgia syndrome and myofascial pain syndrome: Clinical features and muscle pathology. *Arch Phys Med Rehabil* 69:451–454. Reprinted with permission.)

### *Treatment*

The foundation for a treatment plan in FM is patient education. This includes a realistic discussion of diagnosis and prognosis. Patients should be aware that FM is a common syndrome and that although there are no specific laboratory findings to suggest the disease, a diagnosis can be made with a high degree of reliability. Patients should also be made aware that FM is neither life threatening nor degenerative, nor will it cause structural deformities.

An aerobic exercise program of moderate intensity which gradually improves cardiovascular fitness, flexibility, muscle tone, and posture has been shown to significantly decrease pain symptoms in FM patients.[8] The exercise should be instituted gradually and should not be overly vigorous. Too much exercise can worsen the symptoms.

Because stress and a resultant lack of sleep have been shown to aggravate FM, attention to obvious stress factors should be undertaken. Relaxation training, possibly through biofeedback, is also useful. Patients should be encouraged to plan activities, alternate work with rest periods, and find avocational activities that ease tension. Attention to proper posture at work, during home activities, and while sleeping is also important.

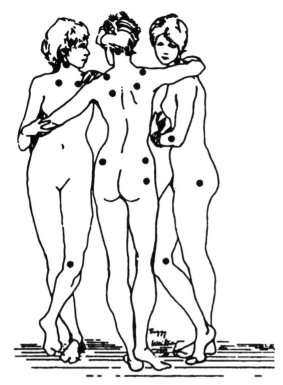

**Figure 20-1.** Tender point locations for the 1990 classification criteria for fibromyalgia (The Three Graces, after Baron Jean-Baptiste Regnault, 1793, Louvre Museum, Paris). See Table 20-2 for details of the tender point site locations. (Wolfe F, et al.: The American College of Rheumatology 1990 criteria for the classification of fibromyalgia. *Arthritis Rheum* 1990;33:160–172. Reproduced with permission.)

Physical modalities such as massage, ice, acupuncture, ultrasound, and transcutaneous electrical nerve stimulation (TENS) may be beneficial in individual patients, but the results are usually temporary.

Medications that have been found to benefit patients with FM in placebo controlled studies include amitriptyline (Elavil) and cyclobenzaprine (Flexeril).[9,10] When taken before bedtime in low doses they increase the time spent in stage IV restorative sleep. Analgesics and nonsteroidal anti-inflammatory drugs (NSAIDs) have limited benefit in the treatment of FM, and narcotics should be avoided as in most chronic pain states. Additionally, patients should avoid ingesting excessive caffeine, as this has been shown to aggravate FM.

## Myofascial Pain Syndrome

Myofascial pain syndrome (MPS) is a syndrome of regional complaints often accompanied by trigger points and uncommonly by autonomic symptoms. The regional complaints are of an aching, sore, and stiff muscle or group of muscles. The patient sometimes reports that pain, numbness, or tingling radiates distally or to the head. Similarly, autonomic symptoms such as vasoconstriction, sweating, pilomotor response (gooseflesh), or a feeling of coldness may be noted. These complaints are rare, however.

MPS is extremely common, and an element of the syndrome is found accompanying a wide variety of other problems ranging from cervical strain to postoperative pain.

All patients with MPS have regional pain. It is usually present as an acute or subacute problem, although it can become chronic. Both sexes are affected equally, and it is not associated with sleep disturbance (except sometimes due to trouble finding a comfortable position), generalized fatigue, or other disease.

Trigger points are a subject of controversy in MPS. Some argue that the condition can only be diagnosed if such points are present. Others deny that they exist. The truth probably lies somewhere between these extremes. When present, trigger points refer symptoms in a pattern characteristic to the muscle in which they are located. The spontaneous pain that the patient is complaining of does not always occur at this same spot. Many patients with MPS have such trigger points, and palpating them causes a referred pain pattern that is highly suggestive of this syndrome. Other patients have only local tenderness at these spots (similar to FM), and a minority have no tender areas at all. Only rarely does palpation of a trigger point cause autonomic symptoms.

Trigger points in the neck and shoulder often refer pain to the head and are causes of headache. They also refer pain into the arm, and may mimic the symptoms of radiculopathy. They can be differentiated from radiculopathy because pressing on the muscle rather than compressing the nerve, such as with a Spurling maneuver (see Chapter 12), reproduces the distal symptoms. Back and pelvic trigger points may refer symptoms to the legs.

**Table 20-2.** The American College of Rheumatology 1990 Criteria for the Classification of Fibromyalgia*

---

1. History of widespread pain

   *Definition*—Pain is considered widespread when all of the following are present: pain in the left side of the body, pain in the right side of the body, pain above the waist, and pain below the waist. In addition, axial skeletal pain (cervical spine or anterior chest or thoracic spine or low back) must be present. In this definition, shoulder and buttock pain is considered as pain for each involved side. "Low back" pain is considered lower segment pain.

2. Pain in 11 of 18 tender point sites on digital palpation

   *Definition*—Pain, on digital palpation, must be present in at least 11 of the following 18 tender point sites:
   *Occiput:* bilateral, at the suboccipital muscle insertions.
   *Low cervical:* bilateral, at the anterior aspects of the intertransverse spaces at C5–C7.
   *Trapezius:* bilateral, at the midpoint of the upper border.
   *Supraspinatus:* bilateral, at origins, above the scapula spine near the medial border.
   *Second rib:* bilateral, at the second costochondral junctions, just lateral to the junctions on upper surfaces.
   *Lateral epicondyle:* bilateral, 2 cm distal to the epicondyles.
   *Gluteal:* bilateral, in upper outer quadrants of buttocks in anterior fold of muscle.
   *Greater trochanter:* bilateral, posterior to the trochanteric prominence.
   *Knee:* bilateral, at the medial fat pad proximal to the joint line.

   Digital palpation should be performed with an approximate force of 4 kg.
   For a tender point to be considered "positive" the subject must state that the palpation was painful. "Tender" is not to be considered "painful."

---

*For classification purposes, patients will be said to have fibromyalgia if both criteria are satisfied. Widespread pain must have been present for at least 3 months. The presence of a second clinical disorder does not exclude the diagnosis of fibromyalgia.
(Wolfe F, et al.: The American College of Rheumatology 1990 criteria for the classification of fibromyalgia. *Arthritis Rheum* 1990;33:160–172. Reprinted with permission.)

As in FM, laboratory, electromyographic, and x-ray studies are normal in MPS (except, of course, when other concomitant conditions aggravate or cause MPS).

### Etiology

MPS may be caused by overwork fatigue of a muscle or by trauma or overstretching of the muscle. It is often caused by the initiation of a new activity or exercise. It can be caused by structural factors such as leg length discrepancy, poor posture, or after injury or surgery when body kinematics have changed. Underlying diseases that cause muscle splinting, such as herniated disk, may also aggravate MPS. In addition, increased muscle tension from anxiety, nutritional problems, chronic infections or allergies, and arthritis may worsen symptoms.

The phenomenon of the trigger point is controversial, and there is no accepted pathologic entity that describes it. It is often said to be an irritable locus within a taut band of skeletal muscle or fascia. It is often described as causing a "jump sign"—pain on palpation that causes the patient to give a

jump and cry out.[11] It is sometimes said to manifest a local twitch response, an involuntary contraction of the palpated fibers. Whether these signs are indeed pathognomonic of the syndrome is not known. What is clear is that palpation of a true trigger point causes symptoms to be referred.

### Treatment

As in FM, patient education plays a vital role in the treatment of MPS. Each patient must take responsibility for complying with the treatment regimen. Structural and postural modifications must be made, if needed, to avoid muscle overwork. Any underlying medical problems such as herniated disk or connective tissue disease must also be addressed.

A reconditioning program, beginning with stretching, aerobic exercise, and then progressive resistance exercises aimed at the affected muscles should be instituted. This reinforces an active role for the patient in treating the condition.

The spray and stretch technique (see Chapter 6) for treating MPS was first introduced in the

1940s.[12] A vapocoolant spray such as fluorimethane is directed over the trigger points parallel to the course of the muscle fibers to cool the muscle. This is followed by stretching. Hot packs are also useful to facilitate relaxation and stretching.

Ischemic compression is a technique of applying a local pressure to the trigger point.[13] This causes an initial ischemia and subsequent reactive hyperemia and can be taught to patients to treat trigger-point symptoms at home. The beneficial mechanisms of the procedure are unknown; it may be that local or reactive hyperemia relaxes the tight muscle and reduces symptoms. In any case, the compression can be applied multiple times daily. It can be performed by hand, by leaning against or lying on a tennis ball, by leaning against door frames, or with special canelike devices to reach the back. It should involve firm, even pressure. Rubbing or massage should be avoided, as they may actually worsen the pain.

Injections of trigger points are advocated in treating MPS. It is unclear what their mechanism of action is in reducing pain, but they certainly cause a remarkable reduction in symptoms in many patients. Some argue that insertion of the needle into the trigger point is as effective as injecting medication. Others advocate injection of sterile saline alone. Most physicians who inject these points use either a local anesthetic or anesthetic-steroid combination. Successful injection usually reproduces the patient's symptoms as it is taking place. It can be followed by ice application or ultrasound treatment. Injections may reduce symptoms enough to allow the patient to more easily perform a stretching and exercise routine.

### Differential Diagnosis

The differential diagnosis for FM and MPS is similar and extensive. It includes rheumatic and non-rheumatic conditions such as rheumatoid arthritis, polymyalgia rheumatica, psychogenic rheumatism, bursitis, tendonitis, metabolic disease, malignancy, hypothyroidism, and viral infection to name only a few. As a rule, these other conditions can be excluded fairly readily by physical examination and laboratory, x-ray, and electrodiagnostic studies.

## Points of Summary

1. Fibromyalgia is a syndrome of generalized pain complaints accompanied by sleep disturbance and fatigue and is more common in women.
2. Myofascial pain syndrome involves local or regional pain complaints and shows no preference for either sex.
3. Fibromyalgia is associated with tender points; myofascial pain syndrome is associated with trigger points (and sometimes with tender points).
4. Fibromyalgia tends to become chronic; myofascial pain usually resolves.
5. Fibromyalgia is treated with moderate aerobic exercise and medication to help normalize the sleep cycle.
6. Myofascial pain is treated with physical modalities, stretching, injections, and strengthening.

## References

1. Yunus M, Masi AT, Calabro JJ, et al.: Primary fibromyalgia (fibrositis): Clinical study of 50 patients with matched normal controls. *Semin Arthritis Rheum* 1981;11:151–171.
2. Wolfe F, Smythe HA, Yunus MG, et al.: The American College of Rheumatology 1990 criteria for classification of fibromyalgia: Report of the Multicenter Criteria Committee. *Arthritis Rheum* 1990;33:160–172.
3. Yunus MB: Primary fibromyalgia syndrome: Current concepts. *Comp Ther* 1984;10:21–28.
4. Wolfe F, Cathey MA, Kleinheksel SM: Psychological status in primary fibrositis and fibrositis associated with rheumatoid arthritis. *J Rheumatol* 1984;11:500–506.
5. Buckelew SP: Fibromyalgia: A rehabilitation approach—a review. *Am J Phys Med Rehabil* 1989;68:37–41.
6. Ahles TA, Yunus MB, Gaulier B, et al.: The use of contemporary MMPI norms in the study of chronic pain patients. *Pain* 1986;24:159–163.
7. Mikkelsson M, Latikka P, Kautiainen H, et al.: Muscle and bone pain threshold and pain tolerance in fibromyalgia patients and controls. *Arch Phys Med Rehabil* 1992;73:814–818.
8. McCain GA: Role of physical fitness training in the fibrositis/fibromyalgia syndrome. *Am J Med* 1986;81(Suppl 3A):73–77.
9. Campbell SM, Galter RA, Clark S, et al.: A double blind study of cyclobenzaprine versus placebo in patients with fibrositis. *Arthritis Rheum* (Suppl) 1984;27:576.
10. Goldenberg DL, Felson DT, Direrman H: A randomized, controlled trial of amitriptyline and naproxen in

the treatment of patients with fibromyalgia. *Arthritis Rheum* 1986;29:1371–1377.

11. Kraft GH, Johnson EW, LaBan MM: The fibrositis syndrome. *Arch Phys Med Rehabil* 1968;49:155–162.

12. Kraus H: The use of surface anesthesia in the treatment of painful motion. *JAMA* 1941;116:2582–2583.

13. Goldman LB, Rosenberg NL: Myofascial pain syndrome and fibromyalgia seminars in neurology. *Semin Neurol* 1991;2;274–280.

## Suggested Readings

Travell JG, Simons DG: *Myofascial Pain and Dysfunction: The Trigger Point Manual.* Baltimore: Williams & Wilkins, 1983.

Yunus MB, Kalyan-Raman UP, Kalyan-Raman K: Primary fibromyalgia syndrome and myofascial pain syndrome: Clinical features and muscle pathology. *Arch Phys Med Rehabil* 1988;69:451–454.

# Chapter 21

# Musculoskeletal Disorders in the Pediatric Population

BARBARA KOCH
PHILLIP R. BRYANT

Musculoskeletal disorders in children often differ from those in adults. The child is more susceptible to certain types of injuries than the adult because of the presence of growth cartilage and the process of growth itself. The specifics of these problems are the subject of this chapter; however, only a few of the disorders most common in children are described in detail.

## Pathophysiology of Pediatric Injuries

Pediatric injuries most commonly occur at the growth cartilage of long bones or at the sites of tendon insertion into bone (apophyses). Injuries are usually due to either high impact or repetitive trauma.

In growing bones, the epiphyseal plate is the weak link and succumbs to stress before the ligaments or joint capsule. For instance, with valgus stress at the knee, a child is more likely to sustain an epiphyseal fracture rather than a torn ligament. The adult, on the other hand, is more likely to incur a ligamentous injury. In most epiphyseal injuries the vascular supply to the growing cells is not compromised; however, in crush injuries there may be such damage.

Apophyses are usually injured by overuse conditions. The tendons insert into the apophyses, which act as points of attachment and which are more rigid than the underlying bone.[1] With chronic repetitive stresses there is microtrauma and injury at the tendon/apophyseal transition. As a result of this microtrauma, a phase of inflammation occurs and brings with it increased vascularity which produces warmth, redness, and even the stimulation of growth. The inflammation affects both the apophysis and the tendon.

Bones in children are softer than in adults and are more prone to deformation than to fracture. When they do break it is often as a greenstick fracture in which the cortex fails on one side but stays in continuity on the other side.

## Pediatric Injuries

### Shoulder Girdle

Dislocations and subluxations of the glenohumeral joint are the most common sports injuries of the shoulder. When they occur in children they almost always become a recurrent problem.[2] Active treatment with an aggressive rehabilitation program may reduce the incidence of recurrence.[3]

Most dislocations occur anteriorly, but posterior and inferior dislocations also occur.

Other disorders of the shoulder girdle which may occur in children are rotator cuff tendonitis and acromioclavicular sprain. Rotator cuff tendonitis is seen most commonly in sports such as wrestling, football, and in throwing activities. Acromioclavicular sprains occur with falls on the shoulder and are often associated with football tackles.

### Elbow

The most common elbow injury seen in young children, usually toddlers, is a dislocation of the head of the radius out of the annular ligament, a condition known as "nursemaid's elbow." This occurs when the arm is forcibly pulled, usually when a child is lifted by one arm or when the person holding the child's hand tries to prevent a fall. It is usually easily reduced by flexing and supinating the elbow. Radiographs should be obtained to rule out associated fracture.

In older children the most common elbow disorders are usually related to overuse from throwing, mainly baseball pitching. The acceleration phase of throwing stresses the medial elbow, and the repetitive motion of pitching strains the attachment of the aponeurosis to the bone. The microtraumatic stresses on the ulnar collateral ligament often create pain before, during, and after the activity. Treatment consists of having the pitcher rest the arm, often in a foam splint that keeps the wrist in slight extension and the elbow in 90 degrees of flexion.[4] At the same time, the athlete is given a course of nonsteroidal antiinflammatory drugs (NSAIDs). The coaching staff needs to reevaluate the child's throwing style, as improper technique may be contributing to this condition. Correcting the pitching motion helps to minimize the problem. A reduction in the incidence of elbow injuries in baseball has come about through changes in rules which limit the number of innings a young player can pitch per game.

In addition to the overuse condition described, a quick throw may also cause an avulsion of the medial humeral epicondyle. There is tenderness and swelling at the medial humerus, and the diagnosis can be confirmed by x-ray film. Treatment is generally through open reduction. Fractures may also occur in the transcondylar or supracondylar area. They typically produce swelling and tenderness at the distal humerus. These injuries are of particular concern in pediatrics since they likely occur through the growth plate. The wide epiphyseal plate in this area makes accurate x-ray diagnosis difficult.

### Wrist and Hand

A common wrist injury is a fracture of the scaphoid bone. This usually occurs due to falling on an outstretched hand. The scaphoid lies next to the styloid tip of the radius, and with the fall it abuts the radius. The child complains of pain during palpation of the anatomic snuff box (see Chapter 16) or on attempting to make a fist. Treatment is with casting. X-ray followup is essential to determine the state of healing. Problems may arise because of the poor blood supply to this bone. This can cause secondary complications of nonunion or avascular necrosis. After the cast has been removed, the athlete should be given a protective splint for competition to prevent reinjury.

Finger injuries generally consist of relatively mild sprains caused by improper catching or dribbling of balls. In addition, ligament avulsion may be seen (see Chapter 16).

### Pelvis

A common injury of the pelvis is a bruise of the iliac crest, often referred to as a hip pointer. Since both abdominal muscles and hip flexors insert on the iliac crest, movement of these muscles aggravates the pain of this injury. Treatment consists of rest and ice, and possible injection of local anaesthetic-antiinflammatory medication. When the child returns to athletics, the area involved should be padded. If the child returns to play prior to complete healing of the injury, a posttraumatic periostitis may develop, and the iliac wing will remain tender. In some cases there may be an avulsion injury of the growth cartilage at the iliac crest. If so, surgical treatment is indicated.

### Hip

A slipped capital femoral epiphysis occurs with minimal trauma which causes the femoral head to slip across the epiphyseal growth plate. This injury occurs mainly in children who are large, obese and sexually immature, usually boys between 13 and 16 years and girls from 11 to 14 years. The child often complains of anteromedial knee pain (referred from the hip) and limps. The examination is characterized by limitation of internal rotation, abduction, and flexion of the hip, with the child letting the leg fall into a position of external rotation. Plain radiographs are the diagnostic tool of choice in making the diagnosis. These patients often require surgery to keep the slip from progressing.

### Knee

A very common apophysitis in young athletes is Osgood-Schlatter disease (see Chapter 18). Inflammation at the attachment of the patellar tendon into the tibia leads to overgrowth and enlargement of the tibial tubercle. The patient complains of pain at the tubercle that occurs with activity and that goes away with rest. There is tenderness over the prominent tibial tubercle.

Sinding-Larsen-Johansson syndrome is another overuse syndrome. It is characterized by pain with jumping and running. In this condition the pain and inflammation are present at the inferior pole of the patella. It is commonly found in basketball players with tight hamstrings.[5]

### Foot and Ankle

Sever's disease is an overuse syndrome of the posterior calcaneal apophysis. It results in pain and tenderness at the insertion of the Achilles tendon similar to the knee conditions just described.[5]

### Back

Stress reactions involving the spine are generally manifest as stress fractures of the pars interarticularis of a lumbar vertebra. This is known as spondylolysis and may be aggravated by repetitive exercise, particularly that involving hyperextension of the lumbar spine, as is seen in gymnastics, high diving, wrestling, football, weightlifting, pole vaulting, and hurdling. Plain radiographs may fail to detect the fracture, but a bone scan is typically positive. The main objective in the treatment of spondylolysis is to rest the area for approximately 6 weeks. Full recovery may take up to 2 years.[6] The role of bracing in the treatment of spondylolysis is controversial.

Spondylolisthesis occurs when, in the presence of spondylolysis, there is forward displacement of a superior vertebra on an inferior one. This condition may be controlled by substituting activities which cause no pain for those that do. However, in the presence of persistent pain, surgical correction may be necessary.[7]

### Scoliosis

Scoliosis, a lateral curvature of the spine, is often an incidental finding when examining children. It is more common in girls. If it is mild and the child is essentially finished with growth, the curvature is not usually of concern. If it occurs in younger children, before the growth spurt, it should be followed closely with x-ray studies every 3 to 6 months. A marked scoliosis, or one that is progressing, may need to be treated with bracing or surgery.

## Medications

Aspirin is generally contraindicated in the pediatric age range because of its relation to Reye's syndrome. Therefore children should be given acetaminophen for pain and other nonsteroidal medication for antiinflammatory effects. Not all of the nonsteroidal medications used in adults are approved for use in children under 14 years of age; tolmetin, naproxen, and ibuprofen are.[8]

## Protective Equipment

Each sport has different areas in which the body needs protection. The reader is referred to other sources for more specific information about protective equipment.[9] However, one important pediatric issue in the use of protective equipment is that it should fit properly. Unfortunately most protective equipment is costly, so teams keep a supply of equipment which is passed on from year to year. This means that the equipment often does not fit properly and therefore does not protect properly.

The eye is a vulnerable organ in many sports and loss of vision is an unacceptable risk; therefore, eye protection is extremely important. The athlete should wear goggles or a helmet especially designed to protect the eyes.

Cervical spine injuries may result in quadriplegia or even death. Since such injuries occur more frequently when the neck is in the flexed position, maintaining normal cervical lordosis through proper equipment and technique is mandatory. Data on sports injury of the head and neck is kept in a national registry, so that serious injuries can be analyzed and rule changes made as needed.

## Anabolic Steroid Use

Anabolic steroid use has been known for three decades to improve athletic prowess in events that require great strength and size. Anabolic steroids, which are derivatives of testosterone, increase muscle mass and create a state of euphoria with increased aggressiveness and lessened fatigue. Given these effects, the adolescent competing in sports is tempted to use anabolic steroids for their physical and psychological effects. School-age athletes and even nonathletes often abuse these drugs. Adverse effects of the drugs include accelerated maturation with changes in physical and secondary sexual characteristics. There is also an increase in low-density lipoprotein cholesterol (which places the child at increased risk of cardiovascular disease) and testicular atrophy. There are also problems of impaired hepatic function, increased incidence of Wilms' tumor, premature epiphyseal closure, worsened acne, and transmission of acquired immunodeficiency syndrome (AIDS) due to sharing of needles for steroid administration. Psychologically the athlete may experience mood swings, aggressive behavior, and irritability.

Peer pressure during adolescence may encourage the use of steroids despite evidence of their deleterious effects. Coaches, counselors, school officials, and medical personnel need to be vigilant for the use of anabolic steroids and strongly discourage this practice.

## Points of Summary

1. Traumatic pediatric injuries occur most commonly at the epiphyseal plate.
2. Overuse syndromes in children commonly affect the apophyses.
3. Bones in children may break as greenstick rather than complete fractures.
4. Aggressive rehabilitation of shoulder dislocations may reduce the incidence of recurrent dislocation.
5. The most common adolescent apophysitis is Osgood-Schlatter disease; others include Sinding-Larsen-Johansson syndrome and Sever's disease.
6. Tolmetin, naproxen, and ibuprofen are approved for use in children.
7. Protective equipment must fit properly to be effective.
8. There is no place for anabolic steroid use in athletics, especially for children.

## References

1. Woo S, Maynard J, Butler D, et al.: Ligament, tendon, and joint capsule insertions to bone. In Woo SL-Y, Buckwalter JA (eds): *Injury and Repair of the Musculoskeletal Soft Tissues.* Park Ridge, IL: American Academy of Orthopedic Surgeons, 1988:133–166.
2. Rowe CR, Sakellarides HT: Factors related to recurrences of anterior dislocations of the shoulder. *Clin Orthop* 1961;20:40–47.
3. Aronen JG, Regan K: Decreasing the incidence of recurrence of first time anterior shoulder dislocations with rehabilitation. *Am J Sports Med* 1984;12:283–291.
4. O'Donoghue D: *Treatment of Injuries to Athletes.* Philadelphia: WB Saunders, 1984:225.
5. Andrish JT: Overuse syndromes of the back and legs in adolescents. *Adolescent Medicine: State of the Art Reviews* 1991;2(1):223–230.
6. Micheli LJ: *Pediatric and Adolescent Sports Medicine.* Boston: Little, Brown & Co, 1984:115–117.
7. O'Donoghue D: *Treatment of Injuries to Athletes.* Philadelphia: WB Saunders, 1984:402–403.
8. Koch BM: Rehabilitation of the child with joint disease. In Molnar GE (ed): *Pediatric Rehabilitation*, 2nd ed. Baltimore: Williams & Wilkins, 1992:293–333.

9. Sanders B: *Sports Physical Therapy*. Norwalk, CT: Appleton & Lange, 1990:289–306.

## Suggested Readings

*Adolescent Medicine: State of the Art Reviews*. 1991;2(1):213–244.

Johnson MD: Steroids. *Adolescent Medicine: State of the Art Reviews*. 1991;2(1):79–90.

Lovell WW, Winger RB (eds): *Pediatric Orthopedics*, Philadelphia: JB Lippincott, 1990.

Micheli LJ: *Pediatric and Adolescent Sports Medicine*. Boston, MA: Little, Brown & Co, 1984.

# Chapter 22
# Geriatrics

RALPH BUSCHBACHER
LOIS BUSCHBACHER

Musculoskeletal disorders in older patients is a subject about which much is written but very little said. Even after tackling volumes of material concerning so-called musculoskeletal and sports medicine in the elderly, readers are often left as confused and frustrated as when they started their endeavor. In truth, it must be acknowledged that there are very few musculoskeletal disorders which are uniquely endemic to the older population. Older patients do have more osteoarthritis, joint replacements, and chronic rotator cuff tears than younger individuals, but these conditions are hardly unheard of in the young. This chapter attempts to shed some light on a few special issues that may arise more often in the elderly. For a more comprehensive explanation of specific disorders, the reader is referred to the appropriate chapters elsewhere in this text.

## Aging, Disuse, and Their Effects on the Body

### The Muscular System

It is nearly impossible to differentiate the effects of aging and of disuse on the human body, as the two are usually intertwined. As people get older they are usually less active. Less activity leads to weakening and disuse atrophy, which makes it even harder to maintain and resume activity. In addition, medical illness, which is more prevalent in the elderly, tends to inhibit regular activity. So what exactly does happen to the body during aging?

First, muscle mass declines. This decline preferentially affects type II muscle fibers.[1,2] The decline in mass is mainly due to atrophy,[3] although loss of fibers also seems to occur.[2] As muscle mass declines, basal metabolic rate and the rate of maximal oxygen consumption are reduced.[4,5] Muscles fatigue more readily and speed of contraction is slowed. The body proportions change, with a decrease in lean muscle mass and a reduction in the muscle/fat ratio.

These changes are largely due to disuse. A person who is active throughout life tends to maintain more muscle mass, strength, and coordination than one who is sedentary.[3] Nevertheless, even regular exercise cannot completely prevent the decline in muscle mass,[6] although the decline is much less than in a sedentary person. The sedentary individual can also regain some muscle mass, strength, and endurance with a training program, even if it is begun late in life.[3,7,8] The results of training, however, are not as spectacular as in younger participants. It seems that while elderly people do experience some muscle hypertrophy with exercise, neural factors such as improved synchronization of muscle fiber firing and recruitment play a relatively larger role in strength gains than in the young.[9]

While some or even most of the declines outlined here may be prevented or reversed with exercise, it is clear that not all can be. As yet, the exact explanations for this are not known, but possibly the cumulative effects of diet, caffeine, smoking, and alcohol use take a toll on the muscular system. Endocrine factors, central nervous system changes, or maturation may also be important.

### Bones

As people age they lose bone mass and body calcium, and their bones remodel themselves more slowly. Bone mass increases up to age 30, plateaus, and then declines with advancing age. This decline is accelerated in women after menopause (see Chapters 23 and 26). As with the loss of muscle mass, these effects appear to be partially due to aging and partially due to disuse. While increasing activity may slow down bone loss or even temporarily reverse it, there is no convincing evidence that even a lifetime of vigorous activity will completely prevent the loss. It may, however, slow down the rate of loss enough so that only a very-long-lived person would suffer the complications of bone loss: osteoporosis and fractures.

### Connective Tissue

Flexibility is an often ignored component of fitness and musculoskeletal health. The inflexible person may be more prone to injury, no matter what the activity. This is because of being less able to tolerate potentially damaging movements, accidents, or falls. In a young inflexible individual there is probably a safe buffer of strength and coordination to avoid most injury due to inflexibility, but in the elderly this buffer may be lost. Falls become more common, and when they occur they are more likely to cause damage.

It is unclear whether or not loss of flexibility is a direct result of aging or just due to disuse. There are probably components of both factors involved. Older people lose some of the elasticity of their connective tissues. Disuse also allows their connective tissues to become contracted and less able to accommodate unusual movement.

### The Nervous System

In addition to losing musculoskeletal health with age, there appears to be a loss of neural control. The aging process includes a slow loss of some brain cells, which appears to decrease fine motor control and coordination. There is also a slowing of nerve conduction, a prolongation of reaction time, a slowing of central nervous system processing, and decreased proprioception and balance. Disuse, of course, exacerbates such losses, but probably is not the only cause of them.

### Other Changes

The body organ systems also exhibit changes with age. This includes a rise in systolic blood pressure due to reduced elasticity of the blood vessels, decreased cardiac output, a decrease in pulmonary vital capacity, a decrease in total body water with an increase in body fat, decreased hepatic and renal function, and decreased gastrointestinal motility, among many many others.

## Diagnosis and Treatment of Disorders

### Degenerative Joint Disease

For an unknown reason joints tend to deteriorate with age in a condition known as degenerative joint disease (DJD), or osteoarthritis. Aging itself does not cause the deterioration, but it is often complicated by it. In early DJD the joint cartilage becomes damaged and tries to heal itself. For a time it may succeed, but as the degeneration outpaces repair, the cartilage loses proteoglycan and chondrocytes, becomes pitted and fissured, and develops erosions. In an attempt to compensate for this decline in structure, the bone underlying the cartilage becomes sclerotic and the bone at the edge of the joint forms osteophytes (spurs).

The degenerative process is found in nearly all elderly persons. In fact, it is not uncommon to see it in people 30 years or younger in some joints. It involves more than just "wear and tear," although this may certainly contribute to the degeneration, especially in an otherwise abnormal joint. There may be complex interactions between genetic predisposition, a history of joint trauma, obesity, nutrition, overuse, and other factors that cause some joints to degenerate. The degenerative process preferentially affects some joints, and spares others. It is not always painful. It is not known why one person with evidence of severe DJD by radiographic evaluation may have few or no complaints while another, with minimal x-ray findings, can be virtually incapacitated by the disorder.

The treatment of DJD is multimodal. Pain is controlled with analgesics or nonsteroidal antiinflammatory drugs (NSAIDs). The NSAID also helps to control inflammation within the affected joints. In some cases intraarticular antiinflammatory steroid injections are necessary. If overused, these agents hasten joint deterioration. Consequently, joint injection should not be done more often than every 2 to 3 months or more than a few times a year in each joint. As a rule, medication is used only when needed, during pain flareups. Some people, however, require long-term pharmacologic treatment and do well with it. Drug side effects are always a major concern, and if possible, other modalities are preferred for long-term care. They include heat or cold application for comfort, energy conservation techniques to prevent flareups, and splinting as needed to provide support. In addition, range of motion and strength maintenance exercises are required to prevent contractures and deconditioning. Regular weight-bearing exercise, interspersed with frequent rest periods, may also be useful to stimulate proper cartilage nutrition as well as to strengthen the periarticular muscles. Such exercise is avoided during periods of acute inflammation.[10]

In severe cases of DJD, with intractable pain and loss of function, joint arthrodesis (fusion), osteotomy (changing the angle of the bone), or arthroplasty (joint replacement) may be necessary. Arthrodesis is currently preferred in the ankle, while joint replacement gives better results in the hips and knees. Younger patients tend to wear out their joint replacements within their longer life spans; elderly patients generally do well with such replacements.

### Neck and Back Pain

Neck and back pain occur in all ages; however, the causes of the pain do vary with age. Young adults may suffer from connective tissue disease such as Reiter's syndrome or ankylosing spondylitis which cause mainly low back and sacroiliac pain. In middle age, common causes of neck pain include myofascial pain syndrome and posttraumatic pain. Back pain is commonly caused by mechanical low back disorder. Herniated disks occur most commonly in this age group. Older individuals may suffer from DJD, osteoporotic fractures, or spinal stenosis.

DJD, described in detail earlier in the chapter, commonly affects the facet joints. These joints are equipped to provide a weight-bearing surface, yet in a lifetime of improper spinal mechanics they may be injured and degenerate. In facet arthropathy pain is often exacerbated by extension or rotation of the spine. Flexion may relieve the symptoms. Treatment consists of instruction in proper back mechanics, strengthening of the back muscles, and NSAIDs. Facet joint injections may be necessary in some cases. When degeneration allows the vertebrae to slip on each other (a condition known as spondylolisthesis), treatment may consist of an isometric flexion strengthening program and possibly lumbosacral orthoses. Such degenerative spondylolisthesis is different from isthmic spondylolisthesis which involves a fracture of the pars interarticularis (spondylolysis) and is found in younger patients.

Osteoporotic fractures are the dreaded end-result of osteoporosis. In the spine they often occur as wedge-shaped compression fractures of the thoracic or lumbar vertebrae. Pain from such fractures generally resolves as the bone heals, usually in a few months. The fracture leaves a deformity which leads to kyphosis. If no neurologic deficit occurs, the acute compression fracture is treated with a short period of rest, analgesics, and return to activity as soon as tolerated. Positions of flexion are avoided. Back braces, which are useful in younger patients with traumatic compression fractures, are usually not tolerated in the elderly.

Spinal stenosis is a narrowing of the vertebral canal due to a buildup of bone. It can occur in both the cervical and lumbar spine. It can also involve the intervertebral foramina where the spinal nerves exit the vertebral canal. It is more likely in those having a relatively small spinal canal.

When stenosis affects the cervical spine it can cause myelopathy, or damage to the spinal cord.

This may produce lower motor neuron signs of damage at the level involved and upper motor neuron signs below the injury. The patient may complain of numbness, weakness, and tingling of the limbs, mainly in the arms and hands. In more advanced cases there may be spasticity, generalized hyperreflexia, and the presence of pathologic reflexes (especially in the lower extremities). Diagnosis can be suggested electromyographically and confirmed with a myelogram, computerized tomography (CT), or magnetic resonance imaging (MRI). Treatment can be conservative with a cervical collar, NSAIDs, and physical therapy to maximize function. If symptoms become significant enough to interfere with activities of daily living, a surgical decompression of the spinal cord may be indicated.

In stenosis of the lumbar spine there may be symptoms of neurogenic claudication, or pseudoclaudication. In true claudication poor arterial blood flow to the legs causes leg pain after a predictable interval of exercise. In neurogenic claudication, the lumbar stenosis causes similar symptoms due to compression of the lumbar spinal contents. Symptoms of pseudoclaudication are more variable than in true claudication. They occur with back extension and during standing (not just walking). The symptoms do not occur during exercise if the spine is flexed, as when riding a bicycle or when walking in a stooped position. This helps differentiate this condition from true vascular claudication, which occurs with any lower extremity activity and which is relieved by rest, no matter what position the spine is in.

Lumbar spinal stenosis can often by treated with a program of lumbar flexion exercise, a corset, and shock-absorbing shoe inserts. Surgical decompression may be necessary in some cases.

When spinal stenosis causes a narrowing of the intervertebral foramina (lateral stenosis), it pinches the corresponding spinal nerves and may lead to radiculopathy. Diagnosis can be assisted by electrodiagnostic studies, oblique spine x-ray films, or CT (to visualize the foramina). Conservative care with NSAIDs, epidural, oral, or nerve root sleeve corticosteroid injection, and physical therapy may be successful. Surgical decompression may be necessary in some cases.[11] In cases of herniated nucleus pulposus concomitant with such lateral stenosis, surgery may be more likely than conservative care to be successful.[12]

In addition to the above conditions, which are relatively more common in the elderly than young patients, the older patient is also at higher risk of developing neck or back pain from cancer metastases, neck pain from rheumatoid arthritis involvement, or posttraumatic pain. The ligamentum flavum in the posterior of the spinal canal is flexible and elastic in the younger population. As a person ages, it becomes less elastic. Thus in a hyperextension injury, such as a flexion-extension (whiplash) motion in a motor vehicle accident, the less elastic ligamentum flavum may pinch the spinal cord, leading to neck pain or, in severe cases, a partial spinal cord injury.

### Shoulder

Almost all disorders of the shoulder described in Chapter 14 can be found in the elderly. The older individual is, however, more likely to suffer specifically from a few of them. Chronic rotator cuff tears are more common, as is impingement syndrome. Treatment is similar to that for younger patients; however, in these more chronic conditions, conservative care is typically more useful than surgery. If surgery is performed, care must be taken to avoid prolonged immobilization. Such immobilization is more likely to cause adhesive capsulitis in the elderly than in the young. Adhesive capsulitis can also be triggered by anything from trauma to myocardial infarction. Often the cause is unknown.

Another condition that may be more common in the older population is rupture of the biceps tendon. This produces a bulge in the anterior arm due to a retraction of the muscle belly. This reduces the strength of the biceps, but most patients do not complain of weakness. Surgery is helpful in a patient who requires full biceps strength.

DJD of the shoulder can cause severe symptoms, which in the elderly can be incapacitating. The humeral head may migrate superiorly and become virtually locked onto the acromion. Surgical care with arthrodesis or, more commonly, total joint replacement usually provides relief of pain and dysfunction.

The shoulder can also be a site of referred pain in the elderly. The primary pathology may lie in the cervical spine, paraspinal and neck muscles, in the brachial plexus, or in apical lung tumors (Pancoast's tumor). Avascular necrosis of the humeral head may occur in patients treated with oral steroid medication.

## Hip

The hip is a constrained joint which is called on to sustain great compressive loads. Consequently, any degeneration and inflammation can lead to symptoms. Pain can be severe and may be present even when the hip is not bearing weight.

Degenerative disease of the hip can often be treated conservatively with NSAIDs, a cane (as described in Chapter 17), and gentle exercises. Hip replacement surgery is a generally well tolerated treatment for more severe cases of DJD.

Fractures of the hip, often due to osteoporosis in the elderly, require assessment and treatment by an orthopedic surgeon and are not discussed further here.

Other causes of hip pain may be trochanteric bursitis, peripheral vascular disease, abdominal or pelvic tumors, or pseudogout (chondrocalcinosis). Avascular necrosis is also a diagnosis to consider in patients treated with corticosteroids.

## Knee and Leg

Knee disorders are probably more common in younger patients than in the elderly. Meniscal tears, cruciate ligament tears, and chondromalacia are common disorders usually seen in a sports medicine setting. The elderly develop a different set of knee disorders, mainly degenerative meniscal tears and DJD.

Treatment of degenerative meniscal tears is usually conservative with NSAIDs and gentle strengthening exercises. Sometimes joint injections, arthrosopic débridement, or even meniscectomy are necessary. DJD of the knee is similarly often treated conservatively with NSAIDs, a cane, joint injections, and exercises. In severe cases, total knee replacement surgery offers a generally effective way to reduce pain and increase function.

Other causes of knee pain in the elderly may include a Baker's cyst, referred hip pain, and pseudogout. Baker's cyst is a posterior outpouch-

ing of the synovial membrane of the knee. If it ruptures it may mimic deep venous thrombosis.

Leg pain can be due to any number of causes in the elderly. One of the most common is intermittent claudication. While not truly a musculoskeletal disorder, it belongs in this book because it mimics musculoskeletal disorders. Claudication is due to arterial disease which causes symptoms of ischemic leg pain after performing a certain amount of muscular activity. Typically the patient reports that pain starts after walking a set distance. The distance remains remarkably constant from day to day. Symptoms are relieved by rest, not necessarily sitting down (differentiating this from pseudoclaudication). Symptoms may be reduced with a progressive exercise program. Surgery is required if the vascular disease progresses to the point of threatening limb viability.

## Foot

The foot is an anatomically complex part of the body that serves as a lever for ambulation and as a platform for standing. Foot problems in the elderly are due to several classes of etiology. One is the anatomic changes in the foot that are a part of normal aging. In addition, there are problems that occur from a lifetime of wearing improper footwear. Other causes include overuse and disease states.

With aging the fat pads on the plantar surface of the foot become atrophic. These pads act as shock absorbers, and their atrophy places increased stress on the rest of the foot. Elderly patients also have more osteoarthritis of the joints of the foot. Medical conditions such as peripheral vascular disease, peripheral neuropathy, and connective tissue diseases take their toll on the foot as well.

Achilles tendonitis is an overuse condition, and can usually be successfully treated with conservative care. Achilles bursitis is an inflammation of the retrocalcaneal bursa, and is often caused by mechanical irritation from shoes. Again treatment should be conservative in most cases.

Painful heel pads probably occur due to heel pad atrophy and are worsened by obesity. The pain in this condition is felt on the major weight-bearing portion of the calcaneus. Plantar fasciitis is a common condition in both young and old patients. It causes pain to be felt at the anterior border of the calcaneus, where the plantar fascia inserts into this bone. It can usually be treated with warm soaks (or ice), NSAIDs, and shoe orthotics.

Acquired pes planus in the geriatric population is often due to posterior tibial tendon rupture. Pes cavus and associated claw toes can be due to a progressive neurologic disease. Treatment should include stretching and strengthening exercises as well as shoe modification.

Hallux valgus is common in the elderly. It is seen more in women than in men and is felt to be due to high heel shoes and narrow toe boxes. Hallux rigidus is usually due to DJD.

Metatarsalgia is commonly seen in those over age 40, especially in women, and is though to be caused by atrophy of the fat pads of the foot as well as by wearing high heel shoes. It can also be caused by trauma in those who stress their feet with poor footwear.

## Falls

Falls are a common and feared condition in the elderly. They can result in fractures that causes morbidity and even mortality. Subsequent deconditioning, fear of further falling, and medical complications such as deep venous thrombosis often start the patient on a gradual decline in activity and quality of life. Falls in the elderly are more likely than in the younger population because of decreased strength, balance, coordination, reaction time, vision, and flexibility. They are also sometimes the first presenting signs of medical conditions such as orthostatic hypotension, syncope, or Parkinson's disease.

Falls in the elderly must be taken seriously. After ruling out dangerous medical reasons for the falls, the patient often benefits from a strengthening and conditioning program as well as possible use of canes or other adaptive equipment.

## Medications

There are a number of bodily changes that occur with aging that affect the pharmacology and side effects of medications used in musculoskeletal medicine. With age come changes in the gastrointestinal system that decrease the absorption of

drugs. This effect is usually fairly minor and in general does not require higher doses of a prescribed drug. There are also changes in body composition in the elderly, as described earlier. A higher body fat content means that fat-soluble drugs are more likely to be stored in body fat. This increases the time required for these drugs to show clinical effects and retards their complete elimination from the body when they are discontinued. A lower body water content makes the serum levels of water-soluble drugs higher in the elderly, and lower serum albumin increases the serum concentration of drugs that normally bind to this protein. The elderly have a reduced capacity to eliminate medications by the two usual methods, hepatic metabolism and renal clearance. In general they are also more susceptible to drug side effects and adverse reactions. Since older patients are often on numerous medications for various illnesses and diseases, they are also more likely to suffer from adverse drug interactions.

**NSAIDs.**    These are probably the most prescribed medications in any age group. In the elderly, they are especially likely to cause problems of stomach ulcers, gastrointestinal bleeding, and acute renal failure. The salicylates cause more metabolic acidosis in the elderly. Sulindac may be less harmful to the kidneys.

**Acetaminophen.**    Acetaminophen is a very safe medication; however, in the elderly it may have an increased serum half-life, and in patients with impaired liver function it may cause further liver damage if ingested in high doses.

**Narcotic Analgesics.**    The elderly have no special problems with this class of drugs except that they may be more likely to experience any of their side effects such as central nervous system depression, respiratory depression, and constipation.

**Corticosteroids.**    Corticosteroids are powerful medications that can suppress the adrenal glands. In older patients, as well as in younger ones, this can create problems in times of bodily stress, such as during surgery. Patients who have been on chronic systemic corticosteroid medication within a year of such stress may need to have steroid supplementation to avoid complications such as shock. Corticosteroids also worsen diabetes and when used chronically can cause or worsen osteoporosis. These are special concerns in the elderly.

**Tricyclic Antidepressants.** Older individuals are more susceptible to the anticholinergic side effects of these drugs. This includes problems of orthostatic hypotension, confusion, dry mouth, urinary retention, and blurred vision.

**Other Medications.** Virtually any drug can have adverse effects, especially in the elderly. Phenytoin may exhibit a higher serum level, and thus a higher level of side effects, in the elderly. Diazepam has an increased half-life and is stored in body fat. Beta-blockers reduce the rise in heart rate with exercise. These effects as well as many others must be watched for when dealing with the elderly population. To maximize safety it is best to use the lowest dose of medication possible, and to increase the dose only slowly as needed. If possible, drugs should avoided altogether.

## Points of Summary

1. Virtually every body system deteriorates with age to some extent; this may primarily be due to disuse as well as the primary effect of aging.
2. Disorders of a different type predominate in the elderly compared to younger individuals.
3. Falls are common in the elderly. They can be due to less of a physical margin of safety or may be signs of medical disease.
4. Medication side effects are generally amplified in the elderly; the lowest doses possible should be used.

## References

1. Kalu DN, Masoro EJ: The biology of aging, with particular reference to the musculoskeletal system. *Clin Geriatr Med* 1988;4:257–267.
2. Larsson L, Sjodin B, Karlsson J: Histochemical and biochemical changes in human skeletal muscle with age in sedentary males, age 22–65 years. *Acta Physiol Scand* 1978;103:31–39.
3. Klitgaard H, Mantoni M, Schiaffino S, et al.: Function, morphology and protein expression of ageing skeletal muscle: A cross-sectional study of elderly men with different training backgrounds. *Acta Physiol Scand* 1990;140:41–54.
4. Fleg JL, Lakatta EG: Role of muscle loss in the age-associated reduction in $VO_{2max}$. *J Appl Physiol* 1988;65:1147–1151.
5. Tzankoff SP, Norris AH: Effect of muscle mass decrease on age-related BMR changes. *J Appl Physiol* 1977;43:1001–1006.
6. Pollock ML, Foster C, Knapp D, et al. Effect of age and training on aerobic capacity and body composition of master athletes. *J Appl Physiol* 1987;62:725–731.
7. Frontera WR, Meredith CN, O'Reilly KP, et al.: Strength conditioning in older men: Skeletal muscle hypertrophy and improved function. *J Appl Physiol* 1988;64:1038–1044.
8. Larsson L: Physical training effects of muscle morphology in sedentary males at different ages. *Med Sci Sports Exerc* 1982;14:203–206.
9. Moritana T, deVries HA: Neural factors versus hypertrophy in the time course of muscle strength gain in young and old men. *J Gerontol* 1981;36:294–297.
10. McKeag DB: The relationship of osteoarthritis and exercise. *Clin Sports Med* 1992;11:471–488.
11. Turner JA, Ersek M, Herron L, et al.: Surgery for lumbar spinal stenosis—attempted meta-analysis of the literature. *Spine* 1992;17:1–8.
12. Saal JA, Saal JS: Nonoperative treatment of herniated lumbar intervertebral disc with radiculopathy: An outcome study. *Spine* 1989;14:431–437.

## Suggested Readings

Elward K, Larson EB: Benefits of exercise for older adults. *Clin Geriatr Med* 1992;8:35–50.
Kerlan RK (ed): Sports medicine in the older athlete. *Clin Sports Med* 1991;10(2).
Payton OD, Poland JL: Aging Process. *Phys Ther* 1983;63:41–48.
Roth SH: Pharmacologic approaches to musculoskeletal disorders. *Clin Geriatric Med* 1988;4:441–461.

# Chapter 23

# Musculoskeletal and Medical Concerns in Women

RALPH BUSCHBACHER
LOIS P. BUSCHBACHER

## Anatomic and Physiologic Differences Between Men and Women

Just taking a quick look around at average people reveals some major differences between the sexes. Other differences lie hidden beneath the skin, but overall men and women are more alike than different. The differences are, however, important and need to be understood to properly treat and train women.

### Anatomy

On average, the adult male is 6 inches taller than his female counterpart. He weighs more, has more bone mass, and has proportionately less body fat. The average sedentary male's body fat is around 10% to 15% of his weight, while that of the average female is around 20% to 25%.

A common misperception regarding women's build is that they have a wider absolute pelvic width than men. Actually, absolute pelvic width in men and women is approximately equal. When measured relative to height, the pelvis is, however, proportionately wider in women, since they are on average shorter. When measured relative to shoulder width, the pelvis in women seems even

wider.[1,2] A woman's pelvis does differ in shape from that of a man, with a wider pelvic inlet to accommodate childbearing.

In both men and women the hips are obviously wider than the position of the feet when standing. Thus it is natural to have a bit of valgus at the knees (knock-kneed). Since the pelvises of men and women are equally wide, and women's legs are on average shorter, it means that the valgus at women's knees is greater. With a greater valgus angle at the knee, the angle at which the quadriceps pulls on the patella is greater in women than in men. They also have a more shallow patellar groove on the femur. Thus, women are usually reported as having a higher incidence of patellofemoral dysfunction. While this may be true, there is not much evidence to support it, especially in well conditioned women.

### Strength

Muscle mass in the average woman is less than in the average man and even with strength training remains smaller. Strength is also generally less. However, strength can be defined in various ways. If one looks at absolute strength, men are stronger. If maximum tension as a function of muscular cross-sectional area is viewed, then there is no difference. When comparing a man and a woman of equal height and weight, the man is stronger because the woman has a proportionately greater percentage of body fat, and thus proportionately less muscle. When comparing a man and a woman of equal height and equal lean body mass there is less difference, especially in the legs.[3,4]

Muscle hypertrophy with strength training is more readily achieved by a man. This is due to the anabolic steroids such as testosterone which he has in greater quantity than a woman. Even in endurance trained athletes, women have only 85% of the muscle fiber area that men have. The muscle composition and number of fibers are unchanged; men just have larger fibers.[4-6]

### Endocrine Differences

The endocrine differences between men and women are marked. Males have more testosterone and related androgens which generate secondary sexual characteristics including muscular hypertrophy, skeletal strength, laryngeal changes, wider shoulders, and a greater stimulation of hematopoiesis. In females the estrogens predominate. They regulate ovarian function and the menstrual cycle. In addition, they stimulate breast development, cause widening of the pelvic inlet, and increase adiposity.

### Oxygen Uptake

$\dot{V}O_2max$, the maximum rate of oxygen uptake, is a general measure of cardiovascular endurance, and on average is lower in women than in men; thus women have a relative physiologic disadvantage in performing aerobic activity. Part of this disadvantage is due to the proportionately greater amount of body fat that women carry. However, even when measuring $\dot{V}O_2max$ relative to lean body mass in subjects with a similar training background, men have 5% more aerobic capacity than women.[7] This may be due to women's lower hemoglobin concentration or to the lower muscle mass they have compared with men. Other as yet unknown sex-related differences may also be responsible.

### Cardiopulmonary Differences

Women are commonly reported to have smaller hearts, a smaller thoracic cage, and a lower blood volume than men. This is said to reduce their maximal oxygen carrying capacity. However, it is unclear from the literature whether or not these differences are absolute or just related to women's smaller physical size. In an investigation of $\dot{V}O_2max$ among adolescent males with varying heart sizes, boys with greater sizes did indeed have greater $\dot{V}O_2max$, but this effect was mainly due to their concomitantly increased body size.[8] There is no reason to believe that this principle does not also apply to girls and women.

Women do have a lower blood hemoglobin range than men (12 to 16 mg/dl and 14 to 18 mg/dl respectively) and this may affect athletic performance. In one study the hematocrit between male and female volunteers was equalized by drawing blood from the men.[9] This tended to lower the men's $\dot{V}O_2max$, though less so than predicted by the reduction in oxygen carrying capacity.

## Women's Response to Exercise and Training

### Strength Training

Almost all of the research in exercise physiology in women has been done for endurance training. Strength training is somewhat different. The object of strength training is to increase muscle mass. Since the absolute strength of a muscle is a function of its cross-sectional area, increasing muscle mass is the only way to increase absolute muscle strength. Women do not respond as well as men to a strength training program. Androgens are needed to stimulate muscle hypertrophy; thus women never attain the sometimes phenomenal increase in muscle mass and strength seen in men. Nevertheless, strength training is valuable for women. Their muscles increase in size to some extent, and they may develop an increase in the synchronization of muscle fiber activity, thus giving them greater functional strength. In addition, strength training may exert beneficial effects on bone mass and overall psychological well-being.

## Endurance Training

Women's response to endurance training is more similar to that of men. When men and women train at similar levels of effort for similar tasks they have nearly identical rates of increases in $\dot{V}O_2$max, at least for up to 7 weeks of training.[10] Their heart rates at submaximal exercise loads also decrease similarly. Absolute $\dot{V}O_2$ is still higher among the men and the maximal $\dot{V}O_2$ attainable by elite athletes also appears to be higher among men.

Endurance training increases slow-twitch (fatigue-resistant) muscle fiber area to a similar extent in both men and women, although the fibers in men are larger.[5,11]

## Medical Issues

### Menopause and Osteoporosis

Menopause involves the cessation of the menstrual cycle with the resultant loss of fertility. Symptoms accompanying menopause include hot flashes and changes in mood and in sleep habits. Estrogen production decreases, leading to an atrophic vaginal mucosa. Estrogen exerts a protective effect on women against atherosclerosis and coronary artery disease. When its production declines women develop more cardiovascular disease. The decline also leads to loss of bone mass, osteoporosis. Women at risk for osteoporosis are white, thin, have had early menopause, and bore few children. Smoking is a risk factor, and caffeine intake might be also. Osteoporosis is a major health problem in elderly women. It leads to hip and vertebral compression fractures.

Estrogen replacement therapy with a variant of the birth control pill is becoming increasingly popular as a method of preventing the effects of decreased estrogen production. Exercise is also useful as an adjunct.

Certainly the effect of exercise in maintaining cardiorespiratory fitness is well documented in men. There is no reason to believe that women would not also benefit from a lifetime of exercise. If started late in life it should be initiated gradually and only after proper medical screening to avoid complications.

Bone mass declines gradually after the age of 30 to 35. The decline is hastened by menopause. Thus it is critical for a woman to have the maximum bone mass possible during her early thirties. Weight-bearing exercises such as running and walking build up bone mass before this age and slow its decline afterward. Thus ideally women should exercise early in life to build bone and late in life to keep it strong. It is unclear whether weight training has the same effect on bone as weight-bearing exercise, but theoretically it should be just as beneficial at preventing osteoporosis.

Once osteoporosis has developed, women should still be encouraged to exercise, except of course while an acute fracture is healing. Even in older women light weight-bearing exercise such as walking is safe and effective.[12] Exercises to be avoided are those that involve jarring motion and those that involve flexion of the back.[13]

### Pregnancy

### Exercise

Pregnancy affects the body's response to exercise. Greater nonmuscular weight decreases exercise efficiency at any given load. A woman's metabolism increases with increasing gestational mass. Thus, greater cardiorespiratory effort is required for a given workload. There is some training effect of the pregnant state and the woman accommodates to the increased stress.

There is no evidence that mild to moderate exercise has any adverse effect on the developing fetus or on the pregnant woman. Strenuous endurance exercise at or above prepregnancy levels has been reported to decrease the birthweight of infants and cause an earlier delivery (by up to 8 days), but there is no evidence of increased birth morbidity.[14] Also, not all studies have demonstrated such an earlier delivery with lower birthweight, especially at less strenuous levels of activity.[15,16] Certainly women with complications of pregnancy such as abnormal bleeding or hypertension and those with cardiopulmonary disease or a history of abnormal pregnancy should not be exercising vigorously. Also bouncing or jarring activity should probably be avoided, especially near term. Women should stay away from activities predisposing them to abdominal trauma while pregnant, and water-skiing should be avoided. Women with twins may also be cautioned that the extra oxygen required by two fetuses might be compromised by overly vigorous exercise. For most women, however, continued moderate activity such as exercise biking, walking, and swimming are reasonable. They may have less excess weight gain, less deconditioning from a previously fit level, and improved psychological well-being. There is no clear-cut safe limit for maximum heart rate during pregnancy. The American College of Obstetricians and Gynecologists recommends that a rate of 140 should not be exceeded during pregnancy.[17] This limit is very conservative and could probably be raised by 10 to 20 beats per minute, especially in women who were physically active prior to becoming pregnant.

### Flexibility

In pregnant women a hormone called relaxin is produced. As its name suggests, it relaxes connective tissue. The allows the pelvic bones to widen during childbirth, but also obviously may weaken some joints. During late pregnancy or the early postdelivery period women should maintain their normal range of motion, but to avoid joint injury they should not pursue a vigorous increase in flexibility.

### Musculoskeletal and Back Pain

Pregnancy induces a number of changes in a woman's body. A larger abdomen and breasts change the center of gravity and the mechanical efficiency of the abdominal musculature and may strain the back. About 50% of pregnant women develop backache,[18,19] often affecting the sacroiliac joints. The incidence of back pain increases with the age of the pregnant woman, with repeat pregnancy, and in women with weak abdominal muscles. If back pain is severe during pregnancy it is often troublesome after delivery. Back pain during pregnancy usually responds well to a period of relative rest.

Changes in posture and body habitus may lead to overuse syndromes and nerve compression. Water is retained and may predispose the woman to carpal tunnel syndrome and other compression neuropathies. In addition, connective tissue weakening due to relaxin may predispose the woman to sacroiliac pain and to other musculoskeletal disorders. These changes may persist for some time after delivery.

There is no good evidence that exercising women are more predisposed to developing prepartum and postpartum musculoskeletal pain than sedentary women. Certainly it seems intuitive that a woman well-conditioned before pregnancy would tend to have a lower risk for such problems.

### Heat

Excessive temperature rise in the pregnant uterus is felt to be harmful to the fetus and may be a teratogenic agent.[20] For this reason any deep heating agent such as ultrasound, microwave, or short wave diathermy is absolutely contraindicated over the pregnant uterus. Therapies such as Hubbard tanks which may raise the core body temperature are likewise contraindicated, as are steam rooms and saunas. Pregnant women should be counseled not to undertake excessive physical activity in a hot climate to which they are not acclimated, in order to avoid any kind of heat stress to the fetus.

### Medications

Before prescribing any medication or using any over-the-counter drug in a woman who is pregnant, the drug's adverse effects should be reviewed. In general, it is best to avoid taking any medications, especially during early pregnancy.

### Gastrointestinal and Urologic Concerns

Few gastrointestinal and urologic differences that involve the musculoskeletal systems exist between men and women. With vigorous activity both sexes can develop hematuria or occult gastrointestinal blood loss. Rhabdomyolysis may occur and can in severe cases cause renal failure. In addition, nausea and diarrhea are relatively common in competitive runners, both male and female, although in women the incidence is somewhat higher.

## Nutrition in Women

Nutrient requirements in women are essentially the same as for men with the exception of iron and calcium. Both men and women should eat a normal varied diet, not too high in fat.

### *Iron Status and Anemia*

Because of iron loss during menstrual bleeding, menstruating women require 50% more iron than men. Iron is not as readily absorbed by the body as many other minerals and vitamins so it is easy for women to become iron deficient. Women have been noted to have lower blood hemoglobin levels and are at greater risk for iron deficiency and secondary anemia than men. One study of the bone marrow aspirates of college women revealed total body iron depletion in 25% of the subjects.[21] Other studies have suggested that athletes, especially long distance runners, may have low iron stores.[22,23] Up to 40% to 50% of adolescent female athletes have iron depletion.[24] Athletes lose the iron in sweat, through gastrointestinal blood loss,[23,25] and through hematuria and rhabdomyolysis. They may also have decreased iron absorption and may ingest less iron than nonathletes.[26]

Iron deficiency has been shown in animal studies to impair muscular performance in endurance exercise. Iron deficiency, even without anemia, may cause animals to tire earlier.[27-29] The reduction in exercise tolerance is due to increased lactic acid production because of depletion of iron-containing mitochondrial enzymes. When the deficiency becomes severe, anemia results. Anemia decreases the oxygen carrying capacity of blood and impairs performance even further. In humans iron repletion in a deficient athlete has been shown to decrease lactate production.[29] No change in $\dot{V}O_2$max has been noted.

Iron deficiency anemia must be differentiated from so-called "sports anemia," in which iron stores are normal. Endurance training has been shown to increase blood volume. If the red blood cell mass remains constant, an increase in blood volume results in hemodilution, thus creating a false picture of anemia. It can easily be differentiated from long-term anemia caused by iron deficiency by measuring body iron stores.

All women need to take in adequate amounts of iron. In active women this is especially important to maximize performance. If iron deficiency is detected a medical evaluation is indicated to rule out any worrisome sources of blood loss.

### *Calcium*

In order to develop optimal bone strength and mass and to ward off osteoporosis, women need adequate amounts of calcium in the diet, estrogen in the bloodstream, and weight-bearing exercise in their lifestyle. Estrogen is by far the most important of these three factors, but adequate calcium intake is also essential. Exercise, though of lesser benefit by itself, acts synergistically with estrogen to develop bone strength and is highly recommended.

Many women have inadequate dietary calcium intake. This is especially so in those who shy away from dairy products for health reasons or because they do not tolerate them, and in those who have low circulating estrogen levels. Estrogen aids in the absorption of calcium from the gastrointestinal tract. Thus menopausal women or those with hypoestrogenic amenorrhea should ingest even more calcium than euestrogenic women to make up for their poorer absorption. Adequate calcium intake, with supplements if necessary, is to be recommended for all women.

## The Breast

In the past few decades as women became more active in many sports, in particular jogging, numerous concerns with regard to the breast were voiced. One of these was that if a woman were to jog, her breasts would sag. Another belief was that if breasts were bruised they might be more prone to cancer. Women have also been concerned about breast pain during and after exercise.

Surveys were done in the mid-1970s by Gillette[31] and by Haycock[32] investigating the types of sports injuries found in women. They both found that the injury profile was about the same for men and women and that breast injuries were the least common. Because some women complain of breast pain during and after jogging, especially just before menstruation, and because of a concern that jogging would increase the amount of or speed the rate of breast sagging, research was undertaken to determine if and what type of breast support could be recommended. Haycock found that women with a cup size of B or greater benefited from a supportive bra to reduce breast movement during running or bouncing activities. This may decrease postexercise breast pain. She recommends a firm, mostly nonelastic material which limits motion in all directions. Seams should be smooth and metal hooks covered.[30] Lorentzen recommended a bra with nonelastic straps and a cup pad in contact sports.[33] An underwire bra is also an option. The issue of exercise and breast sagging is difficult to study because factors besides exercise contribute to breast sagging. They include genetics, breast size, childbearing, body weight, whether or not a woman has had breast implants, and so on. There is no direct evidence that exercise causes breast sagging. However, in cultures where women do not have any breast support they do seem to have more pendulous breasts.[34] It would seem prudent to support the breast during bouncing activities, especially if this results in any postexercise tenderness.

Women with fibrocystic changes are predisposed to developing sore breasts. This is treated with a supportive bra and pain medication as needed.[30]

In contact sports or accidents the breast is sometimes traumatized. Minor bruising is the most common result and can be treated with compression, ice, and avoidance of further injury. If the skin is broken it should be kept clean to avoid infection. If trauma results in a hematoma it should be treated similarly with ice and compression. If the hematoma increases in size, becomes painful, or shows signs of infection, it may need to surgically evacuated. Sometimes a hematoma may leave behind a hard lump or area of calcification. This condition is benign, but the lump may be removed for comfort, feel, and appearance reasons. Serious breast trauma is rare but in high-risk activities may be prevented by adequate padding.

Recently the lay press has focused attention on the risks of breast implants. Implants may rarely be ruptured by trauma and are not recommended in women involved in contact sports. Because the implants increase nonmuscular body weight they reduce exercise efficiency slightly. They also change breast movement during exercise and thus are probably not to be recommended in elite athletes or those who strive for their absolute best performance. Increased support may be necessary after breast implants.

## Gynecologic Issues

### Premenstrual Syndrome

The premenstrual syndrome (PMS) produces mood changes, headaches, and fluid retention in many women a few days before menstrual bleeding. Exercise does not seem to worsen these symptoms and may actually lessen them.[35,36] PMS may, by affecting mood, impair athletic performance.

### Training After Delivery, Surgery, or Dilatation and Curettage

The following recommendations are made by Shangold.[34] They are to be viewed as minimum waiting periods before resumption of activity. These waiting periods are extremely short and only the rare woman will be able to resume activity this quickly. Waiting longer may improve healing, but will of course delay recovery of athletic ability. Exercise should not be pushed to the point of pain.

Following dilatation and curettage or a first-trimester abortion, weight training and aerobic exercise, except water sports, may be resumed the same or the next day; water sports should be avoided until bleeding has ceased. Tampon use also should be avoided until bleeding has ceased.

Following a vaginal delivery or a second-trimester abortion, weight training may be resumed the same day; aerobic exercise, except water sports, may be resumed in 2 days; water sports may be resumed when bleeding has ceased. Tampon use should be avoided until bleeding has ceased.

Following a laparoscopy, aerobic exercise in and out of water and weight training may be resumed after 1 to 2 days.

Following a cesarian delivery or other abdominal surgery (requiring an incision), light aerobic exercise outside of water and light weight training may be resumed in 7 days; intense aerobic exercise (speed work), submaximal weight training, and water sports should be postponed at least 21 days.

## Exercise and Menstruation

Despite the fact that many women feel that menstruation impairs their athletic performance, there is no evidence of a consistent change in athletic performance at different points of the menstrual cycle.[37] Performance may increase in some women in some sports and may decrease in some women in some sports. Occasionally women may perform better during the follicular phase of their cycle and if they are elite athletes, manipulation of their cycle with birth control pills to coincide with major athletic competition is an option.[34] Performance benefits are small, however. Women may train as usual during menstrual bleeding. Women swimmers effectively use tampons during these times.

Much has been written on the adverse effects of exercise on the menstrual cycle. Mild to moderate activity seems to have little effect and may actually help to regulate the cycle. More vigorous training, especially when coupled with weight loss, may result in amenorrhea or infertility. This is usually a reversible effect. Women with amenorrhea deserve a full medical evaluation. Blaming the condition on the exercise without fully evaluating it may ignore a potentially serious underlying problem.

## Chronic Pelvic Pain

Women are more prone than men to developing chronic pelvic pain. This may be less likely in active individuals. The causes are often unidentified but may include a tension myalgia (myofascial pain) of the pelvic floor musculature, pelvic vein varicosities, or psychogenic expression.

## Endometriosis

This condition of abnormal, abdominally located uterine tissue is a relatively common cause of abdominal pain in women. It may first become manifest by such pain occurring during exercise. It is often well controlled by birth control pills but should always be evaluated by a gynecologist. Regular vigorous exercise, especially when started at a young age, may help protect women from developing symptoms of endometriosis. This has been postulated to be due to decreased estrogen production.[38,39]

## Points of Summary

1. Men have more muscle mass than women due to the effects of testosterone.
2. Women respond similarly to strength and endurance training as men, only to a lesser extent.
3. Exercise capacity is reduced in pregnancy.
4. Exercise of moderate intensity during pregnancy is considered safe.
5. Excess rise in body temperature is to be avoided during pregnancy.
6. Premenstrual syndrome may be lessened with exercise.
7. Menstruation does not in general impair athletic performance.
8. Amenorrhea in an exercising woman should not be attributed to exercise unless other, potentially harmful, conditions are ruled out.

## References

1. Wilmore JH, Behnke AR: An anthropometric estimation of body density and lean body weight in young men. *J Appl Physiol* 1969;27:25–31.
2. Wilmore JH, Behnke AR: An anthropometric estimation of body density and lean body weight in young women. *Am J Clin Nutr* 1970;20:267–274.
3. Bishop P, Cureton K, Collins M: Sex differences in muscular strength, in equally-trained men and women. *Ergonomics* 1987;30:675–687.
4. Bishop P, Cureton KC, Conerly M, et al.: Sex differences in muscle cross-sectional area of athletes and non-athletes. *J Sports Sci* 1989;7:31–39.
5. Drinkwater BL: Women and exercise: Physiological aspects. *Exerc Sport Sci Rev* 1984;12:21–51.
6. Schantz E, Randall-Fox W, Hutchinson W, et al.: Muscle fibre type distribution, muscle cross-sectional area and maximal voluntary strength in humans. *Acta Physiol Scand* 1983;117:219–226.
7. Sparling PB: A metanalysis of studies comparing maximal oxygen uptake in men and women. *Res Q Exerc Sport* 1980;51:542.
8. Blimkie CJR, Cunningham DA, Nichol PM: Gas transport capacity and echocardiographically determined cardiac size in children. *J Appl Physiol* 1980;49:994–999.

9. Cureton K, Bishop P, Hutchinson P: Sex difference in maximal oxygen uptake: Effect of equating hemoglobin concentration. *Eur J Appl Physiol* 1986;54:656–660.

10. Eddy DO, Sparks KL, Adelizi DA: The effects of continuous and interval training in women and men. *Eur J Apply Physiol* 1977;37:83–92.

11. Prince FP, Hikida RS, Hagerman FC: Muscle fiber types in women athletes and non-athletes. *Pflugers Arch* 1977;371:161–165.

12. Smith EL, Redden W, Smith PE: Physical activity and calcium modalities for bone mineral increase in aged women. *Med Sci Sports Exerc* 1981;13:60–64.

13. Sinaki M, Mikkelsen BA: Postmenopausal spinal osteoporosis: Flexion versus extension exercises. *Arch Phys Med Rehabil* 1984;65:593–596.

14. Clapp JF III, Dickerson S: Endurance exercise and pregnancy outcome. *Med Sci Sports Exerc* 1984;16:556–562.

15. Slavin JL, Lutter JM, Cushman S, et al.: Pregnancy and exercise. In Puhl J, Brown CH, Vor RO (eds): *Sports Science Perspectives for Women.* Champion, IL: Human Kinetics Books, 1985.

16. Lokey EA, Tran ZV, Wells CL, et al.: Effects of physical exercise on pregnancy outcomes: A meta-analytical review. *Med Sci Sports Exerc* 1991;23:1234–1239.

17. American College of Obstetricians and Gynecologists: *Home Exercise Programs—Exercise During Pregnancy and the Postnatal Period.* Washington, DC: American College of Obstetricians and Gynecologists 1985.

18. Berg G, Hammar M, Moller-Nielsen J, et al.: Low back pain during pregnancy *Obstet Gynecol* 1988;71:71–75.

19. Mantle MJ, Greenwood RM, Currey HLF: Backache in pregnancy. *Rheumatol Rehabil* 1977;16:95–100.

20. Smith DW, Claren SK, Harvey MAS: Hyperthermia as a possible tertogenic agent. *J Pediatr* 1978;92:878–883.

21. Scott DE, Pritchard JA: Iron deficiency in healthy young college women. *JAMA* 1967;199:897–900.

22. Clement DB, Asmundson RC: Nutritional intake and hematological parameters in endurance runners. *Phys Sports Med* 1982;10:37–43.

23. Stewart JG, Ahlquist DA, McGill DB, et al.: Gastrointestinal blood loss and anemia in runners. *Ann Intern Med* 1984;100:843–845.

24. Rowland TW: Iron deficiency in the young athlete. *Pediatr Clin* 1990;37:1153–1163.

25. McMahon LF, Ryan MJ, Larson D, et al.: Occult gastrointestinal blood loss in marathon runners. *Ann Intern Med* 1984;100:846–847.

26. Martin DE, Vroon DH, May DF, et al.: Physiological changes in elite male distance runners training for olympic competition. *Phys Sports Med* 1986;14:152–171.

27. Finch CA, Miller LR, Inamder AR, et al.: Iron deficiency in the rat: Physiological and biochemical studies on muscle dysfunction. *J Clin Invest* 1976;58:447–453.

28. Finch CA, Gollnick PD, Hlastala MP, et al.: Lactic acidosis as a result of iron deficiency. *J Clin Invest* 1979;64:129–137.

29. Nilson K, Schoene RB, Robertson HT, et al.: The effects of iron repletion on exercise-induced lactate production in minimally iron-deficient subjects (abstract). *Med Sci Sports Exerc* 1981;13:92.

30. Haycock CE: How I manage breast problems in athletes. *Phys Sports Med* 1987;15:89–95.

31. Gillette JV: When and where women are injured in sports. *Phys Sports Med* 1975;3:61–63.

32. Haycock CE, Gillette JV: Susceptibility of women athletes to injury: Myths vs. reality. *JAMA* 1976;236:163–165.

33. Lorentzen D, Lawson L: Selected sports bra: A biomechanical analysis of breast motion while jogging. *Phys Sports Med* 1987;15:128–139.

34. Shangold MM, Mirkin G (eds): *Women and Exercise: Physiology and Sports Medicine.* Philadelphia: FA Davis, 1988.

35. Prior JC, Vigna Y, Alojado N: Conditioning exercise decreases premenstrual symptoms: A prospective controlled three month trial. *Eur J Appl Physiol* 1986;55:349–355.

36. Timonen S, Procope B: Premenstrual syndrome and physical fitness. *Acta Obstet Gynecol Scand* 1971;50:331–337.

37. Brooks-Gunn J, Gargiulo J, Warren MP: Menstrual cycle and athletic performance. In Puhl JL, Brown CH (eds): *The Menstrual Cycle and Physical Activity.* Champaign, IL: Human Kinetics Publishers, 1986:13–28.

38. Barbieri RL: Etiology and epidemiology of endometriosis. *Am J Obstet Gynecol* 1990;162:565–567.

39. Cramer DW, Wilson E, Stillman RJ, et al.: The relation of endometriosis to menstrual characteristics, smoking, and exercise. *JAMA* 1986;255:1904–1908.

## Suggested Readings

Puhl JL, Brown CH (eds): *The Menstrual Cycle and Physical Activity.* Champaign, IL: Human Kinetics Publishers, 1986.

Shangold MM, Mirkin G (eds): *Women and Exercise: Physiology and Sports Medicine.* Philadelphia: FA Davis, 1988.

Wells CL: *Women, Sports, and Performance,* 2nd ed. Champaign, IL: Human Kinetics Publishers, 1991.

# Chapter 24

# Principles of Bracing and Prescription of Assistive Devices

PATRICIA PAYNE

While studying in New York City, my father was able to arrange admittance to a special showing of the Treasures of Tutankhamen at the Metropolitan Museum of Art. On display alongside the treasures discovered in the child king's tomb were artifacts from neighboring cultures. A case stood off to the side containing a pair of greaves, which belonged to Philip of Macedonia (Figure 24-1). Known today as the father of Alexander the Great, he was known then as Philip the Lame. One of his greaves was notably shorter than its mate, and in fact was of slightly different construction. Among this warrior's many injuries was a fractured leg, and this particular greave, dating back to the fourth century B.C., doubled as a short leg brace.

This story illustrates a point. Orthotics are as old as mankind. Today their use has greatly expanded following a recent explosion of new orthotic materials and designs. In response, orthotic nomenclature has undergone a rapid expansion and change. All of this can be foreboding to the uninitiated. Basic principles of orthotics and human anatomy, however, remain constant. This chapter attempts to outline these basics.

## Orthotic Prescription

Referred to today as braces, splints, appliances, and most recently orthoses,[1] all of these external devices, when applied to the body, aid function in some way. Orthotics by definition *support* a body part; prosthetics on the other hand *replace* a body part. Often they are thought of as straightening or "setting right" devices, thus the Greek root *orthos*. The term *orthotic* was first officially adopted in 1960 by the limb fitters and brace makers in America, when they formed the American Orthotic and Prosthetic Association from the original Artificial Limb Manufacturers Associations.[2]

### Goals

When considering an orthotic prescription, one must first determine goals. Generally these can be outlined as in Table 24-1. It is easy to see that these goals may overlap. Immediately following an acute injury, for instance, immobilization of the damaged part and pain relief often go hand in hand.

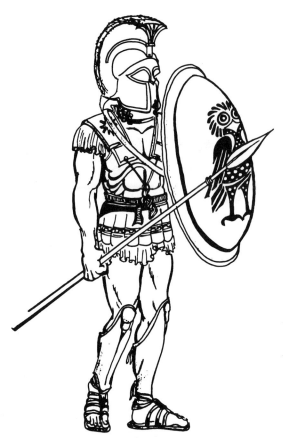

**Figure 24-1.** A pair of greaves. This armor covered the lower leg below the knee. The illustration is typical of the armor worn by the early Greeks around the time of Philip and Alexander.

Continued splinting during the healing phase may help prevent future deformity. When a joint is crossed by the device, however, one must consider initiation of range of motion exercises as soon as possible to prevent soft tissue contracture. This can be accomplished by adjusting wearing schedules, removing the brace for active or passive range of motion as indicated, or by fabrication of an articulated joint.

It could be easily argued that any time the goals of pain relief and correction of deformity are achieved, functional improvement is a logical consequence. When considered as a goal by itself, however, functional improvement also encompasses those orthotic applications which attempt to restore a proper balance to the motion across a joint. One way this is done is by mechanically substituting for lost muscle function. Examples of dynamic braces which function this way are the lower extremity dorsiflexion assist orthosis and the upper extremity wrist driven prehensile orthosis (WDPO) (used when the finger flexors are paralyzed but the wrist extensors remain intact) (Figure 24-2). Static braces may also be used to restore balance through prevention of unwanted motion. Such is the case when an ankle-foot orthosis (AFO) is prescribed to position a spastic equinovarus foot in neutral. This is frequently seen in hemiplegia (whether in spastic cerebral palsy, or following stroke or traumatic brain injury).

### Principles

Once orthotic goals have been established, there are some general principles which should be followed (Table 24-2). The brace should be easy to don and doff. Its construction should be lightweight, while still meeting durability requirements. It should be as unobtrusive as possible, while still fulfilling functional needs. While plastics, air casts, and neoprene sleeves provide advantages over traditional metal braces in these areas, they are not appropriate in every case.

### Cost

Cost must always be considered. With the advent of low-temperature thermoplastics, many therapists have expanded their practice to include brace fabrication, often citing it as a cost-saving measure. While such splint making has long been practiced by therapists with special expertise in the treatment of upper extremity pathology, and more recently in the field of pediatrics where material strength and durability requirements may be lower,[3] its efficacy in addressing more permanent lower extremity bracing needs is questionable.

**Table 24-1.** Goals of Bracing

| |
|---|
| Pain relief |
| Prevention or correction of deformity |
| Immobilization |
| Improved function |
| Prevention of reinjury |
| Support of a weakened part |

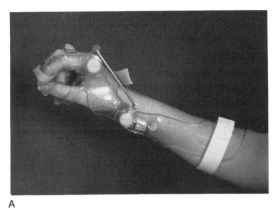 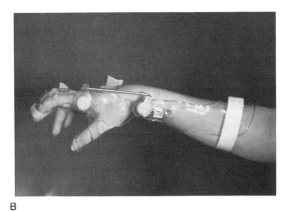

A    B

**Figure 24-2.** Wrist driven prehensile orthosis (WDPO) is used to restore a functional grip following paralysis of the finger flexors. Active wrist extension results in opposition of the thumb. The degree of wrist extension necessary to drive finger closure can be adjusted by a ratchet type lock on the side. *A*, Closed; *B*, Open.

Bracing needs of durability, reliability, and function should be met at the lowest cost possible. While the long-term needs may sometimes be better served by prescription of an initial trial brace, this is not always the case. Long-term cost containment is most often achieved by employing a team approach and ensuring an adequate job of patient assessment, biomechanical analysis, and goal setting at the outset. Prefabricated braces are available and may meet all the requirements specified by the referring team. When a permanent custom-molded brace is the best choice, fabrication by a certified orthotist is often preferable. The American Board for Certification (ABC) in Orthotics and Prosthetics, Inc. was established in 1948 for the purpose of testing and credentialing professionals in the field. It awards the titles CO, CP, and CPO for certified orthotist, prosthetist, and prothetist-orthotist, respectively. The ABC's national office is located in Alexandria, Virginia, and may be contacted for a list of credentialed individuals in different parts of the country. (American Board for Certification in Orthotics and Prosthetics, Inc., 1650 King St., Suite 500, Alexandria, VA 22314).

### Patient Assessment

In addition to defining biomechanical problems, evaluation of the patient's individual physiology is important. Such evaluation must include a thorough assessment of the sensory status of the area to be encompassed by the brace. Accurate contouring helps distribute forces[4] but if the part to be braced has impaired sensation, additional precautions in brace construction may be necessary. Vascular status should be assessed as well. Prescription of a vacuum-formed plastic orthosis, which provides intimate skin contact, may not be appropriate in the presence of fluctuating edema.

**Table 24-2.** General Principles of Brace Construction

| |
|---|
| Ease of donning |
| Cosmesis |
| Comfort |
| Durability |
| Ease of maintenance |
| Cost containment |
| Safety |

### The Orthotic Team

With so many things to consider, orthotic prescription is best tackled by a team of experts. This team should include the physician, orthotist, therapist, *and* the patient. Far too often the patient is omitted from the orthotic team. If compliance is to be ensured, enlisting the patient in the process of goal development is essential. Too many braces are relegated to the closet because the patient was excluded from the decision making process. Ideally, prescription should be conducted in a clinic setting, where team members can openly confer and jointly assess function.

### Nomenclature

The Committee on Prosthetics and Orthotics of the American Academy of Orthopaedic Surgeons has developed technical analysis forms for orthotic prescriptions. (The four-page lower extremity assessment form is shown in Figure 24-3.) In doing so, they have effectively placed the emphasis on a sound biomechanical analysis, and led the way toward a standardized nomenclature which makes sense (Table 24-3).[5] When utilizing these forms, the type of control to be provided across the joint is indicated by a key. Therefore *A* is used to designate a mechanical assist provided to the motion in question, as with a Klenzac dorsiflexion assist ankle joint (Figure 24-4), and *L* is used to designate an optional lock, as is found across the knee joint of a Knee-ankle-foot-orthosis (Figure 24-5). In this way, emphasis is placed on anatomic location and the motion to be controlled, rather than on specific materials or the disease entity. Separate forms are available for upper and lower extremity assessment and prescription.

This approach further serves to illustrate the importance of the assessment team. Identification of specific characteristics of a disease process which may influence orthotic prescription becomes the responsibility of the physician. Detailed analysis of the pathomechanical condition to be corrected may be carried out by the therapist, while material and specific brace construction decisions are often best left to the certified orthotist.

**Table 24-3.** Abbreviations Used for the Lower Extremity Technical Analysis Form Developed by the American Academy of Orthopaedic Surgeons

| | | |
|---|---|---|
| FO | = | Foot orthosis (shoe insert) |
| AFO | = | Ankle-foot orthosis |
| KAFO | = | Knee-ankle-foot orthosis |
| HKAFO | = | Hip-knee-ankle-foot orthosis |

The first letter of the joint or anatomic region directly contained by the brace forms the abbreviation. An example of upper extremity application is WHO for wrist/hand orthosis, and in spinal orthotics a TLS is a thoracic/lumbosacral brace.

### Biomechanics

Discussion of basic biomechanical principles involved in bracing should start with a review of a few definitions of the physics involved (Table 24-4).

All orthotics function by applying an external force to a specific body part. They are often applied using the three-point principle (i.e., a single corrective force is counterbalanced by a more proximal and a more distal force, both applied in the opposing direction). Forces can be described as either compressive or distractive. Shear forces are generally to be avoided, as they typically result in friction between the skin surface and the brace. This can lead to blister formation and eventually skin breakdown. When forces across a joint are out of balance they produce motion on the joint's axis, which is termed a *moment*. Orthotic devices typically use compressive forces to stabilize or direct motion. Distractive forces are most commonly used to stretch contracted tissues.

When a force is applied to a body part, pressure results within the soft tissue intervening between the brace and the underlying skeleton. This pressure should always be kept at a minimum to avoid ischemic problems. Since pressure equals force/

**Table 24-4.** Physical Definitions

| | |
|---|---|
| Force: | Equivalent to an object's mass multiplied by its acceleration, $F = ma$. It may be thought of as a push or pull applied to a body part. |
| Pressure: | Concentration of force per unit area, $P = F/A$. A fundamental principle is to increase the area over which a force is applied in order to reduce pressure. |
| Moment: | The tendency of a force to produce rotation about an axis, $T = F \times D$ (distance). It is synonymous with the term *torque,* and is measured in newton-meters. |
| Lever arm: | The distance between the application of force and the axis of rotation. Since $F = T/D$, the greater the distance, or the length of the lever arm, the lower the force required to produce a given torque. |

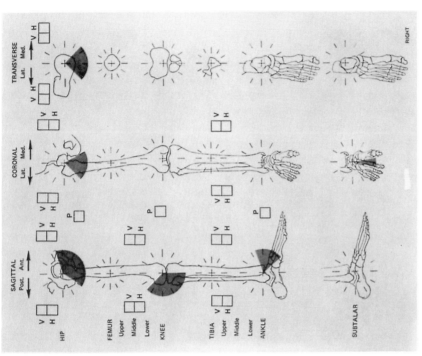

**Figure 24-3.** *A* to *D*, Technical analysis form for the lower extremity. (American Academy of Orthopaedic Surgeons: *Atlas of Orthotics*, 2nd ed. St. Louis: CV Mosby, 1985. Reproduced by permission.)

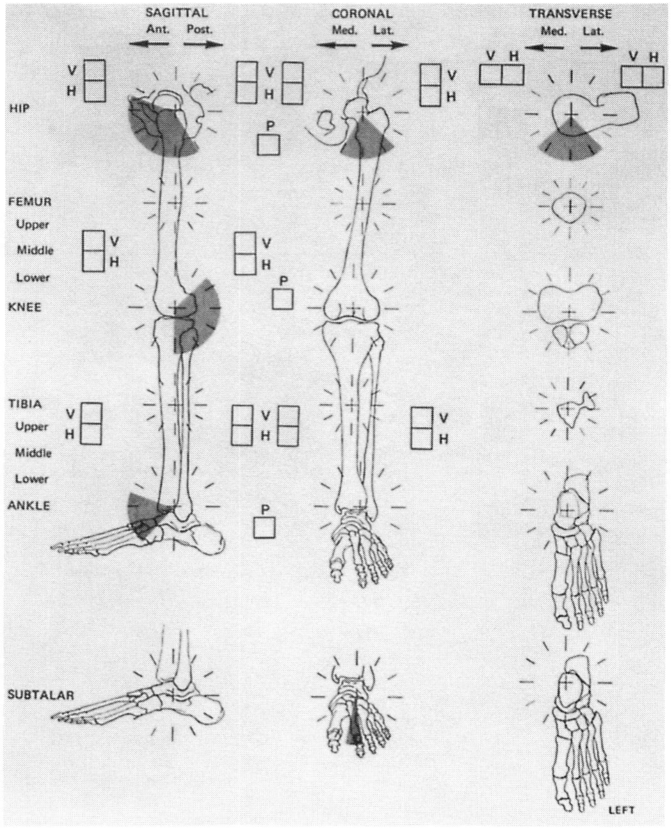

Summary of Functional Disability _____

Treatment Objectives:
Prevent/Correct Deformity ☐    Improve Ambulation ☐
Reduce Axial Load ☐    Fracture Treatment ☐
Protect Joint ☐    Other ___

**ORTHOTIC RECOMMENDATION**

| LOWER LIMB | | FLEX | EXT | ABD | ADD | ROTATION Int. | ROTATION Ext. | AXIAL LOAD |
|---|---|---|---|---|---|---|---|---|
| HKAO | Hip | | | | | | | |
| KAO | Thigh | | | | | | | |
| | Knee | | | | | | | |
| AFO | Leg | | | | | | | |
| | Ankle | (Dorsi) | (Plantar) | | | | | |
| FO Foot | Subtalar | | | | | (Inver.) | (Ever.) | |
| | Midtarsal | | | | | | | |
| | Met.-phal. | | | | | | | |

REMARKS:

Signature _____ Date _____

KEY: Use the following symbols to indicate desired control of designated function:

F = FREE — *Free motion.*
A = ASSIST — Application of an external force for the purpose of increasing the range, velocity, or force of a motion.
R = RESIST — Application of an external force for the purpose of decreasing the velocity or force of a motion.
S = STOP — Inclusion of a static unit to deter an undesired motion in one direction.
v = Variable — A unit that can be adjusted without making a structural change.
H = HOLD — Elimination of all motion in prescribed plane (verify position).
L = LOCK — Device includes an optional lock.

D

SAGITTAL    CORONAL    TRANSVERSE
Ant.   Post.    Med.   Lat.    Med.   Lat.

HIP

FEMUR Upper / Middle / Lower

KNEE

TIBIA Upper / Middle / Lower

ANKLE

SUBTALAR

LEFT

C

**Figure 24-3.** (*Continued*)

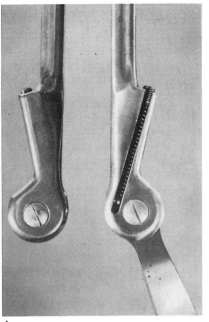

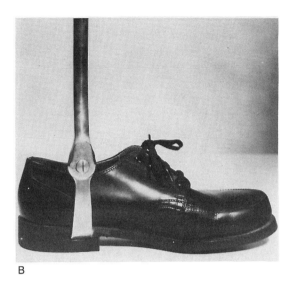

A

B

**Figure 24-4.** Klenzac dorsiflexion assist ankle joint: *A,* A posterior channel is spring loaded. The spring is compressed during heel strike which mimics eccentric function of the dorsiflexors as weight is accepted in initial stance phase. Recoil of the loaded spring aids dorsiflexion necessary for toe clearance during swing phase. *B,* Klenzac joint attached to a shoe.

area, pressure can be reduced by increasing the surface area of tissue that is in contact with the brace. This in turn is best accomplished by intimate fit and contouring of the brace surfaces. Another way to decrease pressure is by increasing the lever arm of the device. A longer lever arm decreases the force necessary to achieve a desired result.

Concern for the control of pressure warrants further consideration of underlying bony architecture. Gray makes an important distinction between functional (biomechanical or corrective) and accommodative orthoses.[6] He points out that if the underlying bony architecture does not remain flexible, attempts at correction will only lead to excessive pressure and are doomed to fail. This

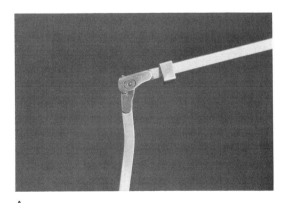

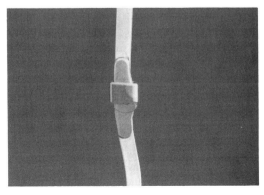

A

B

**Figure 24-5.** Knee droplock. This is commonly used to control flexion across the knee. The ring drops over the joint by gravity, or with manual assistance when the knee is fully extended. *A,* Open; *B,* closed.

fact is true for both upper and lower extremity bracing, and is especially pertinent in the arthritic condition. If the principal goals of using an orthosis are stabilization and distribution of forces, then it must typically accommodate deformities, rather than attempt to correct them. Examples would be in the weight-bearing forces of the lower extremities or the prehensile forces of the upper extremities.

### Materials

Over the last decade, metal and leather have been largely replaced by thermoplastics as the materials of choice. Thermoplastics soften when heated and harden when cooled. They are divided into high and low temperature types, depending on whether they can best be molded above or below 80°C (180°F). Low temperature thermoplastics have the advantage of being directly moldable over the patient's skin or over an intervening garment such as a stockinette or a glove. The disadvantage is less strength and durability as compared with high temperature thermoplastics. For this reason, low temperature thermoplastics are best suited to upper extremity, pediatric, and short-term orthotic use.

Among the high temperature thermoplastics, polypropylene is often the plastic of choice for lower extremity bracing because of its strength, light weight, and durability. Low-density polyethylene may be required when greater flexibility is sought, for example in upper extremity orthotics or for edema control. Co-polymer, which is polypropylene with 10% polyethylene added, offers some advantages of both high and low density thermoplastics.

In the presence of uncontrolled fluctuating edema, metal side bars (single or double uprights) are preferable for AFO construction. Aluminum is generally the material of choice for such appliances because of its qualities of high durability combined with a light weight. As the volume of an extremity changes, a form-fitting plastic brace would run an increased risk of pressure development, especially along the trimlines (edges of the brace). The use of metal upright supports can provide the necessary stability as well as spacing between the patient's limb and the brace, and accommodates a reasonable change in volume.

Compressible foams are often used to line the inside of plastic braces for improved comfort. Included among these are Pelite, Plastizote, Aliplast, and Spenco. Densities of these foams may be high or low depending on the compressibility desired (the amount of force necessary to deform the surface). Plastizote is easily moldable to the bottom of the foot and works well when used as an insert in an extra-depth shoe, for instance, to improve comfort of the arthritic foot, or the safety of a diabetic foot. Once it "bottoms out" from the pressures of weight bearing, additional layers of ⅛-inch Plastizote may be added to the base of the insert.

### Lower Extremity Bracing

Ambulation is the chief function of the lower extremities. Since the act of walking has often been described as a series of prevented catastropies,[7] problems often arise. Lower extremity bracing is most commonly prescribed to assist ambulation, but it can also be used to reduce pain, stabilize, or support body weight. Volumes have been written on lower extremity bracing alone. They cover topics as diverse as a simple shoe modification, such as with a Solid Ankle Cushion Heel (SACH heel) (Figure 24-6), to an ischial weight-bearing hip-knee-ankle-foot Orthosis. Lower extremity braces may be termed static or dynamic, depending on whether or not they incorporate movable joints. Some additional bracing principles which are specific to the lower extremity are included in Table 24-5.

Abnormal biomechanics, along with the effects of bracing, are often studied in motion analysis laboratories. Such laboratories have confirmed the belief that problems of lower extremity alignment

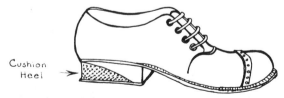

**Figure 24-6.** SACH orthosis. A compressible material is used in the posterior heel of the shoe. This provides shock absorption at heel strike, mimicking the eccentric role of the dorsiflexors during weight acceptance. These are often indicated after ankle arthrodesis, or any time sagittal plane motion across the ankle is locked by the orthotic.

**Table 24-5.** Principles of Lower Extremity Bracing

1. The normal plantar contours of the foot should be incorporated (including support of the three normal arches).
2. A subtalar neutral position of the foot should be maintained. (This generally results in a vertical or near vertical hindfoot.)
3. The foot should be positioned flat on the floor during midstance of the gait cycle.
4. All mechanical joints should be congruent with anatomic joints.
5. Metal side bars and plastic trimlines should conform to the contour of the limb.
6. Normal toe-out is approximately 15 degrees of external rotation.

during the stance phase of gait are often best addressed at the joint below (or distal) to the level of dysfunction. Once the foot contacts the floor, initiating the stance phase of the gait cycle, lower extremity posturing follows a distal to proximal progression. Abnormal pronation of the foot results in internal rotation of the tibial segment above. This may be addressed with a good biomechanical shoe insert such as a UCBL (University of California at Berkeley Laboratory) (Figure 24-7).[8]

Excessive pronation with abduction of the foot, such as is seen in the planovalgus foot of the spastic diplegic child, further leads to an increased forward tilt of the tibial segment. This occurs as the center of mass is displaced forward and the lower leg "rolls over" the medial border of the foot where the longitudinal arch has collapsed. Poor control of sagittal-plane tibial alignment in a case

such as this results in a crouched posture with exaggerated stance-phase knee flexion. In such cases, crouch control may be attained by use of a low-profile ankle-foot orthosis which incorporates a supramalleolar design (Figure 24-8). The mechanism involved is one of preventing unrestrained forward inclination of the tibia by preventing a collapse over the medial border of the foot. It requires stabilization of hindfoot valgus, restoration of the medial longitudinal arch, as well as control of external rotation of the foot on the tibial segment.

It is clear that one must understand the pathomechanics involved in each individual case. Obviously, a crouch arising from hamstring contracture would not be improved by brace prescription. When quadriceps or calf group weakness is identified as chief contributors to a crouch, or if actual buckling occurs across the knee, a floor reaction AFO (FRAFO) (Figure 24-9) may be indicated. Set in a position of plantarflexion, it creates a knee extensor moment once the foot is positioned flat on the floor during midstance. All AFOs are capable of affecting knee position without crossing the knee joint itself.

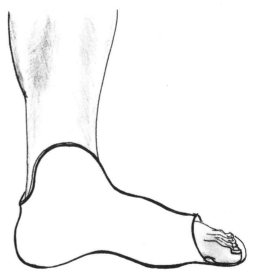

**Figure 24-8.** Supramalleolar ankle-foot orthosis. The trimlines extend above the malleoli for improved medial and lateral stability. By cutting the posterior trimline down to the superior border of the calcaneus, sagittal plane motion of dorsiflexion and plantarflexion may be left free.

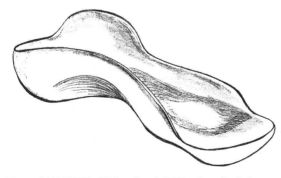

**Figure 24-7.** UCBL (University of California at Berkeley Laboratory) shoe insert is used for correction of flexible hindfoot and forefoot deformities.

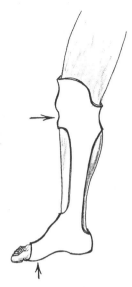

**Figure 24-9.** FRAFO—floor reaction ankle-foot orthosis. Construction characteristics include a high pretibial shell and a solid ankle joint set in mild plantar flexion (5 to 10 degrees). It provides an extensor moment to the knee joint during stance phase, by transmitting the floor reaction forces beneath the footplate to the anterior tibial shell, restricting forward translation of the tibia.

## Upper Extremity Bracing

The primary role of the proximal upper extremity is to position the hand in space so that it can best perform its functions. Because of the specialized nature of the upper extremity, and the dexterity demands placed on the hand, there are some ad-

**Table 24-6.** Principles of Upper Extremity Bracing

1. The functional position of the wrist is in approximately 30 degrees of extension.
2. Prevention of edema is of paramount importance.
3. Extensor injuries should generally be splinted in neutral (resting) position, except in burns.
4. Flexor injuries should be splinted in flexion, except in burns.
5. Avoid unnecessary immobilization.
6. Dorsal splinting interferes least with the the tactile function of the palm.
7. Volar splinting provides better support to the palmar transverse arch.

ditional orthotic principles which should be kept in mind. These are outlined in Table 24-6.

A myriad of upper extremity splint types exist. As with the lower extremity, they may be divided into two general categories, static and dynamic.

### Static Splints

Static splints for the upper extremity are most typically used to rest an inflamed joint or tendon (Figures 24-10 and 24-11). They are also used to prevent deformity following a burn or in a spastic condition. Maintaining the optimal position for healing following surgical repair is another important use.

Static splints run the gamut from a simple three-point pressure splint used to prevent hyperextension of the proximal interphalangeal (PIP)

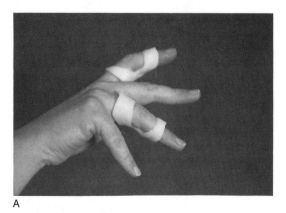

A

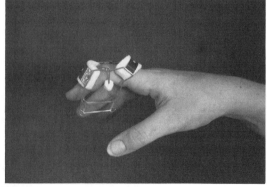

B

**Figure 24-10.** Static and dynamic splints. *A,* Static swan-neck correction splint which prevents hyperextension of the proximal interphalangeal (PIP) joint. *B,* Dynamic brace, utilizing rubber bands to actively resist hyperextension across the PIP joint.

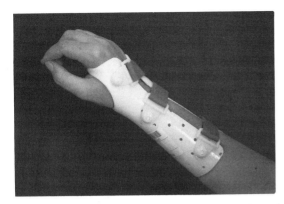

**Figure 24-11.** Static cock-up wrist splint supports the wrist in 30 degrees of extension. These may be custom molded, prefabricated with polyethylene with an open-cell foam liner, or prefabricated with a metal stay encased in a comfortable fabric with lace closure.

joint in a swan-neck deformity (see Chapter 16), to a wrist-hand orthosis which supports the wrist in an extended position of function, often referred to as a cock-up splint. It is important not to immobilize unnecessarily, especially when dealing with the upper extremities. A simple trough or gutter splint used to immobilize a single finger is preferable to taping fingers together, and a cock-up splint to immobilize the wrist should end proximal to the distal volar crease of the hand in order to avoid interference with metacarpophalangeal (MP) joint flexion.

### *Dynamic Splints*

Dynamic splints for the upper extremity (see Figure 24-10B) often employ the use of elaborate outriggers to which rubber bands or spring wires may be attached to assist or resist certain finger motions. They may of course be used solely for traction across a single joint, such as a PIP flexion traction splint which utilizes a three-point pressure system to actively move the joint into further flexion. For more detailed study, an excellent review of upper limb orthotics is included in the text *Orthotics Etcetera.*[2]

## Assistive Devices

Discussion here is limited to ambulatory aids, more specifically to those that distribute weight-bearing forces onto the upper extremity and increase the base of support during stance phase of the affected lower limb. This group of devices includes canes, crutches, and walkers.

Following acute injury or disability, gait training follows a typical progression from pregait exercises, first on the mat and then in the parallel bars, to the use of a walker or crutch walking, and finally to canes. All assistive devices should be adjusted in height so that the elbows are in approximately 20 to 30 degrees of flexion (as a general rule, these devices should be held at the level of the greater trochanter). This allows for optimal functioning of the triceps muscle group. Walkers provide maximal support and balance with a large and stable base of support. They may be wheeled (rolling walkers), or standard without wheels. Rolling walkers may be held in front of the patient, as traditionally works best for the elderly population, or they may be posterior rolling walkers (Figure 24-12). This second type works very well in children

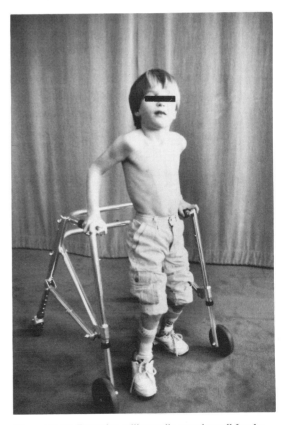

**Figure 24-12.** Posterior rolling walker works well for the pediatric cerebral palsy population to promote extension of the trunk.

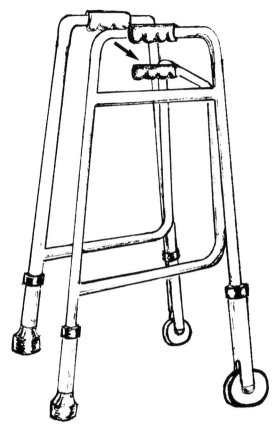

**Figure 24-13.** Hemi-walker. Assistive device typically used when only one upper extremity is functional and a wide base as well as forward support is desired. Arrow points to central support grip.

with cerebral palsy because the alignment of the handgrips is more posterior, thus promoting extension of the trunk, as opposed to the forward trunk lean often associated with front walker use. Hemi-walkers (Figure 24-13) are another style of walker. They have one hand grip mounted along the middle of the front crossbar. These devices are used in adults with hemiplegia who are limited to one functioning hand.

Crutches represent the next step in gait training, as they provide less stability than a walker. Crutch use requires stability and balance skills on the part of the patient. In turn, crutches allow for a higher level of functioning, as negotiation of uneven surfaces including ramps, curbs, and stairs is made easier. Crutches generally provide greater stability than canes, because they have two points of contact with the body. For this reason, they can

also support a greater percentage of body weight. Two general groups of crutches exist, axillary (Figure 24-14) and forearm (Figure 24-15). Axillary crutches allow for the greatest transfer of body weight off the stance-phase lower extremity. Weight, however, should be borne by the hands and not the axilla to avoid nerve damage (a space of two fingerbreaths should be left between the patient and the axillary pad of the crutch). Forearm crutches, which may have a pivoting forearm cuff (Figure 24-15) or a platform to strap into, have the advantage of being shorter and more easily transported. Functional use of the hands is greatest when a pivoting cuff is used, as in the aluminum forearm orthosis (Canadian crutch). A platform crutch (Figure 24-16) is often prescribed if the hands or

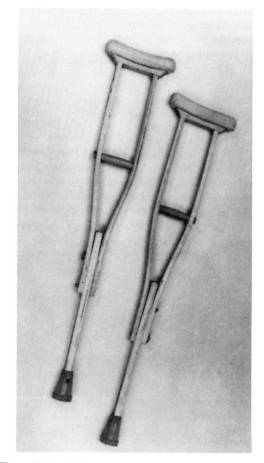

**Figure 24-14.** Axillary crutches. Because contact with the ground is limited to a single point for each crutch, they more easily adapt to uneven terrain and stairs. They also, however, require greater coordination on the part of the patient.

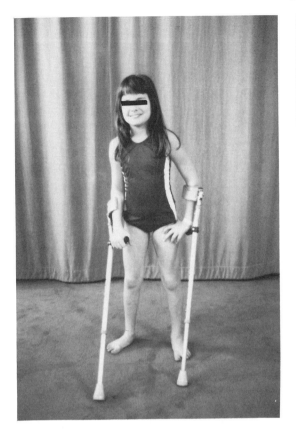

**Figure 24-15.** Forearm crutches, with forearm cuff.

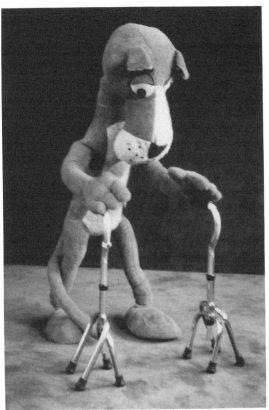

**Figure 24-17.** Low-profile quad cane.

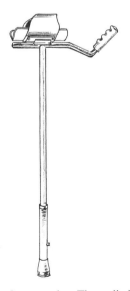

**Figure 24-16.** Platform crutches. These eliminate weight-bearing stresses across the joints of the hand and wrist. They are often useful in the arthritic population.

wrists are unable to accept weight-bearing stress, which is common among those with arthritis.

Canes are typically used in patients who require the least amount of assistance or relief from lower extremity weight-bearing forces. Straight canes represent the simplest design. They consist of a straight shaft with a single point of contact with the floor and a handle at the top. Many varieties of handles exist, ranging from a simple curved top to a plastic grip which is form-fit to the hand and adjustable for comfort of the weight-bearing angle of the wrist.

Addition of extra legs to the base of a cane provides greater stability by increasing the base of support. In a quad cane this is accomplished through the addition of four legs to the base. Different styles of quad canes are available, allowing one to choose from either a narrow or wide base. They may also be termed high or low profile depending on whether the legs originate close to the ground (low profile) (Figure 24-17) or di-

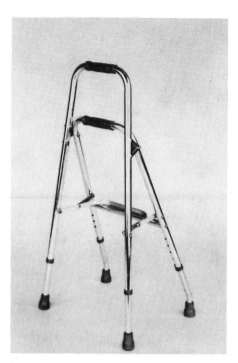

**Figure 24-18.** Hemi-cane is held to the side by the uninvolved upper extremity.

rectly from the shaft itself, up higher off the ground (high profile).

A hemi-cane (Figure 24-18) (sometimes termed a pyramid cane) also has four legs and is free-standing. It generally folds and differs from a walker by its ability to be held by one hand and off to the side. Like all canes, it is held in the hand opposite the affected lower extremity to allow for a more efficient shift of the center of mass toward the sound side.

## Points of Summary

1. When complex pathomechanics are involved, orthotic prescription is best tackled by a team approach.
2. Thermoplastics have become the materials of choice for most orthotics. They are not appropriate in all situations, and metal and leather are still useful in some circumstances.

3. Many prefabricated orthotics are available for both the upper and lower extremities. When custom molding of a permanent orthosis is needed, the patient should be referred to a certified orthotist.
4. Prescription of an appropriate assistive device depends on the amount of weight-bearing relief and balance assistance sought, as well as the status of upper extremity function.

## References

1. Redford JB (ed): *Physical Medicine and Rehabilitation: State of the Art Reviews* 1987;1(1):1–10.
2. Redford JB (ed): *Orthotics Etcetera,* 2nd ed. Baltimore: Williams & Wilkins, 1980:vii.
3. Cusack BD: *Progressive Casting and Splinting for Lower Extremity Deformities.* Tucson, AZ: Therapy Skill Builders, 1990:213–218.
4. Stoner EK: Orthotics. In Krusen FH (ed): *Handbook of Physical Medicine and Rehabilitation,* 2nd ed. Philadelphia: WB Saunders, 1971:97–114.
5. McCollough NC: Biomechanical analysis systems for orthotic prescription. In Bunch WH (ed): *Atlas of Orthotics,* 2nd ed. St. Louis: CV Mosby, 1985:34–75.
6. Gray G: Taking It to the Top: A Progressive Seminar in Abnormal Foot Biomechanics and Related Proximal Dysfunction, October 1989, Course Syllabus, pp 80, 125.
7. Wilson AB: *Lower Limb Orthotics.* Philadelphia: Moss Rehabilitation Hospital, pp. 1–20.
8. Henderson WH, Campbell JW: UCBL Shoe Insert: Casting and Fabrication, University of California Berkeley Laboratory, Technical Report Series, No. 53, August 1967:1–22.

## Suggested Readings

Hislop, H (ed): *Principles of Lower Extremity Bracing.* Alexandria, VA: American Physical Therapy Association, 1967.
Kottke FJ, Lehmann JF (eds): *Krusen's Handbook of Physical Medicine and Rehabilitation,* 4th ed. Philadelphia, WB Saunders, 1991:580–592.
Redford, JB (ed): *Orthotics Etcetera,* 2nd ed. Baltimore: Williams & Wilkins, 1980.
Redford, JB (ed): *Physical Medicine and Rehabilitation, State of the Art Reviews* 1987;1(1).

# Chapter 25
# Chronic Pain

PHILLIP R. BRYANT

Chronic pain is one of the more challenging experiences encountered by clinicians. Typically, the chronic pain syndrome is described as long-standing (usually greater than 6 months), with non-specific or multiple pain complaints and often with no definite identifiable etiology. It is accompanied by a prolonged or persistent maladaptive behavioral response to actual or perceived pain. Pain permeates every aspect of the lives of those suffering from this syndrome. It often affects the lives of those with whom they work or live as well, usually in a disruptive fashion. These individuals focus on their pain to the exclusion of other aspects of their lives.

Treating chronic pain requires the focused efforts of an interdisciplinary team, including the primary physician, physician consultants, psychologists, social workers, and physical/occupational therapists. It is important that the patient's family members are involved in both the short- and long-term management strategies. Not only is it important to identify the appropriate participants on the team, it is also imperative that the team be closely coordinated. This helps ensure that disjointed therapy or repeated trials of ineffective care are avoided.

Chronic pain patients often have multiple factors impacting directly or indirectly on their symptoms. In addition to their subjective pain, they invariably suffer distress or other psychological pain. Their social and vocational interactions may also play a prominent role in perpetuating their symptoms. Dysfunctional family units and lack of family support, secondary gain, use of pain as an avoidance behavior, loss of a job or career opportunities, and financial hardships all adversely affect the patient's coping skills. An interdisciplinary team with insight into these complex interactions is necessary if optimal management is to be achieved.

## Physiology of Pain

Skin, subcutaneous tissues, and internal organs are innervated by a variety of sensory receptors. Some carry very specific information about tissue damage and localization of pain, while others carry more general information to the spinal cord and brain. In the spinal cord the afferent message of pain is modulated and sent to the thalamus and cerebral cortex. All along this path of transmission the incoming information is modified by other afferent inputs, by the state of arousal, and by the emotional state of the person.

In acute pain the incoming information alerts the subject to what is happening. In more chronic states the information is less specific and begins to interact to a greater extent with the emotions.

Pain sensation is transmitted over both fast and slow nerve fibers. The fast fibers provide information about the precise location and intensity of nociception. Slow fibers carry messages of a more diffuse nature.

It is unclear why some people develop chronic pain. There may be subtle changes in the way their nervous systems process incoming nerve signals; there may be emotional or sleep disorders; there may be secondary gain. In any case, chronic pain does occasionally develop, sometimes after seemingly trivial injury.

### Rationale for the Treatment of Pain

In 1965 Melzack and Wall proposed their gate control theory of pain.[1] They postulated that messages of slow pain could be blocked at the spinal cord level by stimulating other nerve fibers, for instance through touching or rubbing. While the original theory has been modified, the basic principles may still be valid. Various forms of treatment, ranging from massage to transcutaneous electrical nerve stimulation, are prescribed on the presumption that they help to "block" the gate to pain.

When pain is a long-standing problem it begins to affect the emotions, sleep cycle, and personality of the sufferer. Often the original trauma or disorder that triggered the pain is healed while the pain persists. This chronic pathologic pain process cannot be treated by healing a specific site of injury, such as a back strain, since the injury is no longer the primary cause of pain. Lasting relief cannot be obtained with narcotic medications either. Instead, a multifaceted approach must be used to help restore emotional health, proper sleep, return to normal daily activities, and to break the pattern of pain behavior. What follows are descriptions of some of the therapeutic interventions used to treat pain.

## Therapeutic Modalities

### Transcutaneous Electrical Nerve Stimulation

Electrical stimulation was first used therapeutically by the Egyptians who used electric eels to treat headaches and gout.[2] Transcutaneous electrical nerve stimulation (TENS) is usually used with high-frequency, low-intensity electrical stimulation. The basis for using low-intensity stimulation is to selectively activate the low-threshold (larger) cutaneous fibers. High frequency is used because it has been found to be more effective.[3]

Another alternative TENS technique utilizes low-frequency, high-intensity stimulation. This is felt to be effective by raising the levels of endogenous opiates in the central nervous system.

Transcutaneous stimulation is a noninvasive, safe modality. It is the most popular and practical means of providing therapeutic electrical stimulation, although direct implantation of electrodes on the nerves has been used in selected cases. When using a TENS unit, an electrical stimulus is delivered by means of electrode pads. The intent is to stimulate large, fast-conducting afferent nerve fibers. These fibers "block the gate" of the slower-conducting pain fibers. In some cases TENS application provides long-term relief of pain.

A number of different electrode pads are available for use with TENS. They include self-adhesive and electroconductive pads, as well as carbon rubber and small button electrodes. The electrodes are typically used with an electroconductive gel. Allergic responses to either the pads or the gel sometimes occur.

TENS has been applied in both acute and chronic pain conditions. It has been used with variable success in acute and chronic low back and neck pain, phantom limb pain, and diabetic neuropathy. Other conditions warranting a trial of TENS include reflex sympathetic dystrophy, peripheral vascular disease, postoperative pain, postherpetic neuralgia, osteoarthritis, and rheumatoid arthritis. It has also been used during labor, although its use in this capacity has not been definitively established to be safe. Until formally proved safe, it is advisable to avoid electrode placement over any part of the abdomen during pregnancy.

There are a number of contraindications to the use of TENS. These include avoidance of use in patients with pacemakers and in those with cardiac arrhythmias or other cardiac disease unless cleared by the patient's primary physician or cardiologist. Additional precautions include avoidance of electrode placement in the area of the carotid sinus or mouth, and over rashes, broken skin, infected sites, or anesthetic regions.

### Heat

Heat is generally prescribed to improve blood flow to an affected area, decrease discomfort, enhance relaxation, and/or prepare patients for range of motion or soft tissue therapy. It is delivered in various forms, including moist hot packs, infrared lamps, whirlpool, paraffin baths, diathermy, and ultrasound.

Heat produces the following physiologic responses: increased blood flow, increased metabolic activity, decreased body fluid viscosity, increased extensibility of collagen tissue, and alteration of pain threshold. Heat appears to have an analgesic effect in some cases and may reduce muscle spasm and joint stiffness. It also has a sedative effect on some patients.

Heat therapy, of course, does carry the risk of burns. For this reason, it should not be administered in those patients who are incapable of recognizing or responding to heat-induced tissue damage, such as unconscious or mentally incompetent patients. Even patients without cognitive deficits may be unaware they are developing a burn injury until the damage has been done, or they may fall asleep during the heat application and not have it removed in sufficient time to prevent injury. It is important, therefore, to always be alert to the possibility of burn injury anytime heat therapy is administered.

### Cryotherapy

Cryotherapy may be applied in the form of ice, cold water, vaporizing liquids, vapocoolant sprays, refrigerated units, or chemical packs. It has been used with substantial success in the acutely injured patient, particularly for swollen joints and acute muscle spasms. It is prescribed primarily to help reduce the swelling associated with edema and hemorrhage, while simultaneously providing a local analgesic effect. Cryotherapy is also said to reduce tissue compartment pressures following trauma. In addition, metabolic activity is reduced locally at the site of application. If such therapy is sustained or sufficiently cold, systemic cooling and reduction of metabolic activity also occur. Cooling is also useful in inhibiting clonus and spasticity.

Cryotherapy has been used with notable success in chronic back pain. It is reportedly at least as effective as moist heat and TENS application in offering relief to patients with chronic low back pain.

It should, as a general rule, be avoided over prominent nerves; at ischemic sites; in the presence of cold intolerance, Raynaud's phenomenon and disease, and cold allergy; and with insensate skin.[4]

### Acupuncture

Although acupuncture is not routinely prescribed or even universally accepted as a viable mode of treatment, it is at least worth mentioning. It is well established that the Chinese instituted the practice of acupuncture over 2500 years ago. Like spinal manipulation, it has its staunch advocates and equally adamant skeptics.

It is unclear what the mechanism of action of acupuncture is in relieving pain. One hypothesis, based on the gate control theory, purports that acupuncture stimulates large sensory afferent fibers and suppresses pain perception. An alternate hypothesis recognizes that acupuncture needle insertion may be a noxious stimulus. This stimulus, in turn, may result in the production of endogenous, opiate-like substances which offer variable degrees of pain relief.[5] The fact that acupuncture analgesia is reversed by naloxone and by hypophysectomy supports this idea.[6] Placebo effects are also a probable mechanism of action. It is interesting to note that acupuncture sites, myofascial trigger points, and muscle motor points share a similar distribution.

Acupuncture has been used with apparent success in a wide variety of painful conditions, including chronic pain syndromes. It can be performed as a dry needle technique, or it can be coupled with an electric stimulator (electroacupuncture).

### Biofeedback

Biofeedback provides immediate feedback information to a patient by the use of devices which amplify muscle action potentials, assess galvanic skin resistance, continuously monitor skin temperature, or detect changes in pulse, blood pressure, and respiratory rate. Both auditory and visual feedback can be provided. By creating this feedback from body functions not normally under conscious control, it allows the patient to develop such control. The goal is to train the patient to voluntarily self-regulate abnormal physiologic states which may be contributing to the chronic pain symptoms. Biofeedback is perceived as an active method in pain management because patient participation is required.

### Therapeutic Exercises

Chronic pain patients typically engage in little or no formal or regular exercise. They are often not motivated to perform exercises, ostensibly due to their pain. Some are openly defiant at any attempt to institute such a program on the assumption that it will only exacerbate their pain. Despite this challenge, it is important that the interdisciplinary team involved in caring for this group of patients understand that gently progressive mobilization is critical to helping these patients return to an active lifestyle and in preventing the complications of immobilization and deconditioning. Work hardening programs have become a popular and often effective means of preparing patients to return to their occupation in an appropriate physical condition.

Chronic pain patients often complain of some exacerbation of their symptoms after initiating an exercise program. This is expected in patients who have been immobilized and deconditioned for extended periods of time. These patients require reassurance and encouragement to initiate and continue the exercise activity. Occasionally a particular form or intensity of exercise may truly aggravate the patient's condition. Careful serial assessment to detect objective evidence of injury, particularly musculoskeletal problems such as joint or tendon swelling, is necessary to ensure that a given exercise program is not causing complications. Again, close cooperation and communication between physicians and therapists is vital and improves the likelihood that the chronic pain patient will cooperate successfully in an aerobic conditioning program. The goal is to assist the patient in improving general physical strength and endurance. Perhaps of greater importance are the goals of improving the patient's sense of well-being, self-esteem, and confidence. This invariably helps these individuals to better cope with their chronic pain symptoms.

### Behavior Modification

In selected cases, a formal behavioral modification program may be the most effective means of addressing the chronic pain syndrome. It is based on the principle of operant and respondent conditioning, and is designed to alter the perception of pain and to reduce pain behaviors. Such a program may be especially useful in those patients whose lifestyle and home and work environment serve to perpetuate maladaptive behavior. An inpatient interdisciplinary behavioral modification program, coupled with a gradually progressive physical reconditioning program, improves one's chance of providing lasting therapeutic benefit for this group of patients. The primary goal of such a program is to improve the patient's ability to cope with pain, not necessarily to completely alleviate it. The program usually involves establishing a contract for each therapeutic intervention anticipated. For example, a physical and/or occupational therapy contract should indicate what type, duration, and intensity of exercises are expected over the course of the program. There is particular emphasis on providing positive reinforcement of appropriate coping behavior. On the other hand, there is a neutral response or negative reinforcement for chronic pain complaints or behavior.

### Psychological Counseling

It is important to be aware of the spectrum of psychological disturbances often experienced by chronic pain patients. These include sleep disturbances, alterations in appetite, decreased libido, decrease in physical activity with associated deconditioning, resentment, anger, depression, and anxiety. With progressive worsening and persistent symptoms, somatic preoccupation, withdrawal from social interaction, and feelings of helplessness and hopelessness, as well as dependency on narcotic medications may develop. Despite a sense of anger and resentment for health care providers who appear ineffective in "curing" their pain, these patients often develop a dependency on the medical system. Psychological counseling is an important component in their treatment.

## Medications

Medications effective in treating acute pain, such as nonsteroidal antiinflammatory drugs (NSAIDs) and narcotic analgesics, are typically ineffective in treating chronic pain. Narcotics lead to drug dependence which exacerbates the personality change in chronic pain and worsens pain behavior. When possible, the chronic pain patient should be kept off all drugs. Occasionally sleep disturbance can be treated with tricyclic antidepressants, and at times adjuvant medications such as anticonvulsants are used to help treat the pain. In special cases, such as reflex sympathetic dystrophy, ganglion block or antiadrenergic medication is also useful.

## Chronic Pain Conditions

### Fibromyalgia

Fibromyalgia (see Chapter 20) is characterized by sleep disturbance and chronic, diffuse, poorly localized discomfort. Proper rest and relaxation maneuvers, balanced nutrition, aerobic conditioning activities, physical therapeutic modalities, nonsteroidal analgesics, and tricyclic antidepressants have been used with variable success for this condition.

### Reflex Sympathetic Dystrophy

Reflex sympathetic dystrophy (RSD) refers to the burning pain which occasionally occurs after nerve injury or trauma (see Chapter 16). It has been attributed to hyperactivity of the sympathetic nervous system. The patient may develop muscle atrophy, hyperhidrosis, vasotropic changes of the affected extremity digits, local hair loss, and bone demineralization. In early treatment it is particularly important to institute physical therapy for gently progressive range of motion and strengthening exercises. This is accompanied by NSAIDs and a desensitization program. Sympathetic nerve blocks with a local anesthetic may also be effective.

### Phantom Limb Pain

Phantom pain has been attributed to deafferentation and subsequent neuronal hyperexcitability after a limb amputation. It is usually localized to a selected region of the amputated limb. Multiple therapeutic modalities including TENS, cryotherapy, desensitization, local anesthetic injections, acupuncture, and hypnosis have been tried with variable success. Tricyclic antidepressants, anticonvulsants, nonsteroidal antiinflammatory medications, and chlorpromazine have all been tried, also with variable success.

### Postherpetic Neuralgia

Postherpetic neuralgia is felt to be due to a reactivation of latent varicella virus. Viral inflammation occurs at the level of the dorsal nerve root and ganglion. It causes a severe, paroxysmal burning, aching, and/or lancinating pain in the distribution of the affected nerve. The pain is often intractable. Treatment with oral steroids, amantadine, vidarabine, alpha-interferon, levodopa, adenosine monophosphate, clomipramine, carbamazepine, and tricyclic antidepressants have all been attempted with relief in some but not all patients.[7] Capsaicin has been applied topically with some success as well, although significant pain relief may be delayed up to 3 or 4 weeks. Additional interventions with varying benefits include TENS and epidural steroid injections. Nerve blocks and cryoanalgesia are usually limited to transient relief only.[7]

### Cancer Pain

Cancer pain can present with a broad spectrum of intensity from mild to unbearable. The pain may be intermittent or continuous. Treatment usually requires the input of multiple disciplines and must be individualized to achieve optimal pain relief. Narcotic medications remain the drugs of choice for relief of intractable pain due to cancer. It is important that these patients have access to recreational therapy and retain, if practical and feasible, independent functional skills, endurance, and strength so that their quality of life can be preserved for as long as possible.

## Conclusion

Care of chronic pain patients is a challenging, labor-intensive effort. There is an increased recognition that beyond the physical symptoms, multiple psychosocial factors and behavioral components contribute to the chronic pain syndrome. Multiple disciplines, including physical and occupational therapists and psychologists, play a critical role in providing properly administered and timed therapeutic intervention. When therapists, physicians, and other members of the interdisciplinary team coordinate their efforts, the potential for a successful outcome is greatly enhanced.

## Points of Summary

1. Chronic pain is a condition that encompasses emotional, behavioral, and psychological disturbances, not just physical injury.
2. The gate control theory of pain helps to provide a rationale for many current modalities used in treating pain.
3. Chronic pain must be treated with an interdisciplinary approach to address the complex behavioral and emotional issues it involves.
4. TENS units are useful in treating some patients with chronic pain.
5. Standard pain medications, especially narcotics, are to be avoided in the chronic pain patient.

## References

1. Melzack R, Wall P: Pain mechanisms: A new theory. *Science* 1965;150:971–979.
2. Frampton V: Transcutaneous electrical nerve stimulation and chronic pain. In Wells PE, Frampton V, Bowsher D (eds): *Pain Management in Physical Therapy*. Norwalk, CT: Appleton & Lange, 1988:89.
3. Bowsher D: Modulation of nociceptive input. In Wells PE, Frampton V, Bowsher D (eds): *Pain Management in Physical Therapy*. Norwalk, CT: Appleton & Lange, 1988:30–36.
4. Basford JR: Physical agents and biofeedback. In DeLisa JA (ed): *Rehabilitation Medicine: Principles and practice*. Philadelphia: JB Lippincott, 1988:265–266.
5. Walsh NE, Dumitru D, Ramamurthy S, Schoenfeld LS: Treatment of the patient with chronic pain. In DeLisa JA (ed): *Rehabilitation Medicine: Principles and practice*. Philadelphia: JB Lippincott, 1988:716.
6. Mehta M: Current views on non-invasive methods in pain relief. In Swerdlow M (ed): *The Therapy of Pain*, 2nd ed. Lancaster, England, MTP Press, 1986:123–125.
7. Gershkoff AM: Pain in neuropathy. *Physical Medicine and Rehabilitation: State of the Art Reviews* 1991;5(1):57–58.

## Suggested Readings

King JC, Kelleher WJ: The chronic pain syndrome. *Physical Medicine and Rehabilitation: State of the Art Reviews* 1991;5(1):165–186.

Walsh NE, Dumitru D, Ramamurthy S, et al.: Treatment of the patient with chronic pain. In DeLisa JA (ed): *Rehabilitation Medicine: Principles and Practice*. Philadelphia: JB Lippincott, 1988:708–725.

# Chapter 26

# Fitness for Life: The Role of Exercise in Treating and Preventing Illness

LOIS P. BUSCHBACHER
RALPH BUSCHBACHER

In recent decades there has been a surge of interest in exercise and fitness. Simultaneously, medical research has begun to identify the benefits of being fit with regard to disease prevention, treatment of particular diseases, and effects on quality of life and longevity. Exercise benefits the cardiovascular, skeletal, and metabolic systems. In addition, it aids in weight control, affects weight distribution and appearance, and lends to a sense of well-being. Probably most importantly, it enables the individual to better meet the normal demands of everyday living.

## Fitness

One can find numerous definitions which describe fitness. Many of these describe a certain quality of life. The President's Council on Physical Fitness, for instance, defines a fit person as one who is able to perform vigorous work without undue fatigue and yet have energy left over for avocational pursuits.[1] Other definitions of fitness are more quantitative and include measures of muscle strength and endurance, body composition, flexibility, and cardiovascular-respiratory capacity.

## Muscle Strength and Endurance

Strength is defined as the maximum force (torque) that can be exerted by a muscle. This force is proportional to the cross-sectional area of the muscle. Therefore, the individual with the largest muscle girth is able to generate the greatest absolute force. Other factors, however, contribute to functional strength. These include the synchrony of motor unit firing (see Chapter 2), learning, hormonal levels, and psychotropic factors.

Muscle strength may be measured in three ways: isotonic, isometric, and isokinetic. Isotonic (constant tension) movement is performed when muscle is used to move a joint in an arc at unchanging torque. Torque, however, changes with body position and muscle length, even with a constant weight. Thus using free weights and most weight machines is not true isotonic exercise. Cam-varied resistance, utilized in some weight machines, such as Nautilus, compensates for body position and muscle length effects and more closely matches a true isotonic exercise.

An isometric (constant length) contraction is static; the joint does not move (though the muscle shortens slightly). An example is holding a baby in one's arms or pushing against a wall. Heavy weight training approximates isometric exercise.

Isokinetic (constant speed) exercise is when the joint moves through an arc at an unchanging speed, regardless of the muscle tension involved. There are special machines, such as Cybex and LIDO, which allow for this type of movement, and these are sometimes used therapeutically.

When a muscle shortens it is called a concentric contraction, and when it allows itself to lengthen it is called an eccentric contraction. An example of this would be a biceps curl. As the elbow bends, the contraction is concentric and as it straightens it is eccentric. For more extensive information on these exercises and their therapeutic use see Chapter 7.

Isotonic exercise is best used in demonstrating the concept of strength and endurance. Maximum strength is the maximum weight that can be moved through an arc one time only (1RM). When the weight is decreased it can be moved through the arc more times. The number of times the motion can be repeated is a measure of endurance.

In the early post–World War II period De-Lorme and Watkins developed a method for gaining strength.[2] This is known as the DeLorme technique. One first determines the 10 repetition maximum (10RM) of the individual. This is the maximum amount of weight that the subject can lift ten times. The program then consists of three sets of lifting the weights. In the first set, one lifts 50% of the weight ten times. This is followed by lifting 75% of the weight ten times, and finally 100% of the weight ten times. Another method for strengthening is the Oxford method in which one does ten repetitions at the 10RM weight, then ten repetitions at 75% of that weight, and finally ten repetitions at 50% of the weight. There are other variations of these programs as well.[3]

When a strengthening program is undertaken, gains in the amount of weight that can be lifted are seen within the first 6 weeks. This is not initially accompanied by hypertrophy of the muscle. Electromyographic studies have shown that there is, however, improvement of muscle firing synchrony.[4] Thus functional strength improves even before muscle mass increases. With continuation of the activity there is an enlargement of the existing muscle cells, called hypertrophy. New cell growth occurs,[5] but it is not generally believed to contribute significantly to the increase in muscle mass.[6]

A sex difference is notable in strength training. This is due to the effects of androgens, such as testosterone, which are found in higher levels in males as compared with females. Women do increase strength and muscle mass with weight training, just not to the same extent as men do.

Muscular endurance is the ability of a given muscle to perform an activity repetitively at submaximal load. Endurance exercise is the alternating use of large muscle groups such as the pelvic and thigh muscles and is performed to improve the functioning of the cardiovascular and respiratory systems. In general, endurance type exercise is what has been studied for its effects on health and disease. Strength training, while perhaps desirable to improve function and physique, does not seem to have as much of an overall health benefit as endurance training. What follows is an overview of some of the beneficial aspects of exercise on health.

## Hypertension

Hypertension is a disease affecting up to 25% of the American population. It is a risk factor for atherosclerotic and cardiovascular disease including myocardial infarction and stroke. It often goes undetected, as there are few symptoms associated with mild to moderate elevations in blood pressure. Routine blood pressure screening is recommended, and an elevated blood pressure must be found on three separate occasions for the diagnosis to be made. Mild hypertension is defined as a diastolic pressure ranging from 90 to 104; moderate is from 105 to 114, and severe is 115 or more.

Two basic types of hypertension exist: essential (or idiopathic) and hypertension due to a discernible cause such as renal artery stenosis or pheochromocytoma. The majority of people have essential hypertension and in 70% or more it is mild.

Endurance exercise at moderate intensity is felt to benefit individuals with mild-moderate essential hypertension.[7,8] These people can sometimes decrease their systolic and diastolic blood pressures, perhaps by about 10 mmHg, with moderate exercise. When one is diagnosed as having mild hypertension, the first line of treatment can be conservative and nonpharmacologic. That is, an aerobic exercise program is prescribed along with other lifestyle changes including weight loss (if needed), behavioral modification, cessation of smoking, reduction of alcohol intake, and diet changes. If this fails, then pharmacologic treatment may be instituted. In moderate hypertension medication is usually prescribed initially along with the other modifications noted above, including exercise. Exercise may in some cases allow a reduction or discontinuation of the medication at a future date. Severe hypertension usually requires medical as well as behavioral and exercise changes.

The American College of Sports Medicine recommends that aerobic exercise done at 60% to 85% percent of maximal heart rate be done three to four times a week for 20 to 60 minutes in normotensive adults.[9] There is some evidence that exercise near the upper limit of this range of heart rate may actually worsen hypertension;[10] thus exercise of moderate intensity, possibly with a target heart rate range of 50 to 65 is probably most beneficial in the hypertensive patient. Also, isometric exercise, to which heavy weightlifting is similar, causes sometimes marked increases in blood pressure during the exercise and may cause a sustained rise in blood pressure as well. It is thus usually not recommended in the hypertensive patient. Lighter weight/higher repetition and circuit weight training may be safer in hypertensive individuals who wish to pursue some strength training.

The mechanism by which moderate-intensity endurance exercise lowers blood pressure is not yet fully understood, although some believe that it acts by lowering serum catecholamine levels. This theory, as well as how other lifestyle factors and medications interact with exercise, needs further study. Also needing further study is the possibility that exercise testing may be used as a screening tool to identify persons who will later develop hypertension. Early investigation into this area shows promise.[11]

When medications are used to treat hypertension, they often include diuretics, angiotensin converting enzyme inhibitors, beta-blockers, or calcium channel blockers. Of these, the angiotensin converting enzyme inhibitors are probably the best to use in the exercising patient.[12] The calcium channel blockers are also without major contraindications. Diuretics should only be used with caution, as they may cause dehydration and hypokalemia which could be worsened with endurance exercise. The beta-blockers can reduce exercise

tolerance, increase fluid loss, and may cause hyperkalemia.[13,14] They are usually to be avoided in the exercising patient as well.

### Atherosclerosis and Ischemic Heart Disease

Atherosclerosis is the accumulation of fatty plaque in blood vessels which causes a progressive narrowing of the interior of the vessels. This narrowing is particularly dangerous in the vessels of the heart and brain, but also affects the peripheral vasculature. When the narrowing reaches a critical level in the heart, one finds symptoms of ischemic heart disease, such as angina pectoris. Myocardial infarction occurs if the cells of the heart die from lack of oxygen. In the cerebral vessels atherosclerosis can cause thrombotic or embolic strokes. In thrombotic cerebrovascular accident (CVA) a clot disrupts blood flow, and in an embolic event a piece of atherosclerotic plaque (or other mass) dislodges and moves "downstream" to cause a blockage of blood flow. Peripheral vascular disease, a narrowing of the arteries supplying the legs, causes symptoms of claudication and may progress to gangrene and necrosis of the limb. All of these conditions are significant factors of morbidity in Western society. Exercise, as well as other lifestyle changes, can play an important role in preventing them.

The mechanism of action by which exercise helps prevent atherosclerosis is still not completely elucidated, although it does appear to affect some of the risk factors for atherosclerosis. Hypertension is a risk factor, and as already described, exercise may reduce blood pressure. Aerobic exercise also helps in lowering total cholesterol while raising high-density lipoproteins (HDL) with an overall increase in the HDL/low-density lipoprotein (LDL) ratio.[15] Some research indicates that a subfraction of HDL, $HDL_2$, which is thought to be a particularly good inhibitor of atherosclerotic plaque, is enhanced with exercise.[16]

When an exercise program is undertaken, there are predictable changes seen in the heart and vascular system as well as in muscle. Aerobic (endurance) exercise increases the body's maximum ability to take up oxygen, $\dot{V}O_2max$. This is thought to be due to an increase in cardiac output and an increased ability of skeletal muscle to extract oxygen. In high-intensity aerobic exercise there is an increase in left ventricular chamber size which allows for an increase in stroke volume.[17] There also appears to be an increase in myocardial blood supply due to an increase in coronary artery diameter. An increase in myocardial capillary density has been found in exercising animals.[18] Another adaptation to exercise is a lowering of the resting heart rate. This is thought to be due to increased parasympathetic nervous system activity.

Studies which look specifically at whether or not the changes described above are beneficial are difficult to do in humans for ethical and methodologic reasons. However, epidemiologically, those who exercise aerobically on a regular basis do have an increased life expectancy with decreased mortality and less risk of coronary heart disease.[19,20] It can be appreciated that exercise may help prevent ischemic heart disease, but even in the person with established disease, there is still a role for exercise. Exercise and diet changes have been shown to decrease exercise-induced cardiac ischemia in monkeys,[21] and cardiac rehabilitation programs have been shown to improve function in humans with atherosclerotic heart disease.[22] In such patients exercise is optimally accompanied by improvement of diet and other lifestyle changes. Similarly, patients with peripheral vascular disease and claudication can make functional improvements with an exercise program. Whether the disease is to some extent reversible is unknown. There is currently no evidence that exercise prevents stroke or stroke recurrence, but by its general cardiovascular effects it would certainly seem to be beneficial and almost certainly does no harm.

A detailed description of a cardiac or peripheral vascular rehabilitation program is beyond the scope of this chapter. Interested readers are referred to the references at the end of this chapter. It would most likely be advisable that all individuals who have not yet developed atherosclerotic disease or symptoms engage in an exercise program similar to that described for hypertension.

## Diabetes

There are two basic types of diabetes: type I, also known as insulin dependent diabetes mellitus (IDDM), and type II, or non-insulin dependent diabetes mellitus (NIDDM). Both are metabolic disorders in which blood glucose levels are not properly controlled. In IDDM there is an absolute deficiency of insulin, the substance which reduces blood glucose levels and helps cells that need glucose ingest it. This almost always occurs in children, and necessitates supplementation with insulin in all cases. NIDDM occurs most often in adults. In these patients insulin levels are often elevated and peripheral cell insulin receptors are thought to be insensitive to the circulating insulin. These receptors are found on cells including adipocytes (fat cells), muscle cells, and liver cells. Type II diabetics usually have a strong family history of NIDDM and are often obese. They can mostly be treated with oral hypoglycemic medication to reduce blood glucose levels. In this chapter we focus on type II diabetes and the role of exercise in its prevention and treatment. Exercise has little effect on type I diabetics except that by burning calories it may decrease insulin requirements.

Aerobic exercise increases the sensitivity of the receptors on the end-organ cells to insulin, probably as a reaction to glycogen depletion in those cells.[23] Insulin binding to the cells is thus enhanced and may reduce or eliminate the need for medication to control blood glucose levels. Exercise also helps in weight control, and since obesity is felt to be a risk factor for NIDDM, it may aid in prevention of the disease.

When first diagnosed, diabetes may be treated conservatively with a program of exercise and diet modification. The exercise prescription should be for endurance exercise and is tied to a program of patient education. Often patients also require treatment with oral medication. Oral hypoglycemics increase the sensitivity of cell receptors to insulin and may increase secretion of insulin by the pancreas. If they are not successful in treating the disease then insulin shots are sometimes necessary. Care must be taken in the diabetic on oral medication as well as one receiving insulin shots not to cause an excessive drop in blood glucose levels. Such a drop may occur several hours after vigorous exercise; thus exercise in the evening is to be avoided so as not to cause hypoglycemia at night while the patient is sleeping.

The diabetic patient is at risk for numerous complications. These include retinopathy, renal failure, neuropathy, hypertension, and accelerated atherosclerosis. Whether or not exercise helps reduce the risk for these associated conditions is unknown.

## Obesity

Obesity is most practically defined as weight greater than 20% over ideal body weight. It is associated with an increased risk of cardiovascular disease and metabolic disease as well as increased risk of osteoarthritis. Height and weight scales are frequently used in general practice to determine obesity, but percentage of body fat is actually more predictive of the risks of the condition.

Obesity is a common occurrence in the United States; up to 25% of the population is obese. One only needs to watch television or pick up a magazine to see the myriad diets, exercise programs, and fads directed at obese individuals to appreciate how much of a problem obesity is in our society. Obese people often try to lose fat and most do, but the majority who lose it by diet or fad do so temporarily and later regain their previous weight. This section deals with the role of exercise in treating obesity.

Obviously, body weight is determined by caloric intake and energy usage. When more calories are taken in than are used up, weight increases. Dieters usually try to lose weight by attacking the intake part of the equation, but what may happen during dieting is that the body conserves energy instead of expending it. Thus weight loss is slow, difficult, and may be temporary. Some researchers believe that there is a body-fat set point, much like a thermostat, which attempts to keep body fat constant. People can try to fight their set point and may win temporarily, but over the long haul they usually fail. What may be instrumental in losing weight permanently is to move the set point to a new level, and it is in this resetting process that exercise may be most beneficial.

When dieting, the body's basal metabolic rate decreases. This reduces baseline energy consumption and is one reason why sustained weight loss is difficult to achieve with dieting alone. Exercise, on the other hand, tends to have a sustained effect of raising the basal metabolic rate.[24] This, in addition to the calories utilized by the exercise itself, helps bring about a slow, steady weight loss. The sustained increase in metabolic energy expenditure becomes a nearly permanent state in a regularly exercising individual. Thus exercise, even without dieting, can bring about a loss of body weight. When the exercise is combined with dieting, the opposing effects on resting metabolic rate tend to cancel each other out and the metabolic rate tends to stay constant.[25] This holds true mainly for a moderate reduction in caloric intake. If the diet is severe enough, it may simulate starvation, and metabolic rate drops.

As one exercises, changes in body composition occur. Exercise tends to favor a loss of body fat while increasing lean body mass.[26] Since lean body mass is more metabolically active than fatty tissue, it tends to increase baseline energy consumption even further. However, in order to maintain these body changes, physical activity must be continued.

Exercise, not dieting alone, brings about a more sustained loss in weight.[27] Thus when treating obesity, one ideally combines a moderate caloric restriction with modest aerobic activity. Long-term adherence to this change in lifestyle is necessary, and behavioral adaptations may be required. Patients must be advised that regular exercise brings about a slow, sustained loss of fat. The loss of fat is maintained for as long as regular exercise is continued. Dieting, without exercise, is probably worthless as a way to lose weight permanently. The type of exercise recommended varies with the interests and abilities of the patient. In general, any endurance exercise is beneficial, although swimming, whatever its other benefits, has been shown not to be a particularly effective way to lose weight.[28]

## Osteoporosis

Osteoporosis is a common disease found primarily in postmenopausal white and Oriental women. It is associated with considerable morbidity and mortality and is a major health issue among the elderly. The greatest complication of osteoporosis is bone fracture, the most common being vertebral, radial (Colles'), and hip fractures. Osteoporosis can be due to medical diseases such as hyperthyroidism, chronic obstructive pulmonary disease, Cushing's disease, or malabsorption syndrome. It may also be caused by drugs such as anticonvulsants, glucocorticoids, or heparin. However, at least 80% of people with osteoporosis have no known cause. This section discusses the role of exercise in prevention and treatment of primary osteoporosis. Further discussion of the topic can be found in Chapter 23 on women's issues.

Osteoporosis is defined as a decrease in absolute volume of normal bone matrix and mineral. With this decrease comes an increased fragility of bone with susceptibility to fracture. The bone loss is primarily from trabecular bone, and must be fairly advanced to be detectable on routine radiographs.

Bone density peaks between the ages of 30 and 35. Thereafter, there is a slow, steady decline in density. In women the decline becomes more rapid once menopause is reached and estrogen levels drop.

Risk factors for osteoporosis include being female, being white or Oriental, having a lean body build, alcohol ingestion, cigarette smoking, nulliparity, prolonged amenorrhea, low calcium intake, and possibly excessive caffeine ingestion.

Stressing bone, usually by weight-bearing activity but also by some other activities, improves skeletal health. Bone is constantly remodeling itself to better be able to tolerate the stress. Thus inactivity, as found in the bedridden patient or with casting, or weightlessness in astronauts results in a loss of bone mass. Activity, on the other hand, increases bone mass, usually in the bones involved in bearing the body's weight but also sometimes in other bones that are stressed (such as in a tennis player's arm) or in bones that are far removed from the stressor.[29,30] Intermittent bone compression, not static loading, appears to be necessary to increase bone mass.[31]

This information leads one to conclude that weight-bearing activity can prevent osteoporosis. There is one caveat for women, however. With extreme activity there may be a decrease in estrogen production which effectively negates the benefits of loading the bones. Women who exercise to the point of developing amenorrhea are creating a situation similar to the postmenopausal state. And even women who do not develop amenorrhea may be causing a hypoestrogenic state with excessive exercise. On balance, however, exercise appears to be of benefit to the majority of women. When an exercising woman develops amenorrhea it is inappropriate to automatically blame the condition on the exercise. These women deserve a full medical evaluation to rule out other potentially harmful causes of the condition.

The exercise prescription which should be recommended to increase bone mass and to prevent its loss is weight-bearing activity such as walking, jogging, or aerobics. The activity should be undertaken at least three times a week (preferably more) for 30 to 60 minutes. Swimming, an otherwise excellent aerobic activity, does not significantly affect bone mass and therefore is not recommended as prophylaxis for osteoporosis. It would make sense to recommend an overall weight training program to increase bone mass in non-weight-bearing bones, although studies proving such a benefit have not yet been done. Young women should exercise to increase their bone mass before it starts to decline. In the postmenopausal woman weight-bearing exercise appears to slow down the loss of bone mass. More studies need to be done to fully determine how much effect such exercise has and whether it augments estrogen supplementation. Most likely exercise is able to prevent or reverse osteoporosis only partially. Adequate calcium intake and postmenopausal estrogen replacement are probably required as well, at least in some women.

### Exercise and a Sense of Well-Being

It is generally accepted that exercise improves one's sense of well-being. There are numerous subjective reports of this in both the clinical and the lay literature, and much has been written about the "runner's high." In 1984 the National Institute of Mental Health conducted a workshop dealing with exercise and its effects in both the healthy population and in those with mental illness. The consensus was that:[32]

1. Physical fitness is positively associated with mental health and well-being.
2. Exercise is associated with the reduction of stress emotions such as state anxiety.
3. Anxiety and depression are common symptoms of failure to cope with mental stress, and

exercise has been associated with a decreased level of mild to moderate depression and anxiety.

4. Long-term exercise is usually associated with reductions in traits such as neuroticism and anxiety.

5. Severe depression usually requires professional treatment, which may include medication, electroconvulsive therapy, and/or psychotherapy, with exercise as an adjunct.

6. Appropriate exercise results in reduction in various stress indices such as neuromuscular tension, resting heart rate, and some stress hormones.

7. Current clinical opinion holds that exercise has beneficial emotional effects across all ages and in both sexes.

8. Physically healthy people who require psychotropic medication may safely exercise when exercise and medication are titrated under close medical supervision.

These principles are still valid today. Although it is generally accepted that vigorous exercise is associated with an improved sense of well-being, the mechanism is poorly understood.

It may be that exercise increases the serum levels of antidepressant neurotransmitters, endogenous opiates, or that it simply distracts participants from their usual worries.[32] It may also reduce muscle tension and help regulate the sleep cycle. Whatever the mechanism, it does seem to work. Future investigation is needed to tell us exactly why.

Most studies on the effects of exercise on well-being involve aerobic type activity, yet there are subjective reports that strength training also produces a sense of well-being and even euphoria. In the film *Pumping Iron*, Arnold Schwarzenegger reports that he finds the sensation of "the pump" during weightlifting equivalent to orgasm. This is yet another area which may deserve further investigation.

## Points of Summary

1. Moderate-intensity aerobic exercise may help to control mild to moderate essential hypertension.

2. Intense exercise and heavy weightlifting may be contraindicated in hypertensive patients.

3. Exercise improves the HDL/LDL ratio to one more favorable to prevent coronary artery disease.

4. Aerobic exercise may help to control non-insulin dependent diabetes, probably by increasing the sensitivity of cell receptors to insulin.

5. Aerobic exercise increases the basal metabolic rate and favors a loss of body fat.

6. Regular weight-bearing exercise may help in preventing osteoporosis, at least to some extent in some women. It is probably most effective when combined with adequate calcium intake and estrogen replacement therapy.

7. Regular exercise leads to an improved sense of well-being.

## References

1. President's Council on Physical Fitness: *Adult Physical Fitness: A Program for Men and Women*. Washington, D.C.: U.S. Government Printing Office, 1979.

2. DeLorme TL, Watkins AL: Techniques of progressive resistance exercise. *Arch Phys Med Rehabil* 1948;29:263–273.

3. deLateur BJ, Lehmann JF: Therapeutic exercise to develop strength and endurance. In Kottke FJ, Lehmann JF (eds): *Krusen's Handbook of Physical Medicine and Rehabilitation*, 4th ed. Philadelphia: WB Saunders, 1990:480–519.

4. Moritani T, deVries HA: Neuronal factors versus hypertrophy in the time course of muscle strength gain. *Am J Phys Med* 1979;58:115–130.

5. Gonyea WJ, Sale DG, Gonyea FB, et al.: Exercise induced increases in muscle fiber number. *Eur J Appl Physiol* 1986;55:137–141.

6. Tesh PA: Skeletal muscle adaptations consequent to long-term heavy resistance exercise. *Med Sci Sports Exerc* 1988;20:S132–S134

7. Hagberg JM, Seals DR: Exercise training and hypertension. *Acta Med Scand Suppl* 1986;711:131–136.

8. Tipton CM, Matthes RD, Marcus KD, et al.: Influences of exercise intensity, age, and medication on resting systolic blood pressure of SHR populations. *J Appl Physiol* 1983;55:1305–1310.

9. American College of Sports Medicine: *Guidelines for Graded Exercise Testing and Exercise Prescription*. Philadelphia: Lea & Febiger, 1990.

10. Tanji JL: Hypertension. I. How exercise helps. *Phys Sports Med* 1990;18:77–82.

11. Tanji JL, Champlin JT, Wong GY, et al.: Blood pressure recovery curves after submaximal exercise: A predictor of hypertension at ten-year follow up. *AJH* 1989;2:135–138.

12. Tanji JL: Exercise and the hypertensive athlete. *Clin Sports Med* 1992;11:291–302.

13. Gordon NF, Kruger PE, Van Rensburg JP, et al.: Effect of β-adrenoceptor blockade on thermoregulation during prolonged exercise. *J Appl Physiol* 1985;58:899–906.

14. Gordon NF, Van Rensburg JP, Russell HMS, et al.: Effect of beta-adrenoceptor blockade and calcium antagonism, alone and in combination on thermoregulation during prolonged exercise. *Int J Sports Med* 1987;8:1–5.

15. Williams PT, Krauss RM, Wood PD, et al.: Lipoprotein subfractions of runners and sedentary men. *Metabolism* 1986;35:45–52.

16. Haskell WL: The influence of exercise training on plasma lipids and lipoproteins in health and disease. *Acta Med Scand Suppl* 1986;711:25–37.

17. Maron BJ: Structural features of the athletic heart as defined by echocardiography. *J Am Coll Cardiol* 1986;7:190–203.

18. Ljunqvist A, Unge G: Capillary proliferative activity in myocardium and skeletal muscle of exercised rats. *J Appl Physiol* 1977;43:306–307.

19. Paffenbarger RS Jr, Hyde RT, Wing AL, et al.: Physical activity, all-cause mortality, and longevity of college alumni. *N Engl J Med* 1986;314:605–613.

20. Powell KE, Thompson PD, Caspersem CJ, et al.: Physical activity and the incidence of coronary heart disease. *Annu Rev Public Health* 1987;8:253–287.

21. Kramsch DM, Aspen AJ, Abramowitz BM, et al.: Reduction of coronary atherosclerosis by moderate conditioning exercise in monkeys on an atherogenic diet. *N Engl J Med* 1981;305:1483–1489.

22. Brammel HL: Rehabilitation of the cardiac patient. In DeLisa JA (ed): *Rehabilitation Medicine: Principles and Practice.* Philadelphia: JB Lippincott, 1988:671–687.

23. Bogardus C, Thuillez D, Ravussin E, et al.: Effect of muscle glycogen depletion on in vivo insulin action in man. *J Clin Invest* 1983;72:1605–1610.

24. Thompson JK, Jarvie GJ, Lahey BB, et al.: Exercise and obesity: Etiology, physiology, and intervention. *Psychol Bull* 1982;91:55–79.

25. Donahoe CP Jr, Lin DH, Kirschenbaum DS, et al.: Metabolic consequences of dieting and exercise in the treatment of obesity. *J Consult Clin Psychol* 1984; 52:827–836.

26. Hill JO, Sparling PB, Schields TW, et al.: Effects of exercise and food restriction on body composition and metabolic rate in obese women. *Am J Clin Nutr* 1987;46:622–630.

27. Dahlkoetter J, Callahan EJ, Linton J, et al.: Obesity and the unbalanced energy equation: Exercise versus eating habit change. *J Consult Clin Psychol* 1979; 47:898–905.

28. Gwinup G: Weight loss without dietary restriction: Efficacy of different forms of aerobic exercise. *Am J Sports Med* 1987;15:275–279.

29. Jones HH, Priest JD, Hayes WC, et al.: Humeral hypertrophy in response to exercise. *J Bone Joint Surg* 1977;59A:204–208.

30. Dalen N, Olsson E: Bone mineral content and physical activity. *Acta Orthop Scand* 1974;45:170–174.

31. Camay A, Tschantz P: Mechanical influences in bone remodeling: Experimental research on Wolff's law. *J Biomechanics* 1972;5:173–180.

32. Morgan WP: Affective beneficence of vigorous physical activity. *Med Sci Sports Exerc* 1985;17:94–100.

## Suggested Readings

Bjorntorp P, Krotkiewski M: Exercise treatment in diabetes mellitus. *Acta Med Scand* 1985:217:3–7.

Bouchard C, Shepard RJ, Stephens T, et al. (eds): *Exercise, Fitness, and Health: A Consensus of Current Knowledge.* Champaign, IL: Human Kinetics Books, 1990.

Drinkwater BL: Osteoporosis and the female athlete. In Sutton JR, Brock RM (eds): *Sports Medicine for the Mature Athlete.* Indianapolis: Benchmark Press, 1986: 353–359.

Morgan WP: Affective beneficence of vigorous physical activity. *Med Sci Sports Exerc* 1985;17:94–100.

Pollock ML, Wilmore JH: *Exercise in Health and Disease: Evaluation and Prescription for Prevention and Rehabilitation,* 2nd ed. Philadelphia: WB Saunders, 1990.

Tanji JL: Exercise and the hypertensive athlete. *Clin Sports Med* 1992;11:291–302.

# Chapter 27

# Musculoskeletal Issues in Persons with Physical Disability

SHARON GEER RUSSO

Lengths of stay for patients in trauma and rehabilitation centers are becoming shorter because of changes in health care delivery along with technologic and pharmaceutical advances in medical management. Many of these individuals benefit from continued rehabilitative services as outpatients in their community. Mandates for improving societal accommodations through assistive technology and removal of physical barriers will increase the number of physically disabled citizens who are active in the community. Persons with physical impairments may then face new risks for musculoskeletal injury related to the demands of their increased levels of activity. As a result of these changes, community based physicians and therapists may see more individuals with physical disability for ongoing rehabilitation needs along with musculoskeletal concerns secondary to their primary diagnosis.

There are numerous texts and articles that include detailed discussions of physical disabilities and their specific complications (see Suggested Readings at the end of the chapter). Rather than providing a diagnosis-specific review, this chapter attempts to provide the community based physician and physical and occupational therapists with a conceptual framework for analyzing the musculoskeletal issues in the postrehabilitation individual. To correctly evaluate the patient's musculoskeletal complaint, the practitioner must understand anatomic and kinesiologic influences on the involved region as it functions following disability. Different physical impairments require unique strategies for achieving movement. The evaluation approach must include a systematic survey of the biomechanical requirements for movement in combination with the more global assessment of factors such as level of physical dependence, availability of assistance, cognitive and motivational abilities to comply with prescribed treatments, and financial resources to procure necessary therapy or assistive technology. These "nonmedical" considerations are critical to the successful medical management of the musculoskeletal problem, which cannot be treated successfully in isolation from the primary disability.

This model for musculoskeletal assessment is illustrated by applying it to several of the more common complications seen in individuals living with spinal cord injury, stroke, and traumatic brain injury. Possible causative factors related to the context and biomechanics of the individual's movement requirements are explored as a basis for discussing treatment options. Although examples are limited to these three diagnoses, the reader is challenged to apply this level of analysis to other neurologic and orthopedic disabilities that may be encountered in community practices.

## Impact of Physical Disability on the Musculoskeletal System

### Anatomic and Kinesiologic Influences on Function

The practitioner examining an individual with a primary physical disability who presents with a secondary musculoskeletal complaint must determine whether the complaint is a result of recent trauma or the cumulative effect of disability-altered anatomy and kinesiology.

**Joint Alignment.** Impaired neuromuscular control may change joint alignment at rest and during movement due to paralysis or weakening of the muscular components of joint function. A classic example of this is the painful subluxing hemiplegic shoulder. Lack of muscular activity in the flaccid shoulder, or the abnormal resting lengths of spastic muscles, combine with the effects of gravity and positioning to contribute to glenohumeral subluxation.

**Synergistic Force Couples.** Normal synergistic force couples may no longer exist to provide for balanced muscular control of joint stability or motion. The "winging scapulae" of the individual with C5 tetraplegia illustrates the impact of serratus anterior paralysis on the intricate balance of muscle forces in the shoulder girdle. Central nervous system damage may also change the relative activation levels of synergist and antagonist muscles across a joint. Reduced input from any muscle that contributes to normal movement alters the demands on the remaining muscles and in some way affects their motor performance.

**Passive Elastic Properties.** The passive elastic properties of the musculotendinous unit are often restricted following physical disability. This can be due to sarcomere reduction or passive muscle shortening in response to inadequate muscle lengthening stimuli. This is observed when a muscle remains in a shortened position for prolonged periods and results in contracture. Neurologic injury may limit active motion or create an imbalance of muscle activity between opposing muscles around a joint. Neurogenic muscle shortening may then be compounded by the passive effect of gravity on the resting limb, reduced passive stretch effected by weight bearing, and avoidance of discomfort associated with the lengthened position. As a result, weak muscle groups may be further handicapped by having to work against the passive resistance of shortened antagonist muscle(s). This can affect joint excursion as well as speed and efficiency of movement.

**Muscle Performance.** To accomplish a functional task, one must be able to initiate the planned movement, appropriately vary its speed and force, then inhibit or turn off the muscle activity to allow the moving part to change direction or perform the next task. Any or all of these criteria for functional movement may be compromised in individuals with neurologic disabilities. Impaired motor control, whether a result of spasticity, sensorimotor processing problems, or central motor planning deficits, interferes with task performance and may lead to excessive joint stress or soft tissue irritation. In addition, denervation and disuse atrophy reduce the muscle strength available to carry out the planned motions, thus exacerbating the stressors on the muscle fibers remaining.

### Context of Movement

Rehabilitation following a disabling condition emphasizes the relearning of movement to maximize independent function. Motor reeducation seeks to facilitate the return of motor and sensory function to normalize movements for functional use. In many cases, however, this return may be slow or incomplete. The individual must then learn to move about and manipulate the environment using new movement skills to compensate for the impairment. Thus the context of movement, the structural requirements of the neuromuscular and skeletal systems, is often drastically altered from what the individual has known premorbidly. The musculoskeletal system's ability to tolerate the demands of this new mobility over the years often determines the extent to which the person is able to continue functioning at this new level of independence.

*The Upper Extremity: When the
Manipulator Becomes the Mobilizer*

Nonambulatory individuals, such as those with spinal cord injury, suddenly find themselves dependent on their upper extremities for most environmental interactions: mobility, postural stability, as well as the usual, but possibly compromised, manipulation of objects for activities of daily living. While the hip joint's configuration and congruity, along with its thick ligamentous support, provide optimal stability for weight-bearing functions, the shoulder complex is primarily stabilized by muscular forces. Its anatomic structure is simply not designed to assume the weight-bearing functions of the pelvic girdle without some risk of musculoskeletal trauma. The upper extremity is best suited for open chain functions: movements of a free distal extremity on a fixed or stabilized shoulder girdle and thorax.

*Functional Demands on the
Musculoskeletal System*

The mobility demands of the person with a spinal cord injury, or similar impairment, challenge the shoulder girdle to perform in a closed chain weight-bearing capacity for transfers, bed mobility, postural stability, pressure relieving lifts, and bracewalking if appropriate. This necessitates uncustomary co-contractile strength and motor control to support and mobilize the body's weight on the distally fixed upper extremity. Muscles are called upon to perform reverse actions, now pulling the bony origin toward the insertion. In lifting the body on the arms for a transfer, for example, the anterior deltoids pull from their origin along the lateral clavicle to assist in pulling the shoulder girdle and, through muscular linkages, the thorax forward to raise the hips from the seat surface.

Any disability which affects the balance of muscle forces around the shoulder, either directly by impairment or indirectly through selective hypertrophy, potentially leads to musculoskeletal complaints. Of particular importance to the examining practitioner (because of the potential for corrective intervention) are imbalances created through functional hypertrophy. By identifying muscular imbalance and the activities that have caused one muscle group to be stronger and possibly less flexible than its opposing counterpart, the clinician and the individual can develop strategies to regain a proper balance. This alone may correct joint and soft tissue alignments to resolve the musculoskeletal dysfunction. A case study later in this chapter illustrates this concept.

*Quality of Movement*

Movement in a disabled individual may exhibit poor control in either force production or gradation, joint translation, or velocity of motion. The effort needed to coordinate movement may be increased due to spastic hemiplegia or asymmetric denervation. The individual often comments on how heavy the involved limbs feel and how quickly fatigue becomes a factor in movement efficiency. Often there is excessive co-contraction, in place of smooth reciprocating activity, between agonist and antagonist muscle groups. Thus, excessive energy expenditure, abnormal joint alignment, increased joint compression forces, slowed velocity, and impaired coordination result.

One aspect of movement which does not change following a disability is the constant force of gravity. The musculoskeletal system affected by disability, however, may not be able to counteract gravitational effects on movement or joint alignments. Progressive postural deformities and associated discomfort develop if not properly addressed.

## Musculoskeletal Evaluation
of the Person with Physical Disability:
Practical Considerations

For the practitioner who has limited contact with neurologically disabled clients, there are a few unique considerations to be given to the medical management of this population.

*Office Accessibility*

If the office environment is not accessible to patients with impaired mobility due to physical or sensory disabilities, the practitioner may wish to seek out the services of a consultant who is familiar with accessibility issues, specifically as related to the requirements of the Americans with Disabilities Act (ADA). Persons with disability must often exert a great deal of effort, physically and logistically, to arrive at the physician's or therapist's office, so it is important that avoidable obstacles do not hinder their access to these services. It is important to ensure that the facility's waiting areas, examination rooms, hallways, and bathrooms welcome the mobility-impaired patron.

### Patient Handling Techniques

Once inside the examining room, the patient may require special consideration during the examination process. If the individual is in a wheelchair, the practitioner may benefit from beginning the examination while the patient is still in the wheelchair. Seating posture, functional mobility skills, and their demands on the region of musculoskeletal complaint should be observed. If the evaluation necessitates patient transfer onto an examination table, the practitioner will make great strides toward patient rapport and trust by asking the patient to explain what assistance is required and if there are any precautions to be heeded. Many individuals will be able to transfer independently or only need supervision for safety in the unfamiliar setting. Others may require maximal to total physical assistance, at which time proper body mechanics and additional manpower should be enlisted. The presence of spasticity should be given special consideration. Spasticity, if not anticipated, may create additional physical demands during movement of the patient. The individual should be able to inform the clinician of the intensity and direction of spasticity patterns, what stimulates them, and the best method of minimizing their effect. Avoiding sudden movements when handling the patient often minimizes the severity of the spasticity and reduces the chance of injury to all involved.

### Evaluation Methods

Some of the evaluation methods typically employed during the musculoskeletal examination may require an additional level of care in the presence of neurologic dysfunction. Passive range of motion and joint mobility testing of paralyzed extremities should be done cautiously in light of potential osteoporosis or soft tissue impingement. Manual muscle testing in muscles exhibiting the influence of spasticity (increased deep tendon [muscle stretch] reflexes, increased resistance to passive movement, or impaired volitional movement control) remains of questionable validity.[1] The ability to identify accurately the source of pain complaints may be impeded by altered conduction or processing of sensory stimuli.

As with all patients, much can be learned through the skillful patient interview. Questions related to recent changes in activity, assistive devices, perceived level of function, and even personal care attendants may provide insight into factors contributing to the presenting musculoskeletal complaint.

### Examples of Musculoskeletal Issues in Physical Disabilities

Rather than listing musculoskeletal problems specific to individual diagnoses, this section is organized around structural dysfunctions that often cross diagnostic categories. Case examples drawing from clinical experience with three neurologic populations: spinal cord injury (SCI), cerebrovascular accident (CVA), and traumatic brain injury (TBI) are used to illustrate the conceptual framework presented earlier.

### Muscle Imbalance Around a Joint

Unbalanced activity in muscles contributing to a particular joint's movement and stability may result in trauma, dysfunction, and discomfort at the joint or in the surrounding muscle or soft tissue. This imbalance can be caused by (1) spasticity; (2) asymmetric neurologic recovery; (3) varying degrees of denervation of musculature surrounding a joint (due to different spinal levels of muscular innervation); and (4) functional hypertrophy of muscle groups that serve a primary role in patient mobility and simultaneous weakness in muscles playing a less active role. The individual may seek medical attention for a variety of pathologies resulting from chronic muscular imbalance. Changes in joint and soft tissue alignment due to muscular imbalance may assist in clarifying the diagnosis.

*Neurogenic Musculoskeletal Imbalance*

Spasticity preferentially affecting one muscle group surrounding a joint, unopposed muscle activity created by asymmetric motor recovery, and partial innervation of a joint's musculature can all create an imbalance impacting on motor control at that joint. If not addressed appropriately, the spastic or predominating muscle can quickly become shortened, resulting in soft tissue contractures and joint malalignments. Decreases in passive elasticity of the musculotendinous unit make normal joint alignment difficult and, in some cases, painful.

> *Case Study:* Ambulation in a patient with a CVA is complicated by increasing gastrocnemius spasticity on the involved side. His swing phase of gait is characterized by absent propulsion at toe-off (despite apparent hyperactivation of the plantarflexors), inadequate dorsiflexion for toe clearance, equinovarus posturing of the foot, along with additional deviations proximally. Stance on this limb begins with absent heel strike, the foot contacting the ground along its lateral border, and poor translation of the tibia over the foot due partially to gastrocnemius and soleus resistance to passive ankle dorsiflexion. One of the most visible results of this complex series of events at the ankle is hyperextension of the knee at midstance.

Analysis of the muscle function and biomechanics related to this hemiplegic gait pattern reveals that the knee hyperextension is not a direct result of the gastrocnemius contractile activity pulling the knee into extension. Rather it is caused by an abnormal torque being created at the knee because of the plantarflexed position of the ankle (Figure 27-1). Proprioceptive and protective sensation is often compromised, so the patient may not complain of pain. One would expect increases in ligamentous instability, lack of articular integrity, and associated pain resulting from chronic knee hyperextension; however, longitudinal studies of such changes in this population are lacking.

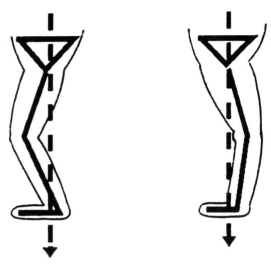

**Figure 27-1.** (*Left*) At midstance, with normal ankle dorsiflexion range, a knee flexion moment is created. (*Right*) With limited dorsiflexion, a knee extension moment results.

There may be several factors involved in knee hyperextension in the patient with hemiplegia. In addition to ankle plantarflexion just described, this individual may be hyperextending the knee volitionally to improve its perceived stability when muscular control of the loaded knee is inadequate. By use of an adequate biomechanical assessment and through systematic trials of various interventions (e.g., orthotics, biofeedback, motor retraining), the clinician must determine how best to normalize joint alignment to reduce potentially destructive joint stresses and improve ambulatory function. A detailed study of gait and orthotic management in the hemiplegic population is beyond the scope of this chapter; the interested reader is referred to the reading list at the end of the chapter.

*Functional Muscular Imbalance*

Muscular imbalance resulting from functional hypertrophy is an indirect result of the primary disability. Hypertrophy of the anterior shoulder and chest musculature, for example, often occurs in wheelchair users. These muscles become hypertrophied and shortened as they are under constant stress to produce the forces required to propel a wheelchair, along with being prime movers in other activities such as transfers. Posterior shoulder and scapular muscles, such as rhomboids, posterior deltoids, and middle trapezius, though active, may become relatively weaker than their anterior counterparts. In situations where there is increased demand on these posterior muscles, they may suffer muscle spasms and pain related to muscle fatigue.

> *Case Study:* A T10 paraplegic presents 7 years post-injury with palpable tender nodules along the spinal border of the right scapula. Postural examination reveals thoracic kyphosis, forward shoulders with abducted scapular position, and excessive cervical lordosis. Flexibility is limited by tight pectorals and anterior deltoids. She reports that she has been active in wheelchair basketball for years and is now participating in competitive wheelchair tennis. She is right-hand dominant. Strength testing of her posterior shoulder and scapular muscles reveals muscle strength in the 4− to 4+ range (see Chapter 11). Anterior muscle groups are normal.

After a thorough evaluation, the clinical hypothesis was that this patient's tennis stroke had created new demands for muscular force output and endurance in the scapular muscles on the right. During tennis, her upper extremity moved into marked shoulder extension, abduction, and scapular retraction. The weaker posterior muscles contracted against the resistance of the tight anterior muscles, leading to muscle fatigue and painful muscle spasms. She was instructed in a program of stretching for the tight muscles and low-load, high-repetition, antigravity strengthening for the posterior musculature. Within several weeks, her symptoms resolved, and she was able to resume competitive wheelchair tennis.

### Skeletal Complications

#### Postural Abnormalities

When the patient reports pain in the axial musculature of gradual onset that is exacerbated by activity or upright positions, a careful assessment of postural alignment may reveal potential sources of the complaint. If abnormal posture is observed, one must determine if the deformity is fixed or flexible in order to initiate the appropriate intervention. A flexible deformity can be corrected either actively by the patient or passively through manipulation by the examiner. A fixed deformity cannot be corrected and thus requires compensatory interventions.

The source of the problem and the site of intervention are often in the configuration of the wheelchair. The wheelchair configuration, for any patient, is critical to avoiding mechanical pain syndromes caused by improper postural alignment. To interact with the environment, the wheelchair-seated individual assumes a posture that affords a horizontal gaze. If positioned in a wheelchair in which the seat is horizontal to the floor and meets the back at an angle of 90 degrees, the person with impaired trunk control will have difficulty maintaining an upright posture. This individual typically scoots the hips forward in the chair, requesting assistance if needed. This sacral-sitting posture moves the trunk's center of mass posterior to the hips to provide trunk stability. A postural chain of events beginning with a posterior pelvic tilt, lumbar flattening, thoracic kyphosis, and eventually cervical lordosis is created to achieve horizontal gaze. Prolonged sitting posture of this nature may result in sacral decubitus ulcers and cervical or low back pain.

Lateral deviations such as pelvic obliquities and scoliosis can be caused by asymmetric trunk muscle activity as seen in CVA, TBI, or incomplete SCI patients. If not muscular, the cause may be related to skeletal asymmetries such as leg length discrepancies in the ambulatory patient. Pelvic obliquities due to fractures or surgical procedures involving the ischial tuberosities or overlying soft tissue may also be a cause of deviations.

The guiding principles in managing any of these postural deviations are to correct flexible deformities and to compensate for those that are fixed. Correction of abnormal anterior-posterior spinal curves in the nonambulatory individual can occur through appropriate wheelchair configuration. Wheelchair designs have advanced to offer great adjustability for postural tilt-in-space so that horizontal gaze can be maintained (Figure 27-2). Various buildups can be incorporated into the seat cushion design to correct or compensate for pelvic

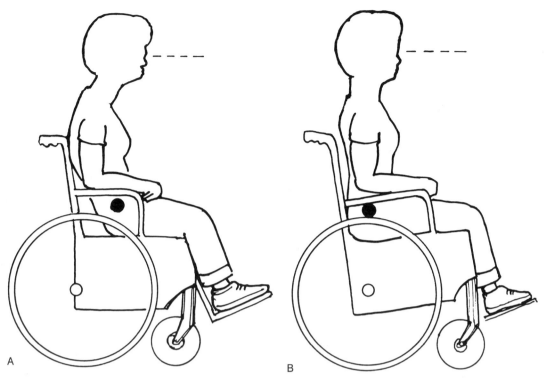

**Figure 27-2.** *A*, In a person with impaired trunk control in a standard wheelchair, horizontal gaze and postural stability are attained at the expense of poor postural alignment. *B*, In an adjustable tilt wheelchair, horizontal gaze and trunk stability can coexist with good postural alignment.

obliquities. After positioning the pelvis in a position of neutral tilt, one can determine the need for external lateral supports. However, proper pelvic position and gravitational assist through a slight posterior tilt of the chair is often all that is needed to ensure functional sitting balance in the wheelchair. The patient and caregivers should ensure that the proper sitting position is maintained. A properly configured seating system is only effective if the individual is properly positioned in the wheelchair.

*Osteoporosis, Pathologic Fractures,
and Heterotopic Ossification*

These skeletal complications are mentioned to alert the primary physician and treating therapists to the increased risk of posttraumatic skeletal injury in patients with neurologic impairments. Ragnarsson reports that osteoporosis, the loss of bone mass due to a negative calcium balance, occurs during the first 6 months following SCI in all bones below the level of the lesion.[2] This loss of bone mineral content in persons with SCI, which Biering-Sorenson reports as averaging 25% below normal in the femoral neck and shaft and 50% below normal in the proximal tibia, predisposes these individuals to pathologic lower extremity fractures.[3]

Ingram,[4] Ragnarsson,[2] Comarr,[5] and Eichenholtz[6] report the incidence of lower extremity fractures to range between 4% and 6% in the spinal cord injured population. These rates may be slightly below actual incidence, with underreporting being a result of absent sensation and reduced mobility. Caution should be taken when initiating any activity, such as bracewalking or functional electrical stimulation, which could potentially exceed the load bearing capability of the lower extremity long bones. Reports on medical management of lower limb fractures in SCI vary by author and range from open reduction and internal fixation of certain fractures to nonoperative care using well-padded splints. Proper union and alignment without limb shortening are the main goals in the ambulatory patient. Minimizing deformities created by malunion or rotation helps to prevent excessive tissue pressures at points of contact with the wheelchair seat or footplate.

Heterotopic ossification, the formation of mature bone in abnormal locations, has been observed to be clinically and functionally significant in approximately 10% to 20% of both spinal cord and traumatic brain injured populations.[7] Garland states that most cases of heterotopic ossification following TBI and SCI occur within 2 months of injury, so patients presenting to community-based medical services are unlikely to be suffering from acute heterotopic ossification except in cases of recurrence following surgical resection.[7] Mature periarticular bone, however, may indirectly contribute to other musculoskeletal problems if it interferes with joint motion, creates nerve entrapment,[8] or challenges proper positioning and pressure distribution in the wheelchair.

### Complications of the Weight-Bearing Upper Extremity

#### Shoulder Pain

Shoulder pain is a common complaint in the chronic SCI population. Documented incidence rates range from 30% to 52% in a mixed SCI population.[9,10] Bicipital and rotator cuff tendonitis and impingement syndromes have been identified as the primary sources of shoulder complaints in both the wheelchair-bound and bracewalking populations. Degenerative processes of the articular surfaces are reported to be proportionately less severe in these active individuals than in immobile persons.[11] Observations of the weight-bearing upper extremity during transfers, pressure relieving lifts, and wheelchair propulsion suggest that large forces are required to lift or move loads approaching one's body weight. In addition, the bicipital and supraspinatus tendons are often placed in extreme stretch in the positions of shoulder hyperextension and elbow extension used for such motions. This causes microtrauma to the tendons of the shoulder, and although the individual may remain asymptomatic for some time despite this microtrauma, an inflammatory reaction may ensue and result in pain and reduced

mobility.[12] The highly repetitive nature of the upper extremity load-bearing movements in SCI has been compared with the cumulative trauma suffered by industrial workers performing repetitive job tasks.[13]

Shoulder pathology in quadriplegics may differ from that of paraplegics as a result of muscle imbalance created by paralysis and spasticity. As discussed earlier, these factors may further alter normal joint alignment and stability during passive and active movements and create stresses contributing to synovial and capsular inflammation and rotator cuff or bicipital tendonitis.[12] These painful conditions may further increase spasticity and in turn further increase joint stresses and functional disability.

#### Compressive Mononeuropathies

Studies of the prevalence of compressive mononeuropathies of the wrist in chronic paraplegics estimate a prevalence of carpal tunnel syndrome and ulnar mononeuropathies at 20% to 60%. The variability in prevalence is attributed to differences in population demographics and electrodiagnostic protocols used for establishing the diagnoses.[13] Carpal tunnel syndrome is typically associated with high carpal tunnel pressures created by forceful extremes of wrist flexion or extension. Observation of wrist postures during transfers (wrist and finger extension), wheelchair propulsion (wrist extension and radial deviation), and crutch-aided bracewalking (wrist extension and radial deviation) would suggest increased risk for compressive mononeuropathies in these individuals. Davidoff, however, found a poor correlation between the clinical symptoms of nerve compression and electrodiagnostic evidence, thus raising this topic for further study.[13]

#### Respiratory Support of Muscular Activity

Respiratory function is an important component of muscular health and activity. Injuries to the central nervous system may alter an individual's respiratory function either directly through paralysis of respiratory musculature or indirectly through the progressive decline of thoracic compliance for lung expansion. Chronic respiratory complications or compromise should be considered in cases where patients complain of increasing levels of fatigue. Properly fitted abdominal binders can facilitate diaphragm function in patients lacking active abdominal musculature. Training to enhance thoracic cage mobility and accessory muscle activity can increase respiratory function in these populations.

## Impact of Musculoskeletal Dysfunction on Disability

Any secondary musculoskeletal complication of impairment may cause further difficulties. For example, a person with a complete cervical cord injury at the C6 level may be able to accomplish level-surface transfers despite absence of triceps function. By positioning the shoulders in external rotation and using the anterior deltoids to pull the distal humerus forward, the patient locks the elbows in extension in preparation for lifting the body for the transfer. Any complication, such as heterotopic ossification or soft tissue contracture, resulting in restricted shoulder, elbow or wrist extension, or shoulder external rotation could interfere with this function.

The clinician must be sensitive to the far-reaching implications of any secondary musculoskeletal problem that further limits the capacity for independent mobility. Increased functional dependency places greater demands on the individual's support system (family, friends, or attendants). The potential for immobility related complications (e.g., decubitus ulcers) or time lost from work or school is increased if the patient is unable to obtain the added assistance he or she needs.

## Issues Surrounding Therapeutic Intervention

The clinician faced with a musculoskeletal problem in an individual with an established physical impairment can rarely treat it as a simple case. Just as the assessment of the problem requires a systematic evaluation of the broad scope of the patient's lifestyle and mobility demands, consideration must be given to the impact of any interventions on the holistic functioning of this individual. Any pharmaceutical intervention must be made in light of the altered physiologic systems in the neurologically impaired person that may result in untoward side effects. Prescription of assistive technology must be carefully evaluated and monitored for its effect on efficient function, skin integrity, joint stresses, safety, and self-image. For example, a young woman with brain injury resulting in severely impaired trunk control and dependence on a wheelchair for mobility may be prescribed a body jacket to provide external trunk stability and postural symmetry. The orthosis may fit appropriately and accomplish the therapeutic objective of trunk support, but unfortunately may impair wheelchair propulsion, dressing, and the performance of other activities of daily living which were previously accomplished more readily. This illustrates the importance of clinical trials, possibly with "off-the-shelf" devices, prior to the prescription of costly adaptive devices.

Assistive technology, from ready-made devices to custom-made adaptations to sophisticated robotics have an important role to play in providing accommodation for the impaired individual in the home, school, job, and community environments. Referral to facilities experienced in and equipped for assistive technology evaluations and trials may provide viable alternatives to the individual whose mobility or lifestyle is complicated by musculoskeletal problems created by the physical stressors of the disability. Physicians and therapists must judiciously apply technology and therapeutic interventions to avoid further handicapping those that they are seeking to help.

## Points of Summary

1. Individuals with physical impairments may present with musculoskeletal complaints commonly seen in the able-bodied athletic or industrial population. Reliance on the upper extremities for mobility may increase an individual's risk for musculoskeletal injury.
2. The musculoskeletal examination must include a systematic assessment of the biomechanics of the patient's movement patterns in response to the contextual demands of mobility.
3. Muscle imbalance around a joint can result directly from neurologic injury, or in many cases,

indirectly from disproportionate hypertrophy related to functional movement requirements. One must determine if the injury or complaint is a result of altered joint position, limited musculotendinous length, disrupted muscular force couples, or impaired motor control.

4. Intervention must address the movement component that is increasing musculoskeletal stress. Effective treatment often requires assessment and possible modification of wheelchair configuration to promote postural stability and biomechanically efficient mobility.

5. Changes in bone density, autonomic response to exercise, and respiratory function in individuals with neurologic impairment may require a modification of therapeutic exercise programs.

6. With growing support for enablement of the disabled, assistive technology resources will continue to be developed. Careful assessment of individual needs for accommodation, along with a critical evaluation of the available technology, will be necessary to ensure judicious use of these resources.

## References

1. Rothstein JM: Measurement in clinical practice: Theory and application. In Rothstein JM (ed): *Measurement in Physical Therapy*. New York: Churchill Livingstone, 1985:1–46.
2. Ragnarsson KT, Sell GH: Lower extremity fractures after spinal cord injury: A retrospective study. *Arch Phys Med Rehabil* 1981;62:418–423.
3. Biering-Sorenson F, Bohr H, Schaadt O: Bone mineral content of the lumbar spine and lower extremities years after spinal cord lesion. *Paraplegia* 1988;26:293–301.
4. Ingram RR, Suman RK, Freeman PA: Lower limb fractures in the chronic spinal cord injured patient. *Paraplegia* 1989;27:133–139.
5. Comarr AE, Hutchinson RH, Bors E: Extremity fractures of patients with spinal cord injuries. *Am J Surg* 1962;104:732–739.
6. Eichenholtz SN: Management of long-bone fractures in paraplegic patients. *J Bone Joint Surg* 1963;45A:299–310.
7. Garland DE: Clinical observations on fractures and heterotopic ossification in the spinal cord and traumatic brain injured populations. *Clin Orthop Rel Res* 1988;233:86–101.
8. Brooke MM, Heard DL, deLateur BJ, et al.: Heterotopic ossification and peripheral nerve entrapment: Early diagnosis and excision. *Arch Phys Med Rehabil* 1991;72:425–429.
9. Bayley JC, Cochran TP, Sledge DB: The weight-bearing shoulder: The impingement syndrome in paraplegics. *J Bone Joint Surg* 1987;69A:676–678.
10. Nichols PJ, Nordan PA, Ennis JR: Wheelchair user's shoulder. *Scand J Rehabil Med* 1979;11:29–32.
11. Wylie FJ, Chakera TMH: Degenerative joint abnormalities in patients with paraplegia of duration greater than 20 years. *Paraplegia* 1988;26:101–106.
12. Silfverskiold J, Waters FL: Shoulder pain and functional disability in spinal cord injured patients. *Clin Orthop Rel Res* 1991;272:141–145.
13. Davidoff G, Werner R, Waring W: Compressive mononeuropathies of the upper extremity in chronic paraplegia. *Paraplegia* 1991;29:17–24.

## Suggested Readings

Brunnstrom S: *Clinical Kinesiology*, 3rd ed. Philadelphia, FA Davis, 1972.

Letts RM: *Principles of Seating the Disabled*. Boca Raton: CRC Press, 1991.

Perry J: Kinesiology of lower extremity bracing. *Clin Orthop* 1974;102:18–31.

Perry J: The mechanics of walking. *Clin Orthop* 1969;63:23–31.

Rosenthal M, Griffith ER, Bond MR, Miller JD: *Rehabilitation of the Head Injured Adult*. Philadelphia: FA Davis, 1983.

Smidt GL (ed): *Gait in Rehabilitation*. New York: Churchill Livingstone, 1990.

Treischman RB: *Aging with a Disability*. New York: Demos Publications, 1987.

Umphred DA (ed): *Neurological Rehabilitation*. St. Louis: CV Mosby, 1985.

# Chapter 28

# Psychological Components of Musculoskeletal Pain

MARY J. WELLS

Since the beginning of mankind, individuals have attempted to understand and manage the role of pain in human life. Philosophers since Aristotle have pondered the question of whether pain resides in the body or in the mind. The traditional medical view has consistently held that pain is a sensory phenomenon with an organic cause. Modern medicine has based most of its pain treatment on the concept that pain has as its origin a specific underlying cause and can be treated by modifying physiologic processes through either pharmacologic or surgical interventions. This assumption becomes more difficult to maintain when faced with a number of patients who complain of pain without clear underlying tissue pathology. Today, professionals who treat pain are recognizing that it is not linearly related to tissue pathology and that there are other, nonorganic, factors contributing to the pain experience. Pain is not exclusively a physical experience. It is intrinsically connected to the emotional and cognitive realms as well.[1]

## The Psychological Pain Experience

In order to fully understand the psychological pain experience, there are a few concepts that need to be defined. Fordyce[2] differentiated the role of pain, suffering, and legal disability with regard to the treatment of low back pain. Drawing on conceptual formulations developed by Loeser,[3] Fordyce introduced four basic pain dimensions: nociception, pain, suffering, and pain behavior.

*Nociception* is defined as the mechanical, thermal, and chemical events reacting on specific nerve endings which activate the pain fibers that signal the central nervous system that an aversive event is occurring. Essentially, nociception is the activity that occurs within specific peripheral nerve fibers and their synaptic connections.

*Pain* is defined as the sensation arising from the stimulation of perceived nociception. This definition includes central pain states and phantom limb pain. It is important to note that a specific linkage between peripheral nociception and the sensation of pain is not absolute.

*Suffering* is defined as the affective or emotional component of the central nervous system that is triggered by either nociception, pain, or other emotionally aversive events. These could include such things as the loss of a loved one, threat, or fear.

*Pain behavior* is defined as the specific set of activities and behaviors that an individual engages in to show others that he or she is in pain. Keefe and Block operationally identified a number of behaviors including guarding, bracing and grimacing as pain behaviors often seen in conjunction with complaints of low back pain.[4] Pain behavior has been conceptualized as a response to the pain experience, an output system, or a way of communicating to others the extent of distress experienced.

Of these four dimensions of pain, only nociception can be objectively verified in some cases. We believe that a patient is experiencing nociception when tissue abnormalities are detected, whether a tumor or a herniated disk. However, we still cannot verify nociception on a cellular or microscopic level. Pain and suffering are personal and subjective experiences that can only be observed indirectly. Pain behavior, of course, is easily observed and sometimes that much harder to trust.

When an individual initially experiences musculoskeletal pain due to illness or injury, a complex series of psychological and biochemical events are set in motion. The physiologic component of pain, nociception, starts the process. The brain immediately interprets the nociceptive information as pain based on both the event itself and on previous experiences and beliefs about pain. Thus, even from the onset of a pain experience, cognitive factors play a large role in both the understanding of and response to pain.

Following the injury or illness, changes in behavior are initiated by the sufferer. An individual experiencing pain is likely to decrease physical activity. Bed rest is often prescribed when the advice of a physician has been sought. The patient may be told not to engage in activities that increase pain. This leads to a decrease in frequency or total cessation of a number of normal activities, including work, activities of daily living, household chores, or leisure activity. The pain itself acts as an aversive consequence of a number of normally pleasant activities. A person's life can be quickly altered.

In a typical acute pain episode, the aversive events are short-lived. The pain resolves and the individual quickly resumes normal activities. The pain is at best a minor annoyance and at worst, something to maneuver around. For some individuals, however, this does not occur. The pain continues relentlessly. Normal activities are not resumed, and as the individual remains immobilized for longer and longer periods of time, negative physical cycles begin to set in. Muscle guarding results in an increased demand on muscles which often lack the flexibility and ability to manage the increased demands. Deconditioning sets in very quickly following an injury. Deconditioned muscles are unable to manage normal demands of daily living, thus resulting in increased experience of pain and a tendency to decrease activity even more.

Chronic pain has been linked to numerous antecedent factors including early childhood deprivation and trauma, pain models in the family, and other family maladjustment and personality disorders.[5] However, because of flawed methodology, the conclusions drawn from a number of studies are questionable. Most recently, studies suggest that pain is consistently associated with current emotional disturbance and not with previous life functioning.[6–9] Overall, emotional disturbances, particularly depression, are more likely to be consequences than causes of pain.

### Psychological Problems Associated with Persistent Pain

A number of psychological symptoms and problems are associated with persistent or chronic pain. They include affective, behavioral, and vegetative changes as well as a number of cognitive factors associated with belief systems regarding health and health behavior.

### Vegetative Signs

One of the most common complaints associated with chronic pain is sleep disturbance. Pain disrupts both sleep onset and sleep maintenance. It is not unusual to experience nonrestorative sleep. The difficulties begin because an individual has difficulty finding a comfortable position. With position changes and restless sleep, pain reawakens the individual throughout the night. Chronic fatigue decreases pain tolerance and results in even minor injuries being perceived as traumatic events.

Appetite, another vegetative symptom, is often affected. Some individuals experience a significant weight loss. More commonly, however, weight gain is reported. Individuals with chronic pain begin spending more time at home and less time engaged in other activities. They find themselves restlessly snacking throughout the day. This, combined with the decrease in physical activity, leads to an increase in weight. Self-esteem then becomes affected because individuals become uncomfortable with their weight gain and their physical appearance.

Vegetative problems of sleep disturbance and appetite disturbance are also accompanied frequently by changes in sexual desire or libido. Individuals who experience chronic pain often note difficulty in performance of the sexual act. Particularly for the individual suffering from low back pain, sexual activity can be almost intolerable. As chronic pain causes the individual to become more and more uncomfortable participating in a sexual relationship with his or her partner, withdrawal from sexual intimacy occurs and one often notices a decrease in desire as well as difficulty with performance.

### Affective Symptoms

Depressed mood is a common side effect of persistent pain. Patients often complain of feelings of helplessness or hopelessness related to pain control. As the pain continues over time, it is not unusual to hear patients complain of a loss of interest in activities that previously brought pleasure (anhedonia) or feelings of uselessness in the role of breadwinner or active family member. Suicidal thoughts, while rarely acted on, are common.[10]

A number of studies have noted the frequency with which depression accompanies a chronic pain problem. From 30% to 80% of all chronic pain sufferers have been reported in the literature as experiencing depression.[11] Depression has become known as the "handmaiden" of chronic pain. While it is clear that a number of pain patients suffer from a variety of depressive symptoms, the true diagnosis of clinical depression is probably overdiagnosed in chronic pain sufferers.[12]

Patients can also become anxious in response to pain. Fear of reinjury can play a central role in the development of a dysfunctional lifestyle due to pain.[13] A patient may worry that the underlying cause of the pain has not been found or adequately explained and may fear that it is life-threatening or that it will be made worse by activity. A slight increase in pain with activity sets off an extreme response which only compounds the problem.

Another common psychological problem associated with chronic pain is that of irritability. Individuals (or their families) frequently complain of short temper, increased irritability, and loss of anger control. In order to control their outbursts, individuals often withdraw from others. This withdrawal leads to increased isolation and an increased focus on the pain. The effort required to interact pleasantly with others seems overwhelming, even though pain patients are often lonely and would like to have friends.[14]

### Behavioral Changes

Patients often present with a number of behavioral symptoms during clinical examination and in the presence of others who express doubt about the seriousness of the pain problem. Pain behaviors are present in a large number of pain patients and vary in expression and intensity. They can and often do reflect genuine discomfort but are also ways of communicating to others the emotional distress. Waddell and colleagues have demonstrated a number of methods of measuring emotional overlay through careful observation of pain behavior and its relation to anatomic structures.[15,16] Their methods are an invaluable tool to quantify and somewhat objectively identify magnification of the pain problem. Table 28-1 lists a number of commonly observed pain behaviors.

### Cognitions, Beliefs and Expectations

Florence describes the chronic pain syndrome as a perceptual illness.[17] The chronic pain syndrome likely develops as a result of inappropriate perceptions regarding the meaning of pain and the value of various treatment options. Beliefs and expectations about pain and outcome play an essential role in the process of evaluating and treating musculoskeletal pain. Cognitions are defined as the set of attitudes, beliefs, and expectations developed by

**Table 28-1.** Pain Behaviors

| | |
|---|---|
| Sighing | Obvious exaggerated exhalation of breath |
| Grimacing | Obvious facial expression of pain |
| Rubbing | Touching, holding, rubbing affected area |
| Bracing | Stationary position in which fully extended limb supports and maintains abnormal weight distribution |
| Guarding | Abnormally stiff or rigid movement while shifting from one position to another |

(Adapted from Keefe FJ, Bloch AR: *Behav Ther* 1982;13:363–375.)

the individual over time, based on experience and social learning. Cognitions are thought to link external events and emotional response.[18,19]

In a recent study,[20] it was determined that a cognitive behavioral mediation model was useful for understanding the relationship between pain and depression. Results suggested that treatment success in a multidisciplinary pain clinic is moderated less by depression than by the cognitive appraisals (thoughts) and the preferred coping strategies of patients. The presence of depression alone was not found to predict whether or not an individual will respond to cognitive behavioral and interdisciplinary treatment strategies. Rather, influencing the style of coping and using active and skill-oriented activities were more likely to achieve a positive outcome.

Another recent study[21] evaluated coping strategies and pain beliefs. There were three distinct pain belief subgroups in a sample of chronic pain patients. They differed significantly in their use of and perceived effectiveness of pain coping strategies. The vast majority of these patients (70% of the total sample) had beliefs that their pain would be enduring and was of a mysterious nature. The authors characterize this subset of patients as individuals who are convinced that their pain will persist and that there is no adequate explanation regarding their pain. Patients in this subgroup rated their ability to use pain strategies to decrease and control pain lower than patients in the other subgroups. They tended to use a more catastrophic response with less reinterpretation of pain sensations when coping.

### Disability and Return to Work

One of the difficulties with the treatment of chronic low back (and other) pain patients is facilitating return to work. In one study noted, only 35% to 45% of chronic low back pain patients who had undergone treatment were managing a job 1 year after treatment. Epidemiologic data suggests that a person who is out on sick leave for more than 3 consecutive months for low back pain has virtually no chance of return to work. Absenteeism for back disorders accounts for about 25% of all sick leave[22] and chronic pain accounts for 70% to 87% of compensation benefits for workers.[23] In some areas of the United States, up to two thirds of total

compensation benefits are paid out for low back injuries.[24] In as many as 85% of these cases no specific diagnosis can be made.[25]

Psychosocial and psychological factors tend to be underemphasized in assessing pain, especially early on. Despite considerable evidence from a wide body of literature suggesting that nonbiologic factors contribute as much as tissue pathology to the experience of pain and suffering, efforts to assess and quantify psychosocial and psychological factors are not usually made until after the patient has already developed a chronic pain problem. The compensation system itself presents a number of disincentives to return to work. For compensable injuries on the job, the tax free income can provide an incentive to remain at home. Employers are also less likely to rehire an injured worker or to provide "light duty" work. Individuals end up being frightened and confused by the "system" and hear clear messages that they are unemployable in their previous setting and therefore need to stay on continued disability compensation.

The medical system reinforces disability by the continual search for a biologic or physiologic cause of the pain. When it is not found, the patient becomes anxious about occult disease and loses faith in the medical profession. Because medicine is so heavily based in a disease model, the psychosocial factors are often overlooked.

Effective vocational rehabilitation is very difficult to find. Vocational rehabilitation specialists are usually not part of the pain treatment team and often lack the sophisticated knowledge necessary to assist chronic pain patients with their specific needs. Because of their lack of understanding of the chronic pain process, they respond to pain problems as acute and send the patient back to the primary physician until such time as the pain is "cured." This inadvertently perpetuates a disability model.[26]

If an individual is unable to return to work for more than 6 months, the incentive to return to work becomes less and less. It is therefore essential to recognize early chronicity and to treat it effectively prior to the onset of total vocational disability.[23,26]

### Malingering

The malingerer fraudulently presents himself as having nonexistent symptoms in order to obtain some kind of gain, usually financial. He differs from the patient with psychological overlay or symptom magnification because he is consciously manipulating the system. The majority of chronic pain patients are not malingerers. They may exaggerate their symptoms to get attention, but most should not be judged too harshly for this. They have simply been conditioned that this is the only way to get attention. The old saying that the squeaky wheel gets the grease is not without merit.

## Treatment Strategies

There has been a gradually building body of evidence suggesting that the adjunctive use of psychological techniques to treat chronic pain is more effective than physical therapy or medications alone.[27-29] Psychological treatment strategies can include assessment and evaluation, individual and group psychotherapy, and interdisciplinary approaches such as relaxation training and biofeedback.

### Assessment and Evaluation

Most physicians refer patients to psychologists when physical findings are insufficient to explain the extent of pain being reported by the patient. Physicians are traditionally trained in a model that assumes a direct correlation between the extent of tissue damage and the report of pain. Pain reports in the absence of specific physical pathology are assumed to be the result of psychological factors. This is the definition of "psychogenic pain." The psychological evaluation is often requested when functional disability greatly exceeds that expected based on physical findings or when a patient is exhibiting significant psychological distress such as depression or anxiety. Physicians often wait until a patient has become problematic or overly demanding before considering a psychological evaluation. Often the physician is fed up or frustrated with the patient's complaints.

Whether or not there is a clear organic basis for pain, factors including depression, beliefs and expectations, familial reinforcement of pain behaviors, anxiety, and stress response can all contribute to the maintenance and exacerbation of pain and suffering. A psychological evaluation can identify the psychosocial and behavioral factors that influence a patient's report of pain. If ignored, psychological factors frequently impede the recovery process and can interfere with response to treatment and rehabilitation.[30] Table 28-2 delineates appropriate and inappropriate uses for psychological assessment.

### Individual and Group Psychotherapy

Psychological treatment, whether offered in a group or individual format, should include specific content areas. Education regarding pain and function as well as some of the theoretical underpinnings of the gate control theory of pain (see Chapter 25) can increase a patient's understanding of pain responses. Cognitive strategies to alter belief systems and to decrease stress responses should also be standard aspects of treatment, along with strategies to combat depression and related helplessness and hopelessness. Behavioral techniques to modify specific behavior patterns related to movement and exercise can also be employed. Finally, instruction and practice in relaxation techniques should be included.

In an individual treatment format, the therapist has the luxury of fully exploring the relationship between the patient's personality and pain coping

**Table 28-2.** Appropriate and Inappropriate Uses of Psychological Assessment

**Appropriate Uses**

To determine specific psychological and behavioral contributors to a patient's pain and concomitant behaviors, disability, and suffering.

To determine appropriate treatment strategies.

To provide essential information on particular aspects of a patient's psychosocial background and current situation that may be impacting the pain problem.

**Inappropriate Uses**

To determine if pain is organic or functional (i.e., real or psychogenic).

To catch malingerers.

To justify dumping of more difficult patients.

(Adapted from Turk DC: *Pain Management* 1990; May/June: 165–172.

strategies as well as gathering information on previous life experiences that impact the patient's level of distress. Patients with psychiatric illness in conjunction with their pain often respond better to the individual format, at least until good therapeutic rapport has been developed and the psychiatric problem has stabilized.[31]

Group psychotherapy provides a number of advantages over the traditional individual approach, although it is not appropriate for all patients.[32] Table 28-3 lists clinically relevant reasons for considering group psychotherapy as the primary or preferred treatment for pain patients.[33]

The strength of a group experience includes cost-effectiveness as well as specific therapeutic factors of universality, cohesion, and instillation of hope.[34] Patients suffering with pain often feel hopeless, confused, and overwhelmed by their pain. The group experience can counteract those feelings and encourage patients to try out new behaviors they may otherwise resist. More importantly, however, patients can work together in a group to provide each other with support and encouragement and to decrease the sense of isolation and uniqueness so common to the chronic pain sufferer.

*Interdisciplinary Treatment Approaches*

The current trend in treatment of the chronic pain patient and concomitant vocational disability is to provide an interdisciplinary approach.[28,29] These programs combine standard physical therapy with behavioral and psychological approaches consisting of education about pain, relaxation training, and cognitive behavioral techniques, as well as more nontraditional techniques such as Yoga and acupuncture. Such programs have been found to improve patients in terms of functional impairment, use of active coping strategy techniques, decreased medication use, and more effective self-efficacy beliefs.[28,29,31] In one study,[35] these changes were upheld over a 6-month followup with continued use of active coping strategies at a greater level than subjects in a controlled condition. The authors conclude that cognitive and behavioral treatments substantially augment effective physical therapy and traditional teaching.

**Table 28-3.** Clinical Advantages to Group Treatment Format

| |
|---|
| Credible feedback and confrontation from peers |
| Amelioration of sense of social isolation and alienation |
| Avoidance of patient's dependency on therapist |
| More efficient use of therapist's time |

(Adapted from Gentry WD, Owens D: Pain groups. In Holzman AD, Turk DC (eds): *Pain Management: A Handbook of Psychological Treatment Approaches.* New York: Pergamon Press, 1986:100–112.)

**Referral**

It is clear that the way in which physicians convey perceptions of chronic pain treatment impacts the way in which individuals respond both in the short term and in the long run. The process of psychological consultation or evaluation requires the cooperation of patients. Their approach to this treatment is influenced by the way in which a psychological assessment or treatment is presented. If they feel comfortable and confident, they are much more likely to be open in describing their difficulties. If, on the other hand, they are feeling angry, weary, or apprehensive, they are much more likely to be guarded and suspicious of the evaluation process. In some cases, they may refuse a referral or not follow up on a referral made. They may feel that the referring physician thinks they are "crazy" or that the pain is not real because they are being sent to the psychologist. Table 28-4 presents guidelines for making a good referral to psychological services.[36]

**Table 28-4.** Guidelines for Psychological Services Referral

| |
|---|
| • Clearly identify nonmedical consultants. |
| • Acknowledge problem is legitimate. |
| • Provide a positive rationale for referral. |
| • Inform other staff of rationale. |
| • Avoid making cynical comments about referral. |
| • Let patient know if referral is routine. |
| • Personalize the referral. |
| • Inform patient that referral does not imply transfer. |

(Adapted from Cameron R, Shepel LF: The process of psychological consultation in pain management. In Holzman AD, Turk DC (eds): Pain Management: *A Handbook of Psychological Treatment Approaches.* New York: Pergamon Press, 1986:240–256.)

## Early Warning Signs

A treating physician should constantly be monitoring patients for early warning signs of potential long-term problems with pain. Any pain that lasts longer than expected given tissue healing processes should be considered potentially problematic. Other early indicators may include an overreliance on the treating physician or physical therapist (i.e., frequent calls, multiple appointments on an emergent basis with no significant change in medical status), a passive approach to recovery, frequent or increasing reliance on narcotic analgesics, significant decrease in activity, or lack of return to normal activities. Complaints of pain with any or all activity may also suggest that a patient is at risk for chronic pain.

## Points of Summary

1. The psychological pain experience is comprised of four components: nociception, pain, suffering, and pain behavior.
2. A patient's beliefs and expectations about pain, its causes, and its treatment have a profound impact on the outcome of treatment.
3. It is essential to foster self-responsibility for treatment and outcome in the pain patient.
4. Depression and anxiety are most frequently consequences of pain, not causes.
5. Very few pain patients are true malingerers, although many do display pain amplification in their attempts to get their pain taken seriously.
6. Interdisciplinary treatment strategies which include education, exercise, relaxation, and stress management are the treatment strategies of choice for the chronic pain patient and may be beneficial in the subacute patient as well.

## References

1. Turk DC, Holzman AD: Chronic pain: Interfaces among physical, psychological, and social parameters. In Holzman AD, Turk DC (eds): *Pain Management: A Handbook of Psychological Treatment Approaches*. New York: Pergamon Press, 1986:1–9.
2. Fordyce WE: Pain and suffering: A reappraisal. *American Psychologist* 1988;43:276–283.
3. Loeser JD: Perspectives on pain. In *Proceedings of the First World Conference on Clinical Pharmacology and Therapeutics*. London: Macmillan, 1980:313–316.
4. Keefe FJ, Block AR: Development of an observation method for assessing pain behavior in chronic low back pain patients. *Behav Ther* 1982;13:363–375.
5. Crauford DIO, Creed F, Jayson MIV. Life events and psychological disturbance in patients with low-back pain. *Spine* 1990;15:490–494.
6. Gamsa, A: Is emotional disturbance a precipitator or a consequence of chronic pain? *Pain* 1990;42:183–195.
7. Roy R, Thomas M, Matas M: Chronic pain and depression: A review. *Comp Psych* 1984;25:96–105.
8. Gamsa A, Vikis-Freibergs V: Psychological events are both risk factors in, and consequences of, chronic pain. *Pain* 1991;44:2711–2717.
9. Krishnan KRR, France RD, Houpt JL: Chronic low back pain and depression. *Psychosomatics* 1985;26:299–302.
10. Dworkin RH, Gitlin, MJ: Clinical aspects of depression in chronic pain patients. *Clin J Pain* 1991;7:79–94.
11. Romano JM, Turner JA: Chronic pain and depression: Does the evidence support a relationship? *Psychol Bull* 1985;97:18–34.
12. Haythornthwaite JA, Seiber WJ, Kerns RD: Depression and the chronic pain experience. *Pain* 1991;46:177–184.
13. Papciak AS, Feuerstein M: Fear of pain and distress in pain-related work disability. Paper presented at the *98th Annual Meeting for the American Psychological Association*. Boston, MA August 1990.
14. Merskey H, Lau CL, Russell ES, et al.: Screening for psychiatric morbidity: The pattern of psychological illness and premorbid characteristics in four chronic pain populations. *Pain* 1987;30:141–157.
15. Waddell G, Main CJ, Morris EW, et al.: Chronic low back pain psychologic distress and illness behavior. *Spine* 1984;9:209–213.
16. Waddell G: A new perspective to the treatment of low back pain. *Spine* 1987;12:6–32.
17. Florence, DW: The chronic pain syndrome: A physical and psychologic challenge. *Postgrad Med* 1981;70:217–228.
18. Beck AT, Rush AJ, Shaw BF, et al.: *Cognitive Therapy in the Emotional Disorders*. New York: International Universities Press, 1976.
19. Beck AT: *Cognitive Therapy of Depression*. New York: Guilford Press, 1979.
20. Kleinke CL: How chronic pain patients cope with depression: Relation to treatment outcome in a multidisciplinary pain clinic. *Rehabil Psych* 1991;36:207–218.
21. Williams DA, Keefe, FJ: Pain beliefs and the use of cognitive-behavioral strategies. *Pain* 1991;46:185–190.
22. Linton SJ, Bradley LA, Jensen I, et al.: The secondary prevention of low back pain: A controlled study with follow-up. *Pain* 1989;36:197–207.

23. Rucker K, Metzler H, Wehman P, et al.: Pain literature and social security policy. *J Back Musculoskel Rehabil* 1991;1:67–73.

24. Dworkin RH, Handlin DS, Richlin DM, et al.: Unraveling the effects of compensation, litigation and employment on treatment response and chronic pain. *Pain* 1985;23:49–59.

25. Frymoyer JW: Back pain and sciatica. *New Engl J Med* 1988;318:291–300.

26. Brena SF, Turk DC: Vocational disability: A challenge to pain rehabilitation programs. In Aronoff GM (ed): *Pain Centers: A Revolution in Healthcare.* New York: Raven Press, 1987:167–180.

27. Sternbach RA: *Mastering pain: A twelve-step program for coping with chronic pain.* New York: Ballantine Books, 1987.

28. Mayer TG, Gatchel RJ, Mayer H, et al.: The prospective two-year study of functional restoration in industrial low-back injury: An objective assessment procedure. *JAMA* 1987;258:1763–1767.

29. Newman RI, Seres J: The interdisciplinary pain center: An approach to the management of chronic pain. In Holzman AD, Turk DC (eds): *Pain Management: A Handbook of Psychological Treatment Approaches.* New York: Pergamon Press, 1986:71–85.

30. Turk DC: Psychological assessment of patients with persistent pain: Traditional views. *Pain Management* 1990; May/June:165–172.

31. Grzesiak RC: Toward a psychotherapy for chronic pain patients: Some directions. Paper presented at the 12th Annual Meeting of the Society for Behavioral Medicine, Washington, D.C., March 22, 1991.

32. Ettin MF, Heiman ML, Kopel SA: Group building: Developing protocols for the psychoeducational groups. *Group* 1988;12:205–225.

33. Gentry WD, Owens D: Pain groups. In Holzman AD, Turk DC (eds): *Pain Management: A Handbook of Psychological Treatment Approaches.* New York: Pergamon Press, 1986:100–112.

34. Yalom I: *The Theory and Practice of Group Psychotherapy.* New York: Basic Books, 1975.

35. Nicholas MK, Wilson PH, Goyen J: Comparison of cognitive-behavioral group treatment and an alternative non-psychological treatment for chronic low back pain. *Pain* 1992;48:339–347.

36. Cameron R, Shepel LF: The process of psychological consultation in pain management. In Holzman AD, Turk DC (eds): *Pain Management: A Handbook of Psychological Treatment Approaches.* New York: Pergamon Press, 1986:240–256.

## Suggested Readings

Brena SF, Turk DC: Vocational disability: A challenge to pain rehabilitation programs. In Aronoff GM (ed): *Pain Centers: A Revolution in Healthcare.* York: Raven Press, 1987:167–180.

Holzman AD, Turk DC (eds): *Pain Management: A Handbook of Psychological Treatment Approaches.* New York: Pergamon Press, 1986:71–85.

Mayer TG, Gatchel RJ, Mayer H, et al.: The prospective two-year study of functional restoration in industrial low-back injury: An objective assessment procedure. *JAMA* 1987;258:1763–1767.

Sternbach RA: *Mastering Pain: A Twelve-Step Program for Coping with Chronic Pain.* New York: Ballantine Books, 1987.

Turk DC: Psychological assessment of patients with persistent pain: Traditional views. *Pain Management,* 1990, May/June:165–172.

# Index